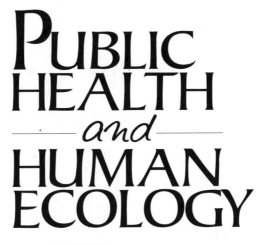

PUBLIC HEALTH and HUMAN ECOLOGY

SECOND EDITION

PUBLIC HEALTH *and* HUMAN ECOLOGY

SECOND EDITION

John M. Last, MD, DPH
Emeritus Professor of Epidemiology and Community Medicine
University of Ottawa
Ottawa, Ontario, Canada

APPLETON & LANGE
Stamford, Connecticut

Copyright © 1998 by Appleton & Lange
A Simon & Schuster Company
Copyright © 1987 by Appleton & Lange

97 98 99 00 01 / 10 9 8 7 6 5 4 3 2 1

Prentice Hall International (UK) Limited, *London*
Prentice Hall of Australia Pty. Limited, *Sydney*
Prentice Hall Canada, Inc., *Toronto*
Prentice Hall Hispanoamericana, S.A., *Mexico*
Prentice Hall of India Private Limited, *New Delhi*
Prentice Hall of Japan, Inc., *Tokyo*
Simon & Schuster Asia Pte. Ltd., *Singapore*
Editora Prentice Hall do Brasil Ltda., *Rio de Janeiro*
Prentice Hall, *Upper Saddle River, New Jersey*

Last, John M., 1926–
    Public health and human ecology / John M. Last. — 2nd ed.
        p.   cm.
    Includes bibliographical references and index.
    ISBN 0-8385-8080-7 (pbk.)
    1. Public health.   2. Human ecology.   I. Title.
    [DNLM: 1. Public Health.   2. Ecology.   WA 30 L349p 1987]
    RA425.L37   1997
    362.1—dc21
    DNLM/DLC
    for Library of Congress   97-7896
                                                       CIP

Acquisitions Editor: Michael Medina
Production Editor: Lisa M. Guidone
Designer: Mary Skudlarek

ISBN 0-8385-8080-7
90000

9 780838 580806

*To students of all ages everywhere
and especially to three young students,
Christina, Peter, and John*

Contents

Preface

The epigraphs for this book define my purpose. I seek to convince aspiring members of all health-related professions, especially my own profession of medicine, that promoting, protecting, and preserving health deserve the highest priority.

To that end, I have described and discussed determinants of health and provided an overview of some present and likely future dangers to health. There are more questions than answers about ways to confront and deal with these dangers, which is as it should be: you, my reader, and I learn best when we work things out for ourselves rather than when somebody else feeds us their version of reality.

I have tried to be brief, but it proved difficult in the chapters on epidemiology—the basic science of public health—and environmental health. There are some changes from the first edition: I have dropped the chapters on Hazards of Health Care and the Future of Health and Health Services, replacing the latter with a new chapter on the health impacts of changes in global ecosystems. The chapters on Communicable Diseases and on Ethics and Public Health Policy are completely rewritten, and the latter is much expanded. The chapters on Food and Nutrition and on Organization of Public Health Services have been brought up to date but are otherwise relatively unchanged. I hope the result is a book that will stimulate and provoke students who can expect to be at the height of their professional careers in the second quarter of the next century.

Why "human ecology"? Ecology is concerned with the healthy interaction of living creatures in a closed system. Human ecology includes humans in this system. Humans interact with each other as well as with other living creatures and these interactions can have important effects on the health of all partners in the complex closed ecosystem of our planet. We ignore this reality at our peril.

John M. Last
Ottawa, December, 1996

Acknowledgments

First, I thank many friends and former students who encouraged me to re-work this book, into which I had poured much feeling 10 years ago but which I had no wish to revise. I though it would be a brain-grinding chore, that I could never recapture the enthusiasm I felt the first time I tackled the subjects I discuss here. I was wrong about that and they were right, so I am grateful to them for pushing me into a task that proved so much more pleasant than I had expected it to be.

I am grateful to all who have helped with this revision by reading drafts, offering corrections and suggestions, and in many other ways. They include Darwish Al Gobaisi, Nick Birkett, Jack Bryant, John Cahill, Betty Flagler, Toby Gelfand, Trevor Hancock, Ron Laporte, Alison Macfarlane, Ian McDowell, Tony McMichael, John Parboosingh, David Phillips, John Powles, Lynne Quon-Mak, Jane Reeves, Doug Scutchfield, Bob Spasoff, Michel Thuriaux, Karen Trollope-Kumar, John Williams, and Rebecca, David, and Dorothyanne Last. Jonathan Last prepared several tables and figures. My editors, Michael P. Medina, John Dinolfo, and Lisa Guidone, at Appleton & Lange have been helpful and supportive throughout. Thanks to Libby Crawford for her copy-editing skills and Heather Ebbs for producing an excellent index.

The entire book was prepared on my home computer system, but I used the photocopying and fax facilities of the University of Ottawa and the Royal College of Physicians and Surgeons of Canada, for which I am very grateful.

My wife, Wendy, has nobly waded through many typescript chapters to check them for sense and typos and, as always, has sustained me in body, mind, and spirit throughout.

JML

"The health of a people is really the foundation upon which all their happiness and all their power as a State depend."

Benjamin Disraeli
(In a speech to the British Parliament, 1877)

"Medical instruction does not exist to provide individuals with an opportunity of learning how to make a living, but in order to make possible the protection of the health of the public."

Rudolph Virchow
(In an address to medical students in Berlin, c. 1890)

"Nothing can be more important to a State than its public health; the State's paramount concern should be the health of its people."

Franklin D. Roosevelt
(In a Report to the New York Legislature, 1931)

The History, Scope, and Methods of Public Health

The goals of medicine, and of public health services, are to promote health, to preserve health, to restore good health when sickness occurs, and to relieve suffering. All four goals are advanced by the practice of public health.

▶ HISTORICAL PERSPECTIVES[1,2]

Humans have evolved via *Homo habilis* and *H. erectus* to *H. sapiens* during the past 4 to 5 million years. *H. sapiens* appeared a mere half million years ago and did not reach full potential until after the last ice age, about 12 thousand years ago. Early humans were hunter-gatherers who used stones and sticks as weapons to kill other animals and each other. They domesticated animals, added agriculture to their skills, and settled in coastal areas and river valleys 10 to 12 thousand years ago. I like to think that women discovered how to domesticate animals and to cultivate crops, while men discovered how to use fire and forge weapons. These skills enabled them to establish permanent settlements, where at first they probably lived in equilibrium with other species that shared their habitat. In all but the most bountiful ecosystems such harmony was evanescent. Trees were felled for fuel and shelter, and excrement and other wastes fouled the environment and were a haven for pests and pathogens. Those early discoveries and innumerable others since spurred the advance of civilizations. At the end of the 20th century our spectacular technical and reproductive success threaten ecosystems we need for survival (see Chap. 11).

We have always had a precarious relationship with disease. The names of some of the great scourges evoke memories of ancient beliefs about their nature and causes. *Influenza* recalls the notion that evil spirits or malign influences cause disease. *Malaria* reminds us of the miasma theory, the belief that emanations from rotting organic matter caused this and other diseases. *Cholera* derives its name from the humoral theory, the belief that diseases were due to imbalances among the vital humors. We speak of "visitations" of plague, acknowledging the notion that it was caused by a wrathful god, punishing us for our misdeeds. Some important diseases have purely descriptive names. *Typhus* means "clouded" and refers to the state of consciousness of the victim; *smallpox* and *yellow fever* describe the effects. These diseases have all shaped our history, contributing to the fall of civilizations and the defeats of campaigning armies.

Throughout history other conditions have sapped the vitality of communities and civilizations. Children have died of diarrhea and respiratory infections, often when already weakened by malnutrition at times of food shortage. In developing nations, 4 million children still die every year from respiratory infections, and 3 million each from diarrhea and vaccine-preventable diseases such as measles (see Chaps. 3 and 9).

The improvements in health that led to our present security against premature death and crippling disability did not begin in the industrial nations until the 19th century, eight to ten generations ago. Declining infant and child mortality rates were followed by a fall in the birthrate. This led to a change in age distribution of the population, an increase in the proportion of older people. Similar changes in the pattern of disease and age distribution began more recently in the developing nations. The results of these epidemiologic and demographic transitions are not all yet apparent, although the most obvious, the hyperexponential increase in numbers of people since the 1950s, has had complex and worrying effects (see Chaps. 9 and 11).

Until the 19th century, there was little known and less done to control disease. Among the best things about human progress since the early 19th century, we should give pride of place to enlarged understanding of causes and ways to control the lethal epidemic diseases.

The slow accumulation of knowledge over many preceding centuries was a necessary foundation for the advances of recent times. The concept of contagion is ancient, signified by exclusion from society of lepers and others with disfiguring stigmata, which were believed to be signs of infection. About A.D. 1400, the Venetians introduced the practice of quarantine, isolating ships that were suspected of carrying contagious diseases. Laws and regulations began to emerge as a way to protect the public against threats to health. Johann Peter Frank, a physician who became director-general of public health to the Hapsburg Empire in 18th-century Vienna, systematized many rules for personal and communal behavior that contributed to better health, in *System einer vollständigen medicinischen Polizey*[3] (1779).

Some understanding of the nature of contagion already existed: Fracastorius, an Italian priest-physician, described several modes of transmission of infectious diseases in *De Contagione*[4] (1546), which appeared 16 years after his mock-heroic poem, *Syphilis sive Morbus Gallicus,* the book that gave the name to this disease. Fracastorius recognized the principal methods of person-to-person spread of disease: direct contact (as with the sexually transmitted diseases), droplet spread, and fomites (i.e., contaminated utensils, clothing, etc.). He recognized that some diseases were transmitted "at a distance" but could not distinguish between vector-borne diseases and those transmitted by a vehicle, such as contaminated water, food, or milk.

Ideas about contagion were reinforced when Antonie van Leeuwenhoek used the microscope (1696) and saw "little animals," some of which he correctly inferred were associated with diseases.[5] Microscopes also advanced understanding about the nature of pathologic processes associated with disease—a necessary prerequisite to rational preventive measures. As medical science progressed, physicians began to widen their horizons, to perceive that diseases had environmental, social, and behavioral causes. Perhaps the first organized effort by the medical profession to control a socially induced health problem was the 18th-century campaign against gin drinking by the Royal College of Physicians of London, vividly depicted in Hogarth's etchings of *Gin Lane.*

The industrial revolution transformed European and North American society, leading to the growth of cities and creating a great demand for labor in factories and mines. Economic and social changes produced a pool of available laborers, comprised largely of the women and children of dispossessed farmers and agricultural workers. The misery and exploitation of these unfortunate people inspired reform movements that had a direct effect on health as social conditions improved. At the same time, industrialization brought wealth and international trade and the ability to pay for imported food, leading to improved nutrition that helped to reduce infant and child mortality rates.

Other important changes were occurring. The new industrial towns lacked sanitation, but expanding medical knowledge and esthetic considerations led to pressure for improvement, and by the end of the 19th century many cities in the industrial nations had installed sewage systems and water purification processes. The epidemiologic observations of John Snow and William Farr, the discoveries of the bacteriologists Louis Pasteur and Robert Koch, and the work of the pathologist-sanitarian Rudolph Virchow in science and politics played a crucial role in all of this. Edwin Chadwick's study of the sanitary conditions of the laboring classes in England,[6] followed by Lemuel Shattuck's similar analysis of living conditions in 19th-century Boston,[7] also contributed. By the end of the 19th century, some of the worst threats to long life and good health had been controlled by applying environmental health measures, reinforced by new laws.

The 20th century brought new approaches to disease control and health improvement. Edward Jenner had shown in 1796 that smallpox could be prevented by vaccinating with serum from the lesions of cowpox (vaccinia),[8] taking the first steps that led to worldwide eradication of this terrible disease by the late 1970s. Other immunizing agents are mostly the results of research and developments in the biomedical sciences since the beginning of the 20th century (Table 1–1).

These advances and the development of chemotherapy and antibiotics led for a time to the virtual disappearance of many previously common and often lethal infectious diseases. By the 1950s the pattern of disease in the industrial nations had begun to change. New public health problems—chronic disabling and life-shortening conditions like arteriosclerotic heart disease, lung cancer, traffic-related injury, emotional disorders—became prominent (Fig. 1–1). Many infectious diseases have remained unconquered until now in the developing world, the habitat for three-quarters of the human race. Moreover, after a brief respite from the 1950s to the 1980s, many common and formerly lethal pathogens (*Staphylococcus, Streptococcus, pneumococcus,* tubercle bacillus, etc.) have returned in antibiotic-resistant strains, and dangerous new pathogens, notably the human immunodeficiency virus (HIV) have emerged (see Chap. 3).

Another expanding frontier of knowledge about health since the early 20th century is scientific understanding of nutrition. Epidemiologic studies have clarified the role of vitamins and essential minerals and the relationship of diet to heart disease, high blood pressure, and gastrointestinal cancer (see Chap. 5). Knowledge of body chemistry has grown: We understand the quality of immune responses, ways in which enhancing immunity can improve health, and how disruption of body chemistry and the immune system can harm it. The intriguing science of psychoneuroimmunology has clarified comprehension of mind–body interactions that contribute to health and disease.

▶ DEFINITIONS

Health[9] is derived from the old English word *hal,* meaning hale, whole, healed, sound in wind and limb. This is quite a good definition of health, but other definitions merit discussion.

The preamble to the constitution of the World Health Organization (WHO) describes health as a state of complete physical, mental, and social well-being, not merely the absence of disease or infirmity. As we rely mainly on measurement of phenomena that indicate degrees of absence of health, this is a poor operational definition. Also, it describes an ideal state rarely attained in the real world, and nobody knows exactly what is meant by "social well-being."

The rise of the health promotion movement, discussed below, led to useful elaboration of the original WHO description of health; this can be paraphrased as follows: the extent to which an individual or a group is able to realize aspirations and satisfy needs and to change or cope with the environment. Health is a resource for everyday life, not the object of living; it is a

TABLE 1–1. **Significant Discoveries in Microbiology**

Disease	Discovery of Agent	Vaccine, etc., Developed
Smallpox	1915 (Noguchi)	c. 1000 Variolation (China) c. 1750 Variolation (Europe) 1796 (Jenner)
Anthrax	1849–1855	1881 (Pasteur)
Rabies	1936 (Webster and Clow)	1885 (Pasteur)
Tuberculosis	1882 (Koch)	1892 Tuberculin 1924 Bacille Calmette-Guérin (BCG)
Diphtheria	1884 (Klebs, Loeffler)	1890–1894 Antitoxin treatment 1912 Antitoxin immunization 1913 Schick test
Cholera	1884 (Koch)	1896 Killed cholera vaccine
Typhoid	1880 (Gaffky)	1896 Immunization
Plague	1894 (Yersin)	1895 (animals) 1906 (humans)
Tetanus	1884–1889	1890 Antitetanic serum (ATS) 1933 Toxoid immunization
Pertussis	1906 (Bordet)	1931–1939
Typhus	1909 (Ricketts) 1916 (Rocha-Lima)	1942 Killed *Rickettsia* vaccine
Gas gangrene	1892 (Welch)	1916 Antitoxin
Influenza	1931 (Smith et al.)	From early 1950s
Yellow fever	1928–1933	1928 (Hindle)
Poliomyelitis	1910 (Landsteiner, Flexner, et al.)	1954 (Salk) 1961 (Sabin)
Measles	1954 (Enders)	1960 Vaccine developed 1963 Vaccine licensed
Mumps	1945 (Johnson and Goodpasture)	1948 Killed virus vaccine 1967 Live virus vaccine
Rubella	1962 (Weller, Neva)	1966 Vaccine developed 1970 Vaccine licensed
Hepatitis A (HAV)	1973 (Feinstone, et al.)	
Rotavirus	1973 (Bishop, et al.)	
Hepatitis B (HBV)	1970 (Dane)	1965 Australia antigen 1978 HBV vaccine
Ebola virus disease	1977 (Piot, et al.)	
Legionnaires' disease	1977 (Fraser, McDade, et al.)	
Helicobacter pylori	1983 (Marshall and Warren)	
Hantavirus	1977 (Johnson and Lee)	
Lyme disease	1982 (Steere, et al.)	
Human immuno-deficiency virus (HIV) disease	1983 (Montagnier, et al.)	
Hepatitis C	1989	

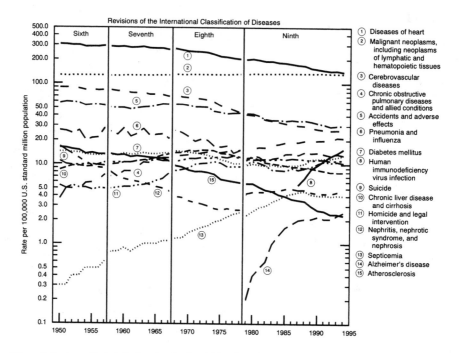

Figure 1–1. Age-adjusted death rates for the 15 leading causes of death: United States, 1950 to 1994. (Monthly Vital Statistics Report. *45(3), September 30, 1996.*)

positive concept, emphasizing social and personal resources as well as physical capabilities.

Here is a definition that acknowledges the aspects of health we are able to measure[10]: Health is a state characterized by anatomic integrity, ability to perform personally valued family, work, and community roles; ability to deal with physical, biologic, and social stress; a feeling of well-being; and freedom from the risk of disease and untimely death.

Public health[9] is the combination of science, practical skills, and values (or beliefs) directed to the maintenance and improvement of the health of all the people.[11] It is a set of efforts organized by society to protect, promote, and restore the people's health through collective or social action. The programs, services, and institutions of public health emphasize the prevention of disease and the health needs of the population as a whole. Public health activities change with changing technology and values, but the goals remain the same—to reduce the amount of disease, premature death, and disease-produced discomfort and disability in the population.

Preventive medicine,[9] also called **community medicine,**[9] is a specialized field of medical practice[12] focusing on the health of defined populations in order to promote and maintain health and well-being and prevent disease, disability, and premature death. In addition to the knowledge of basic and clinical sciences and the skills common to all physicians, the distinctive aspects of preventive or community medicine include knowledge of and competence in: epidemiology; biostatistics; administration, including planning, organization, management, financing, and evaluation of health programs; environmental health; application of social and behavioral factors in health and disease; and the application of primary, secondary, and tertiary prevention measures within clinical medicine.

▶ DETERMINANTS OF HEALTH AND DISEASE

Determinants of health are often classified as inherited (i.e., genetically determined) or acquired, but these boundaries are indistinct. Some "inherited" characteristics (genotypes) are determined by selective patterns of phenotype mortality and survival among previous generations that were exposed to epidemic or endemic diseases such as malaria, smallpox, measles, plague, and influenza. Most "acquired" determinants of health are associated with the physical, biologic, social, and behavioral environment of individuals and populations, and here too the boundaries are indistinct. For example, many aspects of the environment are influenced by human behavior; and exposure to many pathogens—the most important biologic determinants of health—is strongly influenced by the behavior of individuals, communities, cultures, nations, and civilizations.

The most important physical determinant of health is the sun's radiant energy, the spark that started all life as well as the source of potentially harmful solar radiation. Other physical determinants include climate, topography, water supply, and soil chemistry—Hippocrates' *Airs, Waters, Places*—and many other factors, some we are just beginning to understand, like prolonged exposure to high levels of environmental noise. In the near future an important physical determinant of population health may be the global climate, which appears to be changing to produce unprecedented new dangers to health (see Chap. 11).

Biologic determinants of health include naturally and artificially acquired immunity to pathogenic microorganisms, nutritional status, etc. Humans constantly interact with other living creatures that share the same global, regional, and local ecosystem. Another way to define health is as a state of harmony between humans and other creatures that share the ecosystem.

Social determinants include occupation, family, and other social networks and support systems, and again the boundaries are indistinct. We think of education, occupation, and employment status as social determinants, as indeed they are: They are related to income, which is a powerful determinant of health. A sense of self-esteem is part of every person's position in the social system, and this contributes to mind–body interactions that determine individual and, to some extent, community health. Mind–body interactions may contribute more to female than male ill health, because women's impaired sense of self-esteem can be among the consequences of their inferior, subservient status in many cultures.

Behavioral determinants of health include a range of inherent and acquired behaviors. Inherent behaviors include a "language instinct" that is a unique human characteristic and, according to sociobiologists, also include genetically determined social behavior patterns that others, including many geneticists, regard as culturally determined[13]; controversy surrounds the concepts, theories, and empirical observations of sociobiology. Some behaviors enhance and others (such as addiction to tobacco and other harmful substances) endanger health.

Behavioral determinants also include risk-taking behavior. This is a function of how people perceive risk, and it is, among other things, age-related: Adolescent and young adult males typically perceive their own risk of death by misadventure to be low or nonexistent, hence they engage in dangerous recreations and are usually willing recruits in wartime.

It is essential to understand the interactions among determinants of health if we are to intervene intelligently to control health problems. For instance, to prevent adolescent pregnancy and sexually transmitted diseases, we must understand that human sexuality is at least partly an inherent, instinctive drive, that adolescents are risk-takers, and that they tend to ignore or defy parents and other authority figures. Therefore admonitions to refrain from sexual activity ("just say no"), prohibiting education about human sexuality in schools, and impeding understanding of and denying access to effective contraception—the tactics of the religious right wing—are more likely to promote than to prevent adolescent pregnancy and sexually transmitted diseases.

An important class of behavioral determinants of health is a set of characteristics we describe as human values. Our values are influenced by cultural conditioning within the family and in other social groups, by education, by religious beliefs, by past experience, and by many other factors. Health-related human values evolve and change under the influence of expanding knowledge and awareness. Consider diseases resulting from poor hygiene and inadequate sanitation. In the second half of the 19th century, the epidemiologic observations of John Snow, William Farr, and others and discoveries by the bacteriologists Louis Pasteur, Robert Koch, and others convinced the scientific community that germs cause diseases. In an age of improved literacy and political reform, these scientific discoveries soon became part of general knowledge and popular culture. Values changed, and legislation was enacted that mandated environmental sanitation and standards of personal hygiene for food handlers. Since the mid-20th century, evolving scientific and general knowledge about the harmful effects of tobacco smoke have led to another change in values, reinforced increasingly by laws and regulations that discourage or prohibit smoking in many places of public assembly. When I was a medical student in the 1940s, we all smoked. Offering a cigarette was our way of showing friendship when we were introduced to strangers. Now it is as unacceptable to smoke without permission in somebody else's home as it would have been in the late 19th century to cough and spit on the carpet.* When the mode of transmission of acquired immunodeficiency syndrome (AIDS) was worked out, public discussion of sexual practices became socially acceptable. Words like "condom" and "anal intercourse" began to appear in newspapers, condoms were advertised on television, and in the most enlightened European nations, frank discussions and warnings about unsafe sexual conduct, using explicit language, including demotic speech, became commonplace.

Reflecting on these changing values and behaviors in my lifetime led me to suggest a necessary sequence for the control of any public health problem[14]:

- Awareness that the problem exists
- Understanding what causes the problem
- Capability to deal with the problem
- A sense of values that the problem matters
- Political will to control the problem

Discussing progress in public health, Geoffrey Vickers[15] described the two final steps as "redefining the unacceptable"—a phrase that captures well the important role of human values.

In my lifetime I have seen this sequence at work not only with the dramatic change in values, behavior, and regulation regarding the use of tobacco, but also in the use of seat belts in cars, recognition of domestic violence as a public health problem, the rise in popularity of jogging and aversion to high-cholesterol diets, and in many other changes in values, often in response to epidemiologic studies that have identified risk factors for undesirable health outcomes. I pursue further the ethical implications of this in Chapter 10, and in Chapter 11 I discuss urgently needed new changes in values and behavior that are required to mitigate the harmful impact of global change.

Much remains mysterious about determinants of good health. At the end of the 20th century we know that our behavior plays an important part but we are uncertain about many relationships, for instance between the behavior of television characters and that of real people in their everyday lives. Some evidence suggests that "epidemics" of unhealthy or harmful imitative behavior can occur, at any rate among suggestible people. Advertising, which aims to alter behavior, has mainly exerted a more harmful than beneficial influence, leading many people to become addicted to tobacco and attracted to alcohol and commercial products, such as junk foods promoted on television (see Chap. 6).

---

* Thanks to Dr. William Foege for this vivid analogy.

► METHODS OF PUBLIC HEALTH

The historical perspectives, definitions, and the discussion of determinants of health demonstrate the broad scope of public health. As our knowledge increases, we can do more about a widening range of problems; and, as already mentioned, we realize that aspects of life previously taken for granted as normal and acceptable are public health problems. This is happening in the 1990s with increasing recognition of domestic violence as a public health problem.

In the 11th edition of *Maxcy-Rosenau Public Health and Preventive Medicine,* I classified ways to promote and protect health: maintain a safe environment, enhance immunity to infection, behave sensibly, ensure satisfactory nutrition, plan and provide adequately for children, and use health care prudently (Box 1–1).[16] Each of these deserves discussion.

Safe Environment

The 19th-century sanitary revolution was the most important step ever taken by organized communities to enhance health. The sanitary disposal of excreta and the provision of pure piped water removed deadly dangers to the health and survival of weanling and older children and others at every age, who previously had died in huge numbers from all forms of gastrointestinal infections. Improved kitchen hygiene and safer storage and refrigeration of food

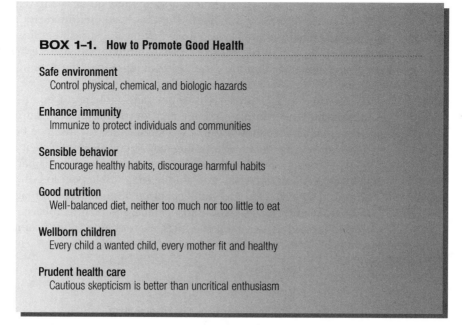

BOX 1–1. How to Promote Good Health

Safe environment
Control physical, chemical, and biologic hazards

Enhance immunity
Immunize to protect individuals and communities

Sensible behavior
Encourage healthy habits, discourage harmful habits

Good nutrition
Well-balanced diet, neither too much nor too little to eat

Wellborn children
Every child a wanted child, every mother fit and healthy

Prudent health care
Cautious skepticism is better than uncritical enthusiasm

had a synergistic effect. Improving economies that led to better housing and smaller families with children more widely spaced contributed to reduced mortality and morbidity from respiratory disease among infants and toddlers, by reducing the likelihood of infection being transmitted from school-age children to younger siblings. (Other factors such as chemotherapy and antibiotics and measles vaccine played a part in more recent years.) The combination reduced the infant mortality rate in the industrial nations from 200 to 250 per 1000 early in the 19th century to about 80 to 100 by 1900 and paved the way for further reductions, to 50 to 60 by the end of World War I, 30 to 40 by the end of World War II. Subsequent reductions to 5 to 10 per 1000 by the late 1990s in the industrial nations are due both to environmental factors (improved living conditions) and the use of immunizing agents and antibiotics (Table 1–2).

New environmental threats have arisen. Atmospheric pollution resulting from combustion of fossil fuels causes respiratory damage and disease and has other serious consequences produced by the "greenhouse effect" (see Chaps. 4 and 11). Contamination of water, air, and essential ecosystems with toxic byproducts of the petrochemical industry and pesticides are equally serious or more so. Some of these new environmental chemical hazards are

TABLE 1–2.   Infant Mortality Rates, Selected Countries and Years[a]

Year	Sweden	United States	Sri Lanka	India
1751	186			
1775	185			
1800	240			
1825	176			
1850	149			
1875	134			
1900	100		170	
1910	75		176	205
1920	63	86	182	195
1930	55	100	175	180
1940	39	47	149	160
1950	21	29	82	127
1960	17	26	70	170
1970	11	16	50	135
1980	7	13	43	120
1993–4	4	8	15	79

[a]Rate per 1000.
Sources: UN Demographic Yearbooks, UNICEF, and WHO Annual Statistical Reports.

poorly understood, but some appear capable of damaging human chromosomes—they may be mutagenic, teratogenic, or carcinogenic, or all of these (see Chap. 4).

Enhanced Immunity

Edward Jenner's discovery in 1796 of the efficacy of cowpox vaccine in preventing smallpox was the first of a long list of immunizing agents. We routinely immunize infants against diphtheria, pertussis, tetanus, poliomyelitis, measles, rubella, and mumps (see Chap. 3). Now we have effective vaccines (i.e., immunizing agents) against about 30 formerly common infections. Immunization protects individuals and communities: Herd immunity reduces the risk of epidemic spread in a population because it reduces the probability that infective organisms will encounter susceptible hosts (see Chap. 3). Ethical problems can arise as formerly common diseases approach elimination and the risks of adverse effects attributable to the vaccine become as great as the risks of getting the disease against which it is used (see Chap. 10).

Behavior

Important public health problems are a result of the way people behave; these are often called diseases of lifestyle. They include all the conditions attributable to tobacco addiction—respiratory and other cancers, chronic obstructive lung disease, and much coronary heart disease. They also include conditions associated with abuse of alcohol and drugs, much of the injury and death caused by traffic crashes and interpersonal violence, certain cancers of the reproductive system, dental caries, obesity, and many other diseases (see Chaps. 6 and 7).

It ought to be a simple matter to reduce the impact of these conditions, but many factors that influence behavior are poorly understood. As noted above, as societies evolve, values alter and behavior sometimes changes. But we do not always know how or why this happens and can only observe change after it has occurred. I discuss this conundrum further in Chapter 6.

Emphasis has moved increasingly toward influencing health-related behavior in a positive direction, i.e., encouraging individuals and populations to behave in healthful ways, such as by taking regular exercise and adhering to healthy diets. This may get better results than attempts to discourage unhealthy habits and behaviors. There is good evidence that exercise is health promoting; this has encouraged health-planning groups to recommend ways to provide more and better opportunities for persons in sedentary occupations to preserve physical fitness by facilitating access to jogging and cycling tracks, etc. Communities in nations all over the world have followed the lead of the WHO-inspired "Healthy Cities" movement that began with Düsseldorf (Germany), Liverpool (England), and Toronto (Canada) in the early 1980s.[17]

Nutrition

Throughout history and for much of the world's population today, food shortages, often severe, have been the normal state of affairs, and nutritional deficiency diseases have been among the most widely prevalent health problems. Vitamin A deficiency remains the commonest cause of blindness in the developing world. Almost a billion people are at risk of iodine deficiency diseases[18]; this causes permanent mental retardation, and it is easily prevented by iodine supplements in cooking or table salt. Nutritional deficit reduces resistence to infection, and infection increases metabolic demand for nutrients, so a vicious circle exists (see Chap. 5). In the affluent industrial nations we see the opposite problem of overnutrition and the diseases it contributes to, e.g., diabetes, obesity, coronary heart disease. This could change rapidly if food security is threatened, e.g., by global climate change (see Chap. 11).

Studies of groups who adhere to dietary restrictions, such as members of religious sects whose rules include avoidance of meat, coffee, tea, alcohol (and tobacco, among strict adherants) have shown that they enjoy lower mortality and morbidity rates from many kinds of cancer and from coronary heart disease compared to persons of other faiths who live and work in the same environment. This supports recommendations for health-promoting diets, another important part of public health policy.

Wellborn Children

Unlike other creatures, we can control our reproductive rate. In periods of high infant and child mortality, the urge to produce many offspring has been unrestrained, but as threats to survival in infancy and childhood receded, voluntary limits on reproductive rates became greater. All cultures have exercised some control over numbers, using methods ranging from abortion, infanticide, and abandoning the weakest, to condoms, contraceptive pills, and other modern means to reduce the risk of unintended pregnancy.

As birth rates fall it becomes more important to ensure that those who are born are healthy. This requires knowledge and application of factors leading to birth of infants in optimum health. Good prenatal care and attention to maternal health and nutritional status help to achieve this. Avoiding exposure of the developing fetus to toxic substances, including prescribed and other drugs, tobacco, and alcohol, is an essential part of good prenatal care.

Genetic counseling can help to prevent unions that would produce infants with lethal inherited disorders such as Tay–Sachs disease. More active interventions are possible as techniques of genetic engineering are refined. Animal and plant husbandry have long relied on empirical methods to breed better strains of corn, hogs, poultry, and racehorses. A few cultures have attempted similar breeding experiments. The pharoahs of ancient Egypt probably practiced their incestuous marital unions for this reason. For several centuries the ruling families of Europe treated their offspring as breeding stock with no observable benefit—indeed, if anything, the reverse. The most recent experiment in human breeding, Hitler's attempt to create a master race, lasted barely half a generation. Probably all such attempts are doomed to failure; we know too little about human genetics to manipulate the gene pool, and human generations are too long for even the longest-lived population geneticist to observe and react to the results of unions. It will be a long time, if ever, before we are capable even of breeding basketball stars, let alone Einsteins. The enthusiasm for "eugenics" that was common among well-meaning public health specialists in the first two decades of the 20th century has evaporated. I think it is unlikely that genetic engineering or the human genome project will change this, although these have profound ethical and moral implications.

Prudent Health Care

Attempting to cure but possessing incomplete knowledge, doctors have often unwittingly harmed some of their patients. Even attempts to protect health by immunizing populations against diseases have sometimes backfired. We express amused horror at the blood-letting, purging, and poulticing of 18th-century medical practice, but recent medical disasters remind us that progress is not always toward human betterment (Table 1–3).

Some physicians remain uncritically enthusiastic about new regimens that have not been adequately tested, but their numbers should diminish in this era of evidence-based medicine (Chap. 2). Randomized controlled trials evaluate the efficacy and safety of innovative therapeutic regimens and procedures, but not always with adequate long-term follow-up. The disastrous epidemic of vaginal cancer in daughters of women who were given estrogens to "prevent" threatened miscarriages would not have occurred if there had been a rigorous evaluation of this (as it turned out) useless as well as deadly treatment. Preventing hazards associated with the provision of health care requires that education of doctors and other health professionals should not be a process in which students' minds are stuffed with ill-assorted facts and poorly digested opinions, but a time to learn how to think logically, rationally, and critically.

▶ HEALTH PROMOTION

Preventive medicine can send a rather "negative" message: We try to stop people doing things that are bad for them, that will harm their health—often things they enjoy, which leads many to disregard our advice. We should instead encourage people to do things that are good for them. The concept of health promotion is positive. It was the subject of a WHO-sponsored conference in Ottawa, Canada, in 1986, which developed the Ottawa Charter on Health Promotion.[19] Health promotion is the process of enabling people to

TABLE 1–3.   **Some Episodes of Adverse Effects of Health Care**

Agent	Year	Consequences
Immunizations:		
Diphtheria immunization	1928	12 out of 31 children died of septicemia
BCG vaccine	1930	207 of 251 newborn babies developed tuberculosis; 72 died
Yellow fever vaccine	1942	28,000 cases, 62 deaths from hepatitis among U.S. servicemen
Polio vaccine	1955	125 cases of paralytic poliomyelitis
Influenza vaccine	1976	160 cases of Guillain-Barré syndrome[a]
Drugs:		
Mercurial teething powders	c. 1890–1951	"Pink disease" (chronic mercury poisoning) affecting many thousands of infants; few deaths
Sulfanilamide	1937	Renal failure; 358 cases, 107 deaths, mostly among children
Chloramphenicol	1946	Aplastic anemia; 200 cases identified in one year (1952) in U.S.; many thousands worldwide, especially in developing countries
Phenylbutazone	1951	Aplastic anemia; 45 deaths in U.K. until 1979
Thalidomide	1956–1961	Intrauterine reduction deformities of limbs; 9000–10,000 cases, about 8000 in former West Germany
Phenothiazines	1953	Tardive dyskinesia; many thousands of cases
Isoprenaline nebulizers	1961	Several hundred deaths of children and young adults in U.K., Australia, New Zealand
Salicylates (for fever in children)	c. 1980	Reye's syndrome
Estrogens	c. 1946–1971	1. Vaginal cancer, genital tract dysplasia in daughters exposed in utero; estimated 10,000 affected in U.S. 2. Postmenopausal endometrial cancer; estimated 15,000 cases in U.S.
Oral contraceptives	1958	Thromboembolic disorders, myocardial infarction, cerebral thrombosis, etc.; estimated 500 deaths per annum in U.S.
Oxygen	1930s	Retrolental fibroplasia in immature and premature infants
Ionizing radiation (x-rays)	Early 1900s	Cancer, leukemia in patients and physicians exposed to radiation; estimated 60–80 excess deaths/yr among physicians, other health workers; "premature aging" of exposed human fetuses
Anesthetic gases (oxides of nitrogen)	1940s	Spontaneous miscarriage, birth defects among offspring of operating room staff
Human Growth Hormone (HGH)	1980	Creutzfeld-Jacob Disease, several hundred cases worldwide due to contaminated HGH

[a] Reappraisal of evidence suggests "swine flu" vaccine was not responsible.
U.K. = United Kingdom; U.S. = United States.

increase control over and improve their own health. It involves the population as a whole in the context of their everyday lives, rather than focusing on people at risk for specific diseases, and is directed toward action on the causes or determinants of health. The aim is to encourage people to behave healthfully, to eat healthy diets, to exercise regularly within the limits of their physiologic capability, to be sociable and helpful toward others, to get regular rest and relaxation. There is good evidence that all these positive actions promote good health, and they are part of national health policies and strategies.

► PRIMARY, SECONDARY, AND TERTIARY PREVENTION

It is customary to distinguish three "levels" of prevention. The aim of **primary prevention** is to maintain health by removing the precipitating causes and determinants of departures from good health. This can be done by eliminating disease agents, as by the eradication of smallpox; by protecting persons and populations from infections, as by vaccinating against infections and pasteurizing milk; by use of dietary supplements such as iodine (iodized salt)[20]; by using safety equipment in hazardous occupations and protecting workers against exposure to toxic substances in the workplace; by effective barrier methods of contraception; by using seat belts or airbags in automobiles and crash helmets for motorcyclists. In epidemiologic language, primary prevention reduces the incidence of disease, injury, and premature death (Box 1–2).

Secondary prevention means the early detection of disease, before it has had time to produce irreversible damage. In epidemiologic language, secondary prevention reduces the prevalence or duration of disease and disability. It is often accomplished by **screening,**[21] i.e., procedures that enable us to

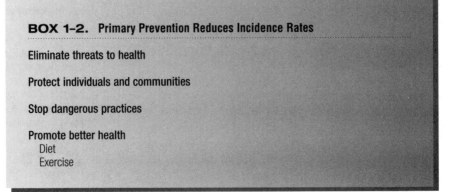

BOX 1–2. Primary Prevention Reduces Incidence Rates

Eliminate threats to health

Protect individuals and communities

Stop dangerous practices

Promote better health
 Diet
 Exercise

detect the early signs and symptoms of disease. We use routine screening tests to detect abnormalities that may be present at birth, e.g., congenitally dislocated hip and inborn errors of metabolism. If congenital hip disease is detected at birth rather than when infants begin to walk, permanently disfiguring limps can be averted. Neonatal detection of phenylketonuria, an inborn error of metabolism, can prevent severe, permanent intellectual damage if dietary treatment begins immediately.

Screening to achieve secondary prevention of disease is an integral part of clinical preventive medicine. The aim is to reverse, halt, or retard the progress of disease by detecting it as early as possible in its natural history (Fig. 1–2). Some screening procedures seek to anticipate the pathophysiologic onset of disease by identifying precursors of disease and taking action to eliminate or correct these. Screening procedures are available at all stages in life (Table 1–4). I discuss the epidemiologic principles of screening in Chapter 2.

Screening must be followed by interventions to deal with the conditions revealed. The Canadian Task Force on the Periodic Health Examination[22] established rules that were elaborated and refined by the U.S. Preventive Services Task Force,[23] which produced a *Guide to Clinical Preventive Services*,[24] the "bible" of clinical preventive medicine (Table 1–5).

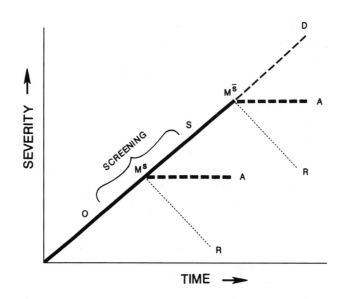

Figure 1–2. Screening and the natural history of disease. **O** = pathophysiologic onset; **S** = symptoms or signs clinically apparent; **M**^{s} = medical care after early screening; **M**$^{\bar{s}}$ = medical care in absence of screening; **A** = disease process arrested; **R** = complete or partial recovery; **D** = death.

TABLE 1–4. **Screening Procedures in Clinical Practice**

Procedure	Target Population
Medical history (questionnaire)	All ages, both sexes
Height and weight	All ages, both sexes
Blood pressure	Men and women over age 20
Chest x-ray	High-risk groups
Tuberculin test	Children, old people
Schick test	Children
Urine	
Reducing substances	All, especially adults
Protein	All, especially adults
Cells	Young females; all over 40
Ocular tension	All over 40

Studies of the costs and benefits of screening programs have shown that the expense is worthwhile for common conditions like cancer of the breast or cervix and for uncommon but permanently disabling conditions like phenylketonuria. As the incidence of a condition declines, the cost of finding a case rises. For example, mass miniature radiography to find cases of tuberculosis is uneconomical when the prevalence of tuberculosis is low; screening for tuberculosis may then be done by using tuberculin skin tests to detect converters, whose close contacts can be investigated—but the HIV epidemic has increased the prevalence of false-negative tuberculin tests among immunocompromised persons with active tuberculosis (see Chap. 3).

There is controversy about the cost-effectiveness of some preventive services.[25] Epidemiologic, statistical, and econometric methods are suggested[26] to establish the monetary and other benefits of interventions. Some services are more efficacious than others; but people feel better if their ailments are dealt with expeditiously and early, and many are reassured by negative tests and are willing to pay for interventions if these are not too costly. Faced with relentlessly rising costs, nations that offer comprehensive health insurance programs must review carefully the budgets they allocate for screening. Such reviews can lead to unpopular policy decisions. Rigorous randomized, controlled trials have shown that mammography at ages below 45 or 50 years is not cost-effective,[27–28] but many women and their doctors believe it is better to be sure than sorry, evidence notwithstanding.

There are well-established approaches for many screening procedures. For example, cytologic examination for early detection of dysplasia or carcinoma of the cervix, a sexually transmitted disease (see Chap. 7), is best practiced among sexually active women with multiple partners or better still, if this is known or can be inferred from local customs and mores, monoga-

TABLE 1–5. Screening Procedures and Developmental Stages

Prenatal Period (Assess pregnant women)
    Genetic disorders (?)
    Blood group incompatibility
    Sexually transmitted diseases
        Syphilis, gonorrhea, herpes, AIDS
    Rubella, toxoplasmosis
    Birth defects
        Neural tube defects, Down's syndrome
    Medical conditions
        Diabetes, hypertension, bacteriuria, pyelonephritis
    Obstetric conditions
        Pelvic disproportion, recurrent or threatened abortion
    Maternal behavior
        Alcohol, tobacco use, neglect or abuse

Infancy (0–18 months)
    Screening routines for phenylketonuria, congenital hip disease, hypothyroidism
    Examination for other defects, e.g., cardiovascular, hearing, visual impairment,
        strabismus, developmental delay or abnormalities

Childhood (18 months–11 years)
    Visual, hearing disorders
    Developmental abnormalities
    Behavior disorders, learning disabilities
    Dental caries
    Posture

Adolescence (12–15 years)
    Tuberculin test
    Dental caries
    Sexual maturation
    Psychosexual development

Adulthood (16–44 years)
    Hypertension
    Diabetes
    Dental caries
    Cancer of cervix
    Family dysfunction

Adulthood (45–64 years)
    Glaucoma
    Hypertension
    Diabetes
    Cancer
        Breast
        Cervix
        Colon and rectum
        Prostate
        Oral cavity
        Lung, bladder, stomach (?)

(continued)

TABLE 1–5.   *(continued)*

Adulthood (65 years and over)
  Sensory impairments (vision, hearing)
  Motor impairments (hips, feet)
  Hypertension
  Diabetes
  Cancer
  Nutrition
  Emotional status
  Intellectual status

AIDS = acquired immunodeficiency syndrome.

mous women whose husbands have multiple partners (Table 1–6). Epidemiologic and sociologic knowledge about the distribution of disease and of vulnerable groups or high-risk individuals enables us to deploy resources efficiently, concentrating on high-prevalence groups.

By whom and where should screening be conducted? Physicians should always be alert to the possibility of detecting as early as possible the presence of known risk factors and any departures from normal, and should accept their responsibility to intervene both to preserve and to restore good health.[29] Surveys show that, on average, two-thirds of the population visit a physician once or more often in the course of a year, and 95 percent of the population visit at least once in 5 years (the other 5 percent almost all enjoy excellent health). Persons who visit a physician in the course of a year in-

TABLE 1–6.   Indications and Procedures for Cervical Cancer Screening

Who?
  All women who are or have been sexually active
When?
  Within 2 years of initial sexual activity
How often?
  Every 3 to 5 years
What groups require more frequent screening?[a]

  Women with multiple sexual partners
  Women whose partners have multiple partners
  Women on the oral contraceptive pill for 5 years or more
  History of vaginal or vulval warts
  Partner's history of penile warts
  Previous abnormal smear
  Heavy smokers

[a] These women mostly require annual smears.

clude most of those who have conditions or precursors that should respond to early intervention, so we might rely on casual, incidental contacts between physicians and their patients as one way for many who require screening to be screened. This assumes that primary care physicians have the time and interest to conduct screening procedures and that the costs are covered, which often they are not. Special screening clinics are then justifiable, but these must provide the relevant interventions or collaborate with practicing physicians who do.

Health promotion and disease prevention in clinical practice requires risk assessment, a logical approach to the person's medical history, targeted physical examination and laboratory tests, and rational use of the information derived. The aims vary and include changing behavior, cessation of smoking and other substance abuse, graded exercises, suitable dietary regimens, etc., according to circumstances and need.[30]

Many primary care physicians practice clinical preventive medicine, i.e., a combination of screening procedures aimed at early detection of disease and counseling and supervision of health-protecting regimens, smoking-cessation, graded exercises, etc. Such programs may be directed toward prevention and control of specific conditions like coronary heart disease, hypertension, diabetes, certain forms of cancer, various occupational diseases, etc.; or they may be all-purpose programs offered by general physicians as part of their service to patients. Intuitively, we might expect specific programs to be more efficient; confirmatory evaluative data are not available.

Fees that impose an economic barrier to needed screening procedures are clearly undesirable; some people, including many high-risk persons who most need screening procedures, are deterred from attending until their disease is far advanced. Furthermore, screening is best combined with counseling about ways to preserve and promote good health; whether this is done by physicians or others, such as dieticians, the time and effort cannot be provided without cost. The economic outlay for screening is recovered if early detection leads to effective treatment that restores health rapidly, so the persons concerned return to the workforce, rather than experiencing prolonged and perhaps terminal illnesses that require costly long-term care.

The growth of for-profit health maintenance organizations (HMOs) in the United States has undermined hopes of building health promotion and disease prevention programs into primary care, because these activities are not regarded as cost-effective. Other nations have escaped this trend.

The aim of **tertiary prevention** is to prevent deterioration and complications from occurring when disease or disability are already established; this is the same as "high-quality health care." It is applied when seriously ill or injured patients are carefully nursed to prevent bedsores, venous thrombosis, and other preventable complications; when bladder care is used to prevent infection; and when diabetics and hypertensives are controlled by treatment aimed at minimizing preventable complications, including those that are hazards of the treatment regimen.

► PUBLIC HEALTH POLICIES

The responsibility of the nation for the health of its citizens has been explicit since lawmakers began enacting legislation on aspects of health protection.[31] This has occurred at different rates and with different emphases in many countries. In the United States, the Constitution does not refer to health as a "right," but presidents and other public figures have taken action that has had direct beneficial effect upon the health of the American people. Tax support is provided for public health and health promotion and for medical and nursing care for the indigent sick. Similar processes have occurred in other nations.

There is a long history of government support for policies to improve health and provision of funds for studies of factors that can improve health. These are the raisons d'être for the U.S. Public Health Service (USPHS), the Centers for Disease Control and Prevention (CDC), and the National Institutes of Health (NIH). See Chapter 8 for details.

In 1974, the government of Canada sponsored the Lalonde Report, a discussion paper that influenced health policy in many nations; this recognized and addressed issues in specific health fields, i.e., biologic, environmental, lifestyle, and health care,[32] and had considerable influence on thinking about ways to improve health, perhaps more outside than within Canada.

The challenge was taken up by WHO. In 1977, the World Health Assembly resolved that the main social target of governments and of WHO should be the attainment by all the people of the world by the year 2000 of a level of health that would permit them to lead a socially and economically productive life, popularly known as "Health for All by the Year 2000." This phrase was a slogan, not an attainable target, but it provided incentives to international and national health planners and policy makers, and progress that otherwise might not have occurred has been made toward improved health.

In 1978 at an international conference in Alma-Ata, in the former Soviet Union, convened by WHO and the United Nations Children's Fund (UNICEF), the delegates agreed that the best way to achieve "health for all" would be to provide primary health care for all people. Those attending the conference unanimously endorsed a far-reaching statement, the Alma Ata Declaration,[33] that merits study by all who care about health.

With WHO support and enhanced activity by UNICEF, much progress has been made toward improving health in the developing world, through the WHO Expanded Programme on Immunization (EPI), tropical disease research (TDR), and stepped-up efforts by the United Nations Development Plan (UNDP), the United Nations Fund for Population Activities (UNFPA), and in recent years, the World Bank. The World Bank's 1993 report, *Investing in Health*,[34] made commitment to health explicit, spelling out the interconnectedness of health and development and promising greater emphasis on health promotion and disease prevention in future donor programs. Many other programs and activities are conducted by nongovernmental organizations. Whereas the main thrust of "Health for All by the Year 2000" has been in the developing nations, many industrial nations have responded to the same challenges, defined health goals and objectives, and set up programs aimed at achieving them. A good example is the "Healthy Cities" initiative mentioned previously. Urban leaders in many nations have improved their local and regional environments, made cities more user-friendly to cyclists and joggers, promoted healthful nutrition, and taken action against indoor air pollution by tobacco smoke.

Nevertheless, *Bridging the Gaps*,[35] the 1995 WHO Report, spelled out clearly the tremendous challenges facing humanity as we approach the next millenium (see Chap. 9). Some challenges have been addressed and progress toward their control has been detailed in triannual reports on the world health situation and programs of work. *Bridging the Gaps* acknowledges the failure in many nations (including the United States and even more so the former Soviet Union and its satellite states) and the sobering realities that face the human community at the end of this millennium.

In the United States, a strategy for health promotion and disease prevention was outlined in 1979 in the surgeon general's report, *Healthy People*.[36] This focused on the nature of the health problems challenging the American people. It was recognized that health improvements earlier in the 20th century had been due primarily to public health measures, i.e., environmental sanitation, immunization, and improved nutrition and housing, with some benefits also resulting from changes in lifestyle. *Healthy People* defined five goals for 1990, one for each of five stages of life (Box 1–3).

In 1980, *Promoting Health, Preventing Disease: Objectives for the Nation*[37] defined specific targets for preventive health services, health protection measures, and activities in health promotion. This specified 226 objectives, arranged in 15 priority subject areas, developed by representatives from na-

---

BOX 1–3. Goals for Five Life Stages

To continue to improve infant health and, by 1990, to reduce infant mortality by at least 35 percent, to below 9 per 1000

To improve child health, foster optimal childhood development and, by 1990, reduce deaths of children aged 1–14 by 20 percent

To improve the health and habits of young people aged 15–24 and reduce death rates by at least 20 percent

To improve the health of adults and, by 1990, to reduce death rates at ages 25–64 by at least 25 percent

To improve the health quality of life of older adults and, by 1990, to reduce the average annual number of restricted activity days by 20 percent

tional organizations and from the public and private sectors. These goal statements were elaborated in several documents, e.g., in a set of implementation plans.[38] Target dates varied; some health objectives were to be achieved by 1990, some by 1995, some by the year 2000.

By 1995, progress toward a few targets was modest at best, and some problems, notably unintended early adolescent pregnancy and sexually transmitted diseases (STDs), had got worse. Daunting new problems—HIV disease, homelessness, rising crime rates, and drug abuse—had emerged.[39]

The fiasco of health reform in 1994 and budget slashing by U.S. federal and state legislators in the late 1990s do not bode well for maintaining the modest gains that were achieved earlier. An alarming trend is cuts made in money and human resources necessary to maintain, let alone expand, essential public health infrastructure. Large outbreaks of food poisoning in the U.S. Midwest in the early 1990s (see Chap. 3) may be harbingers of worse to come if budget-slashing "reforms" continue in future.

The collapse of the former Soviet Union and its satellites and disintegration of the former Yugoslavia into war and genocide have reversed the advance of health in these regions. There has been a dramatic resurgence of vaccine-preventable diseases such as diphtheria and typhoid and sharp increases in infant and child mortality. In much of the former Soviet Union and its satellites, an intractable problem of gross and unprecedented environmental pollution with toxic and nuclear wastes has emerged, revealing dangers to health as bad as or worse than the Chernobyl nuclear disaster, including dangers that threaten nations and people far away. Only massive international efforts and very large financial outlay may restore these damaged communities, and this seems unlikely to happen. Health levels in these parts of what were formerly developed areas appear destined to decline further.[40]

Health promotion and disease prevention initiatives have been more successful in the European Union. Some of the 38 targets originally identified by working groups in the European Region of WHO[41] were to be achieved by 1990, others by 1995 or 2000. Several deserve mention. Prerequisites for health include freedom from the fear of war—"the most serious of all threats to health"; equal opportunity for all; satisfaction of basic needs for food, education, clean water, and sanitation; decent housing; secure work; and a useful role in society (Box 1–4). To achieve these prerequisites, it was recognized, would require political will and public support. All these brave words, of course, were written before the wars in the former Yugoslavia.

However, the nations of the European Union have failed to achieve equity in health, to reduce the gaps in health status between and within countries. In some nations (Sweden, Germany, France) life expectancy has risen, measles, polio, neonatal tetanus, congenital rubella, diphtheria, congenital syphilis, and malaria have been eliminated. Other European region targets— to promote healthy lifestyles, to ensure and enhance the role of the family in supporting healthy living, and to provide improved education in healthy behavior while eliminating or at least reducing health-damaging behavior—

BOX 1–4. Prerequisites for Health

Freedom from fear of war

Equal opportunity for all

Satisfaction of basic needs
  Food
  Education
  Clean water and sanitation
  Decent housing

Secure work and a useful social role

Political will and public support

have only been partially successful. For example, legislating smoke-free public places in France was a failure because almost everyone defied the law. The environment has been restored and improved, with international collaborative efforts to protect environmental quality of air and water and ensure safe disposal of hazardous wastes; housing standards and workplace safety have been improved (except in the United Kingdom, which opted out of legislation enacted in the European Parliament on some aspects of these). But grave concerns have arisen in 1996 about the dangerous levels of pollutants in the Mediterranean, the Baltic, and the North Sea, where many poorly maintained oil platforms are discharging crude oil into the sea, and marine life is threatened by this as well as by overfishing.

In many nations of the European Union, primary health care is emphasized, health resources are more equitably distributed, and there are effective quality assurance procedures, often based on efficient infrastructure of information systems. By 1998, all primary care physicians in France will have computers to support their information systems. Health policies have been formulated to achieve these ends. Health management and health information systems, health work-force development through appropriate educational programs and policies, and health technology assessment are recognized as integral components in public policy for improved health. In The Netherlands, Sweden, and Finland, health planners have looked further ahead, preparing to cope with problems anticipated well beyond the year 2000.[42–44] It is implicit—and often explicit—in documents produced by planning groups in European nations, the United States, and also in India,[45] that emerging health problems differ in nature and quality from those of the past.

Human behavior is the most important determinant of health; this includes the behavior of elected and appointed government officials and industrial and commercial interests. The behavior of transnational corporations is a crucial determinant of future health. For example, transnational timber companies endanger biodiversity and the survival (to say nothing of the health) of indigenous tribes in tropical rain forests. Other transnational corporations have established petrochemical and other polluting industries in developing countries that encourage them by offering a supply of cheap labor and an absence of environmental and occupational safety and health laws and regulations (see Chap. 9).

We have controlled many of the health problems of the past, those that were a consequence of complex interactions between humans and predators, pests and microorganisms, between humans and environments poor in natural resources or deficient in essential minerals such as iodine, problems over which hitherto we had little or no control. What remain, and what has emerged, are problems over which, if we have the will, we can exert more effective control by individual and collective actions.

▶ INDIVIDUAL AND COLLECTIVE RESPONSIBILITY FOR HEALTH

The synergism of individual and collective responsibility for health is clear. To control health problems attributable to the use of tobacco, individuals must make the decision whether to smoke. An important step is to make tobacco products more expensive and less accessible, especially to young starting smokers. Also important are local options that create smokeless zones in public places. The state or nation can help by taxing tobacco products, subsidizing health education campaigns, and legislating to impose sanctions on those who violate laws prohibiting smoking.

Similarly there is a synergistic effect of personal and collective responsibility for reducing traffic-related injury and death. Mandatory seat-belt legislation, individual motivation to use seat belts when driving cars, and effective laws against driving while impaired reinforce increasingly powerful social sanctions against impaired drivers. In U.S. states where legislators have reversed laws requiring motorcyclists to wear helmets, there has been an increase in death rates and permanent disability resulting from brain damage after motorcycle crashes that have become uncommon in states and nations where helmets are required. The United States is alone among the enlightened nations of the world in placing greater value on individual liberty to engage in such destructive behavior than on the right of the community to be protected from harms and costs resulting from these behaviors. No other advanced and peaceful nation has followed the United States down the irrational pathway that leads to the huge, mostly preventable annual toll of deaths caused by firearms.

While shared individual and community responsibility for health is implicit, and sometimes explicit, in policy statements about health promotion in the United States and other countries, the role and responsibility of corporate interests and industrial and commercial enterprises is not well defined. With the rise of transnational industrial and commercial enterprises that move capital and labor to the regions that are cheapest and those with the weakest environmental laws, the only word to describe attitudes is irresponsibility—sometimes to a degree that is reckless, even criminal if there were effective international laws to penalize such behavior. Bismarck recognized well over a hundred years ago that a healthy state is in the national interest because it contributes to the wealth of the state and keeps people contented. Few modern national governments and fewer corporate interests have retained this level of understanding; many still tolerate unsafe working conditions and show little or no consideration for the people and other living creatures who may be damaged by reckless environmental contamination. The role of national and local legislation then is to enforce compliance with safe practices one region at a time. But it is a difficult struggle, especially in nations where lobby groups can sway the votes of legislators and the time horizon of elected officials is a mere 2 years to the next election. The world is in a parlous state of environmental deterioration that requires planning with a time horizon of 50 to 100 years or more (see Chap. 11).

► THE POLITICS OF PUBLIC HEALTH

The preceding paragraphs and other allusions in this chapter have made it clear that steps necessary to protect and improve the public's health may not be universally desired or welcomed. There is opposition, often well-organized by pressure groups or political lobbies. The tobacco industry is the best known. In almost all nations it has been very successful in persuading legislators at every level, from national to local government, to avoid taking action that might reduce cigarette consumption. The meat and dairy industries have reacted aggressively to the suggestion that diets rich in animal fats are harmful to health, and their advertising and lobbying campaigns have had some success. Many polluting industries and industries that engage in work practices dangerous to the health of their workers have political lobbies to argue in support of their unsafe practices and procedures. Labor unions and concerned citizens' groups sometimes form an opposing political force. A different kind of political struggle develops when opponents of fluoridation of drinking water engage in campaigns to "keep the water pure"—a difficult aspiration, politically speaking, for uninformed voters to resist.

Sometimes inexperienced physicians and other public health workers with little political skill may be thrust into situations where their ability to marshall the facts and debate the issues will be severely tested. Obviously it is wise to consider carefully before engaging in debate on such issues. One of the most important roles of national organizations such as the American Public Health Association (APHA) is to advocate health-protecting action in contentious situations such as disposal of hazardous waste and control of indoor air pollution by tobacco smoke, where opposition is powerful and well organized. If physicians or other health care workers find themselves in a position where such political forces may be deployed, they are wise to seek reinforcement from organizations and individuals with advocacy experience.

► ECOLOGY AND HUMAN HEALTH

Not all improvements in health are due to advances of medical science. Ecologic factors account for some past changes[46] and will be responsible for future changes.

The pandemic plague of the 14th century receded for several reasons. The survival of persons who were genetically resistant and their selective breeding produced generations with increased resistance to the plague bacillus, *Yersinia pestis;* this was the same biologic phenomenon as breeding in successive generations of larger proportions of pesticide-resistant mosquitoes and penicillin-resistant gonococci. In the late middle ages, the domestic black rats that carried the fleas that transmit plague were supplanted throughout much of Europe by brown rats, whose preferred habitat was out of doors in orchards and cultivated fields. The increased distance between rats and humans reduced the probability of transmission of *Y. pestis* from rats to humans via the rats' parasitic fleas, so the fulminating epidemics died down. Also about then, building styles in Europe changed; wooden houses were replaced by houses of brick and stone (partly because Europe was running out of suitable trees) and these new houses provided fewer nesting places for rats, adding further to the probability that distance between rats and humans would be greater. Perhaps also *Y. pestis* became less lethal in its effects; historical accounts of the effects of syphilis suggest that this probably happened with *Treponema pallidum,* and it may have happened also with the *streptococcus* of scarlet fever, which appears to have been more lethal in former times (although since the early 1990s, a more virulent strain of *Streptococcus,* the so-called flesh-eating strep, has emerged).

Ecologic changes partly account for the decline of infant diarrhea as a leading cause of death. With the invention of the internal combustion engine, horses were replaced in city streets by automobiles. As the horses departed, there came a rapid decline in the numbers of the ubiquitous flies that formerly bred in heaps of horse manure in streets and stables that were adjacent to most houses. Flies had been an important means of spreading organisms responsible for infant diarrhea. Esthetic considerations as well as concern for domestic hygiene were responsible for another change about that time, the use of screens on windows, to help keep flies out of houses. The combined effect of these changes may have been more important than expanding medical knowledge of causes and methods to control infant diarrhea.

Recent changes in the social environment; the growth of cities; the use of mechanized transportation; the explosion of mass media as the source of information, ideas, entertainment, and political and emotional stimulus; and changes in patterns of work from primarily manual to primarily clerical and service industries have transformed humans from hunter-gatherers into something that may not be so well-equipped by our evolution to cope. Current ecologic changes could influence human health more profoundly than any past changes. Some of these changes are well known and frequently give rise to misgivings about the human situation. There is a widely prevailing attitude toward the environment, epitomized in words like "development" (meaning industrial and commercial development) and "conquest" (as in "the conquest of outer space"). Many people wonder whether the attitudes these phrases imply are healthy for the earth and whether the health of people is secure if the health of the earth is impaired or threatened. Happily, attitudes to exploitation of the world's precious resources are changing: conservation, sustainable development, recycling, responsible waste disposal and have become familiar words, often backed by action. Persistent and diligent actions in these categories can help avert threats to ecosystem health and human health. I return to this theme in Chapter 11 and the Epilogue.

► REFERENCES

1. Sources for the historical introduction include (1) Garrison FH: *History of Medicine.* 4th ed. Philadelphia: Saunders, 1929; (2) Rosen G: *A History of Public Health.* New York: MD Publications, 1958; (3) Singer C, Underwood EA: *A Short History of Medicine.* 2nd ed. Oxford: Clarendon, 1962; (4) Sigerist HE: *A History of Medicine.* New York: Oxford University Press, 1951, 1961; vols 1 & 2. (5) Prinzing F: *Epidemics Resulting from Wars.* Oxford: Oxford University Press, 1916.
2. (1) Henschen F; Tate J (trans): *The History of Diseases.* London: Longman, 1966; (2) McKeown T: *The Origins of Human Disease.* Oxford: Blackwell, 1988.
3. Frank JP; Lesky E (trans): *A System of Complete Medical Police.* Baltimore: Johns Hopkins University Press, 1976.
4. Fracastorius: *De Contagione.* Wright WC (trans): *Contagion.* New York: Putnam, 1930.
5. Dobell C: *Antony van Leeuwenhoek and His "Little Animals."* New York: Russell, 1958.
6. Chadwick E: *Report . . . on an Enquiry into the Sanitary Condition of the Labouring Population of Great Britain.* London: Clowes, 1842; MW Flinn (ed). Edinburgh: University of Edinburgh Press, 1965.
7. Shattuck L: *Report to the Committee of the City of Boston Appointed to Obtain the Census of Boston for the Year 1845.* Boston: Eastburn, 1846 (reprinted New York: Arno Press, 1976).
8. Jenner E: *An Enquiry into the Causes and Effects of the Variolae Vaccinae.* London: Low, 1798 (frequently reprinted, e.g., London: Dawson, 1966).
9. Last JM (ed): *A Dictionary of Epidemiology.* 3rd ed. New York: Oxford University Press, 1995.
10. Stokes J III, Noren JJ, Shindell S: Definition of terms and concepts applicable to clinical preventive medicine. *J Community Health* 8:33–41, 1982.

11. Sheps CG (chairman): *Higher Education for Public Health: A Report of the Milbank Memorial Fund Commission.* New York: Prodist, 1976.
12. American College of Preventive Medicine: Brochure. Washington, DC, 1986.
13. Wilson EO: *On Human Nature.* Cambridge, MA: Harvard University Press, 1978.
14. Last JM: The future of public health. *Nippon Koshu Eisei Zasshi (Japan J Public Health)* 38:10 (suppl 1): 58–95, 1991.
15. Vickers G: What sets the goals of public health? *Lancet* 1:599–604, 1958.
16. Last JM: Scope and methods of prevention. In Last JM (ed): *Maxcy-Rosenau Public Health and Preventive Medicine.* 11th ed. New York: Appleton-Century-Crofts, 1980, pp. 5–8.
17. Hancock T: The evolution, impact and significance of the Healthy Cities/Communities movement. *J Public Health Policy* 14:3:5–18, 1993.
18. Hetzel BS: *The Story of Iodine Deficiency: An International Challenge in Nutrition.* Oxford: Oxford Medical Publications, 1989.
19. World Health Organization: Ottawa Charter for Health Promotion. *Can J Public Health* 77:425–430, 1986.
20. Robbins LC, Blankenbaker R: Prospective medicine and health hazard appraisal. In Taylor RB, Ureda JR, Denham JW (eds): *Health Promotion: Principles and Clinical Applications.* E. Norwalk, CT: Appleton-Century-Crofts, 1982; pp. 67–121.
21. Wilson JMG, Jungner G: The principles and practice of screening for disease. *Public Health Pap* 34. (WHO, Geneva), 1968.
22. Spitzer WO (chairman): *Periodic Health Examination: Report of a Task Force to the Deputy Ministers of Health.* Ottawa: Health and Welfare Canada, 1980.
23. Goldbloom R, Battista RN, Canadian Task Force, et al.: The periodic health examination. 1985 update. *Can Med Assoc J* 134:721–729, 1986.
24. U.S. Preventive Services Task Force: *Guide to Clinical Preventive Services. An Assessment of the Effectiveness of 169 Interventions.* Washington, DC: Office of Disease Prevention and Health Promotion, USPHS, 1989.
25. Russell LB: *Is Prevention Better than Cure?* Washington, DC: Brookings Institution, 1986.
26. Mandelblatt JS, Fryback DG, Weinstein MC, et al.: Assessing the effectiveness of health interventions. In Gold MR, Siegel JE, Russell LB, et al. (eds): *Cost-effectiveness in Health and Medicine.* New York: Oxford University Press, 1996, pp. 135–175.
27. Miller AB: Is routine mammography screening appropriate for women 40 to 49 years of age? *Am J Prev Med* 7:55–62, 1991.
28. Miller AB, Baines CJ, To T, et al.: The Canadian national breast screening study: Breast cancer detection and mortality in women age 40 to 49 on entry. *Can Med Assoc J* 147:1459–1476, 1992.
29. U.S. Public Health Service, Office of Disease Prevention and Health Promotion: *Clinicians' Handbook of Preventive Services: Putting Prevention into Practice.* Washington, DC: U.S. DHHS, 1994.
30. Woolf SH, Jonas S, Lawrence RS (eds): *Health Promotion and Disease Prevention in Clinical Practice.* Baltimore: Williams & Wilkins, 1996.
31. Sigerist HE: From Bismark to Beveridge: Developments and trends in social security legislation. *Bull Hist Med* 8:365–388, 1943.
32. Lalonde M: *A New Perspective on the Health of Canadians: A Working Document.* Ottawa: Health and Welfare Canada, 1974.
33. World Health Organization/UNICEF: *Primary Health Care.* Geneva: WHO, 1978.

34. World Bank: *World Development Report 1993: Investing in Health*. Washington, DC: World Bank, 1993.

35. World Health Organization: *World Health Report 1995: Bridging the Gaps*. Geneva: WHO, 1995.

36. Surgeon-General's Report: *Healthy People*. Washington, DC: U.S. Government Printing Office, 1979.

37. *Promoting Health, Preventing Disease: Objectives for the Nation*. Washington, DC: U.S. DHHS, 1980.

38. *Promoting health/preventing disease: Public Health Service implementation plans for attaining the objectives for the nation. Public Health Rep:* Sept/Oct [supple], 98(9):3–88, 1983.

39. Office of Disease Prevention and Health Promotion, U.S. Surgeon-General: Monthly Reports. Washington, DC. See also *Healthy People 2000: Midcourse Review and 1995 Revisions*. Washington, DC: USPHS, November 1995.

40. Hertzman C: *Environment and Health in Central and Eastern Europe. A Report for the Environmental Action Programme for Central and Eastern Europe*. Washington, DC: World Bank, 1995.

41. *Targets for Health for All*. Copenhagen: *WHO Reg Publ Eur Ser,* 1985.

42. *Summary Outline of the Health 2000 Report, The Netherlands*. The Hague: Department of Health, Staff Bureau for Health Policy Development, 1984.

43. *HS 90: The Swedish Health Services in the 1990s*. Stockholm: Division of Planning and Statistics, National Board of Health and Welfare, 1985.

44. Ministry of Social Affairs and Health: *Health Policy Report by the Government to Parliament*. Helsinki, 1985.

45. Indian Council of Social Science Research and Indian Council of Medical Research: *Health for All—An Alternative Strategy*. New Delhi and Pune: Indian Institute of Education, 1981.

46. Dubos R: *Mirage of Health*. London: Allen & Unwin, 1959.

2

Assessing Public Health, and Other Uses of Epidemiology

Epidemiology is the basic science of public health and preventive medicine. The word derives from *epidemic,* which in Greek means "upon the people"; it evokes the first concern of epidemiologists, to investigate and control epidemics.

► HISTORY

Like much of Western medicine, epidemiology has roots in the Bible and in the writings of Hippocrates. The aphorisms of Hippocrates (4th to 5th century B.C.) contain generalizations that must have been based on careful observation of many cases. The introductory paragraphs of *Airs, Waters, Places* give timeless advice on good environmental epidemiology:

> Whoever would study medicine aright must learn of the following subjects. First he must consider the effect of each of the seasons of the year and the differences between them. Secondly he must study the warm and the cold winds, both those which are common to every country and those peculiar to a particular locality. Lastly, the effect of water on the health must not be forgotten. . . . When, therefore, a physician comes to a district previously unknown to him, he should consider both its situation and its aspect to the winds. . . . Similarly, the nature of the water supply must be considered. . . . Then think of the soil, whether it be bare and waterless or thickly covered with vegetation and well-watered; whether in a hollow and stifling, or exposed and cold. Lastly, consider the life of the inhabitants themselves; are they heavy drinkers and eaters and consequently unable to stand fatigue or, being fond of work and exercise, eat wisely but drink sparely?[1]

Physicians have always been concerned with epidemics, but until late in the 19th century they could seldom do more than observe the victims and record their deaths. John Graunt (1620–1674) is regarded as the founder of vital statistics; he was the first to describe the use of numerical methods, in *Natural and Political Observations . . . on the Bills of Mortality*.[2]

Careful clinical observation, precise counts of well-defined cases, and demonstration of relationships among cases and the characteristics of the populations in which they occur, all combine in the basic method on which epidemiology depends. Modern epidemiologists hold John Snow (1813–1858) in high esteem: He was the first to develop this method and used it to study epidemics of cholera in London in the 1850s, having first logically deduced that cholera must be transmitted in some manner and was not, as was widely believed at the time, caused by a "miasma" or emanation from rotting organic matter. Snow visited the houses where people had died of cholera and found out which company had supplied drinking water, as competing companies often supplied different houses on the same street. He painstakingly collected the facts about sources of drinking water in affected and unaffected households and related these to death rates from cholera, thus demonstrating the mode of transmission 30 years before Robert Koch isolated and identified the cholera vibrio (Table 2–1).

All aspiring epidemiologists should read Snow's book.[3] Aspiring epidemiologists should also read *Vital Statistics*,[4] an edited collection of the writings of William Farr (1807–1883), who was the first compiler of abstracts for the office of the registrar general of England and Wales, a post he held for over 40 years. Farr defined many basic concepts in vital statistics and epidemiology: the concept of person-years; the relationship of death rate to the probability of dying; standardized mortality ratios; the relationships between incidence and prevalence, dose-response relationships, and herd immunity; and the concepts of retrospective and prospective methods of epidemiologic study. He also developed, with his French friend and colleague Marc d'Espigne, the first

TABLE 2–1.   Cholera Mortality in London in the 4-Week Period from July 9–August 5, 1854[a]

Water Company	Houses Supplied	Deaths	Rate per 10,000 Houses
Southwark and Vauxhall	40,046	286	71
Lambeth	26,107	14	5
All others	287,345	277	9

[a]John Snow's "natural experiment" with cholera in London in 1854. The Southwark and Vauxhall Company drew its water from the River Thames downstream, where it was polluted; the Lambeth Company drew water upstream from London, where it was free of pollution. *(From Snow J. 1855[3])*

effective classification of disease, the ancestor of the International Classifica-tion of Disease we use today. He wrote beautifully; I think *Vital Statistics* is among the best textbooks of epidemiology ever written.

Methods of epidemiologic study have evolved since the 1850s. The case-control study was suggested by the French medical statistician PCA Louis (1787–1872) and adopted by WA Guy in studies of the relationship between diseases and previous work history.[5] Cohort studies came into use soon after World War II as a means of identifying risk factors for coronary heart disease, cancer of the lung and other organs, and other emerging public health prob-lems. The use of randomized, controlled trials (RCTs) to demonstrate the effi-cacy of preventive and therapeutic regimens also began in the immediate postwar years. RCTs are now regarded as the "gold standard" in deciding on the best way to control many health problems. Computerized data processing and analysis have greatly enhanced the efficiency of epidemiologic study—though I must add a cautionary note on the risk of being seduced by statistical sophistry and forgetting clinical common sense. Exciting prospects lie ahead: applications of molecular biology in molecular epidemiology; large-scale record linkage studies; capture-recapture methods when denominators are uncertain and the population size is unknown; use of the Internet for instan-taneous worldwide notification of disease outbreaks;[6] and the rise of clinical epidemiology, all discussed in the following pages, are transforming epidemi-ology, giving it even greater relevance than it already enjoys in public health and clinical practice.

▶ DEFINITION

Epidemiology originally meant the scientific study of epidemics, but the defi-nition has broadened with the scope of the discipline. The *Dictionary of Epi-demiology*[7] definition is:

> The study of the distribution and determinants of health-related states or events in specified populations, and the application of this study to control health prob-lems.

These words and phrases require elaboration. *Study* includes observation, surveillance, hypothesis-testing analytic research methods, and experiments. *Distribution* refers to analysis according to time, place, and classes of persons affected. *Determinants* are the physical, biologic, social, cultural, and behav-ioral factors influencing health that I discussed in Chapter 1. *Health-related states or events* include diseases and injuries, causes of death, behavior such as use of tobacco, reactions to preventive and therapeutic regimens, and provi-sion and use of health services. *Specified populations* are those with identifiable characteristics, such as precisely known numbers. *Application to control* makes explicit the purpose of epidemiology—to promote, protect, and preserve good health.

► USES OF EPIDEMIOLOGY

The most important use for epidemiology is surveillance and control of threats to individual and community health. This is an integral part of routine public health practice. Its importance is sometimes underestimated by epidemiologists in university departments who devote their energies to research methodology—to refinement of methods and procedures, etc.—and who teach medical students. Epidemiologic research aims to enlarge our understanding of determinants of health and disease, to define and measure risks. A few epidemiologic researchers have become so detached from the purpose of their calling that they focus only on refinement of methods, rather than the application of these methods to improve the human condition.

Morris defined seven uses of epidemiology: historical study (examining trends over time); community diagnosis; working (i.e., evaluation) of health services; individual chances (risk rating); completing the clinical picture; identifying syndromes; and searching for causes.[8] A few other uses can be added (Box 2–1). Each of these uses deserves brief comment.

BOX 2–1. Uses of Epidemiology

Historical study–Is community health getting better or worse?
Community diagnosis–What actual and potential health problems are there?
Working of health services–Efficacy
                                        Effectiveness
                                        Efficiency
Individual risks and chances–Actuarial risks
                                        Health hazard appraisal
Completing the clinical picture–Different presentations of a disease
Identification of syndromes–"Lumping and splitting"
Search for causes–Case control and cohort studies
Evaluation of presenting symptoms and signs
Clinical decision analysis
Evidence-based medicine

Historical Study

Is the human condition improving, deteriorating, or is it unchanged over time? We can answer this question by the study of trends in community health status, such as infant and general mortality rates or cause-specific mortality and morbidity rates. Value judgments are often involved in interpreting these trends, as further discussed in Chapter 1.

Community Diagnosis

What are the health problems? An important part of the answer to this question depends on being aware that a problem exists. For example, what proportion of children in grade school are becoming addicted to cigarettes, and at what ages? What proportion of drivers and passengers in cars take needless risks, always or never use seatbelts? How widespread is domestic violence? What is the level of knowledge, attitudes, and behavior among the people about these and other risks to health and long life? There are innumerable such questions.

Working of Health Services

Are all necessary services available, accessible, and used appropriately? Is health service staff morale high? Are communications among providers and users satisfactory? What proportion of health care services achieve a satisfactory outcome? Are the costs reasonable? These and many other questions and the need for answers to them have spawned a large industry of health care evaluators who combine in the same team the expertise of epidemiologists, economists, social scientists, statisticians.

Individual Chances

What is the risk that you will die before your next birthday? Is life expectancy the same for a 15-year-old black youth in an urban ghetto and a white youth the same age in an affluent suburb? If not, what explains the risk difference? Do occupational risks differ among underground coal miners, heavy transport operators, white collar workers? Again, if differences exist, how do we explain them? There are innumerable variations on these questions and the answers have important economic and political implications. Risk rating, and even more, risk assessment have become prominent uses for epidemiology.

Completing the Clinical Picture

Patients in an intensive care unit with coronary occlusion are an unrepresentative sample of the clinical spectrum of coronary heart disease, which may present as sudden unexpected death, as a massive life-threatening infarction, or may be symptomless, revealed only at necropsy that discloses a healed infarction. I used the method of "completing the clinical picture" to construct a model of the events that would occur annually in a hypothetical "average family practice": what is known and being treated and what is undetected, undiagnosed, untreated, the submerged part of the "iceberg" of disease, which includes precursors and premonitory states.[9] Construction of such a model is useful both to determine what to look for and to evaluate the effectiveness of diagnostic and screening procedures in clinical practice, e.g., in health maintenance organizations (HMOs), by comparing the observed distribution with what would be expected on the basis of occurrence rates in comparable populations or communities.

Identifying Syndromes

Epidemiologic study enables us to group together the different manifestations of the same underlying disease process, e.g., angina pectoris and acute myocardial infarction, and to differentiate between seemingly identical symptom complexes that are actually due to different disease processes, such as hepatitis A and B or juvenile and adult onset, insulin-dependent and non–insulin-dependent diabetes.

Searching for Causes

This is the most glamorous aspect of epidemiology, whether we speak of epidemiologic investigation of the first known outbreak of "new" conditions like legionnaire's disease, dangerous epidemics such as Ebola virus infection, a cluster of cases of a rare variety of cancer resulting from occupational or environmental exposure to a carcinogen, or as yet unsolved problems like the cause(s) of multiple sclerosis, Alzheimer's disease, and the common kind of hypertension. The techniques of molecular epidemiology have added power to the search for causal pathways in cancer and precision to identification of the microbial strain responsible for an infectious disease outbreak.

Other Uses

Clinical epidemiology and clinical decision analysis have added further uses of epidemiologic methods and procedures to those described by Morris. Evidence-based medicine, the application by clinicians of proved efficacious regimens, relies heavily on the findings of epidemiologic studies, especially those of RCTs. Clinical algorithms spell out the probability that particular combinations of symptoms, signs, and laboratory findings are due to each of several possible diagnoses; once the diagnosis is established, valid evidence from properly conducted epidemiologic studies is applied to identify the best possible way to deal with the condition. This approach is a consummation of the "marriage between quantitative concepts used by epidemiologists to study disease in populations and decision making in the individual case that is the daily fare of clinical medicine."[10]

► QUESTIONS ABOUT HEALTH AND DISEASE: HEALTH INFORMATION SYSTEMS

Many questions about the public health require answers on an ongoing basis. Here are some examples: What are the main health problems of the population? What are people's complaints? What symptoms do they suffer? Why do they seek and use health care services? Which services do they use? What are the reasons for their institutional care? What are their causes of death? How are all these phenomena distributed in the population? How does this distribution compare with that in the past, or in other places? What does health care really cost? To answer these and countless other questions about health, sickness, and health care services, we need a health information system.

A **health information system** is the combination of vital and health statistics from multiple sources, used to derive insights about the health needs, health resources, costs, use of health care services, and outcomes of use by the population in a specified nation, state, municipality, etc. Ideally, a health information system uses all available sources of health-related information and can expand to encompass other data sets; its boundaries are as wide as the imagination of those who design and use it (Table 2–2).

Health and Disease Indicators

The simplest, most absolute indicator of health is its total absence—death. Many other indicators are similarly unequivocal—illness or injury severe enough to need admission to a hospital, an encounter with a physician or other health care worker in a clinic or office, a spell of absence from school or work, or the use of prescribed or over-the-counter medication. Other indicators are derived from "vital" events that are recorded in an official register and appear in due course in official vital statistics—marriages, separations and divorces, births—statistics that are mandated by statute law and used in relation to the periodic population census to obtain a profile of the body politic in almost all states and nations in the world. Vital statistics, i.e., births, marriages, and deaths, are the basis for some of the most comprehensive information about social, economic, and other living conditions in the nation.

Information about health, sickness, use of health care services and the outcomes of use, health-related behavior, individual people's perception of their health status, and much other health-related information of great utility is more elusive than everything revealed by analysis of vital statistics, but it is as important and relevant. Increasing use is made of health insurance data bases, but ethical and legal restrictions on access to personal medical records limit the range of what is possible (see Chap. 10). Administrators of many HMOs and their counterparts in other countries (e.g., in health service trusts in the British National Health Service) have used aggregate data to set standards (masquerading as or supplanting clinical practice guidelines) and use

TABLE 2–2.   Varieties and Some Sources of Health Information

Type of Data	Information	Source
Mortality statistics	Distribution of death rates according to age, sex, location, cause, etc. Derived statistics include expectation of life, life tables	Death certificates
Natality statistics	Age, parity of mother, duration of pregnancy, birth weight, type of birth (single, twin, etc.)	Birth certificates
Hospital discharge statistics	Length of stay, outcome in relation to diagnosis, service, procedures, etc.	Hospital charts (summary or abstract)
Notifiable disease statistics Communicable diseases Occupational diseases Cancer Others	Incidence of communicable, occupational diseases, cancer, others, e.g., birth defects	Notifications, workers' compensation claims, pathology reports, police reports of violence, etc.
Health care utilization statistics	Frequency of patient contacts with health care system Use of prescribed and over-the-counter drugs	Health insurance claims data, economic statistics on drugs, school health reports, etc.
Health status indicators	Frequency of symptoms, complaints, impairments, disabilities	Responses to questions in community health surveys, various agencies for disabled, etc.
Responses to questionnaires	Symptoms, complaints, impairments	Health surveys Insurance claims
Pension statistics, etc.	Disabilities, handicaps (prevalence)	Agencies for disabled
"Behavioral" data	Sales of alcohol, tobacco, etc.	Economic and financial records
Unobtrusive data	Health behavior, patient and provider satisfaction	Broken appointments, staff turnover
	Risk-taking behavior	Traffic violations, etc.
	Antisocial behavior	Graffiti; false fire alarms

these standards to gain access to personal medical records. But if the records are analyzed, it is for fiscal rather than epidemiologic purposes. Health insurance records, for instance in long-established health care plans such as those of the Kaiser Permanente groups, have been a fruitful source of data for analyses of the relationship of processes and procedures to outcomes, e.g., evaluation of breast cancer screening programs.[11]

Much valuable information about many aspects of the health of the American people has come from the surveys conducted by the National Center for

Health Statistics described later in this chapter. Innumerable other sample surveys have been done in the United States and in many other countries, assessing health status, health behavior, use of conventional and unconventional forms of health care, etc. Other kinds of survey examine people's perceptions about their own health status, using various health measurement scales.[12]

Health information systems can also use inferential and unobtrusive data: financial facts on tobacco and alcohol sales; false fire alarms and graffiti (indicators of juvenile misbehavior below the level of criminal activity); calls to the police to settle domestic disputes (indicators of domestic violence); traffic violations, running red lights, jaywalking (indicators of risk-taking behavior); frequency of staff resignations (an indicator of morale in a health service); broken clinic appointments (an indicator of patient dissatisfaction).

▶ RATES

All epidemiology depends on comparisons. For these to be valid, it is not enough to have information only about the number of health-related events that take place in two or more populations; the comparison of health experience between populations must be expressed in the form of rates. A **rate** is:

$$\frac{\text{Number of events (deaths, disease, etc.) in a specified period}}{\text{Population at risk of experiencing the event during that period}} \times 10^n$$

The multiplier 10^n (1000, 100,000, etc.) produces a rate that is a manageable whole number; the events and the population at risk are expressed in the same units of time, usually 1 year. The population at risk is the average number over the specified period.

Vital statistics, i.e., births, marriages, and deaths, are the basis for some of the most comprehensive epidemiologic data. Everyone is born and everyone dies; therefore, statistics based on registration of these vital events truly reflect the experience of the whole population. Death rates especially reveal much of interest and importance about the health of the whole population. Some important vital statistical rates are defined in Table 2–3 (see also Box 2–2).

Population at Risk—The Denominator for Rates

Epidemiologists, demographers, health planners and administrators, public health professionals, and many others need information about the size and composition of the population. In most countries this information is provided by the **census,** a periodic enumeration of the population, originally intended for purposes of taxation and military service. In the United States, the national census is taken every tenth year. Age, sex, and race of the residents of each political subdivision are always ascertained, but in addition many other items of economic interest and of importance for governmental reasons are provided and published in the census volumes. Such information can often be used for epidemiologic purposes. For example, the median

TABLE 2–3.   Important Vital Statistical Rates[a]

	Numerator (Events)	Denominator (Population at Risk)
Birth rate	Live births	Midyear population
Crude death rate	Deaths	Midyear population
Infant mortality rate	Live-born infants who die before 1 year of age	Live births in the year
Perinatal mortality rate[b]	Stillbirths (28 weeks +) and deaths in first 7 days of life	Live births + stillbirths in the year
Maternal mortality rate	Maternal deaths from puerperal causes (i.e., associated with pregnancy, childbirth, and puerperium) within 42 days of delivery	Live births in the year

[a]Expressed as rates per annum; the numerator in each instance is the number of events in a year.
[b]See text for discussion of perinatal mortality rate.

monthly rental by census tracts has been used to estimate the incidence of disease according to economic level. Occupational classifications are also useful.

Between censuses, extrapolations or adjustments made by adding the numbers of births and immigrants and subtracting numbers of deaths and emigrants are used to estimate as closely as possible the numbers in the population at risk. The census gathers much other useful information, e.g., the numbers in each family, their living conditions (sanitation, water supply, car

---

BOX 2–2.   Rates, Incidence, and Prevalence

The three fundamental concepts

Rates are the only valid basis for comparisons

Distinguish between rates and proportions (proportions can rise while rates fall and vice versa)

Incidence = *New* events in a given period

Prevalence = *All* events at a particular time

Rate: What is numerator?

      What is denominator?

      What is time dimension?

ownership, etc.) race, ethnicity, and economic conditions. Though some information is politically sensitive, it can be collected from all but a tiny minority of conscientious objectors, although sentiments against revealing sensitive personal information are growing stronger in many countries (see Chap. 10).

When epidemiologists conduct surveys of population samples they can use an up-to-date list such as registered voters or taxpayers, carry out a sample census in the community to be studied, or use some other suitable sampling method to ensure that the persons included in the survey are representative of the whole population or of specified strata in the population.

Denominator information is available for many special groups, for example, military forces, industrial employees, subscribers to health insurance plans, and schoolchildren. Instead of a complete enumeration of a community or group, a probability sample may be taken and studied as a preliminary to estimating the characteristics of the whole population. If this estimate is used as the denominator for calculation of rates, the confidence limits set by the sample size and frequency of the characteristic must be borne in mind. See later in this chapter for further discussion.

The Numerator for Rates

The vital statistical rates that are of most interest to epidemiologists are various kinds of mortality rates, birth rates, and fertility rates. Numerators for these rates are compiled from the registration certificates of the relevant vital events. Morbidity rates are derived in various ways, frequently from patchy and incomplete records that underrepresent the real numerator, may be distorted in various ways, and may be difficult or impossible to relate precisely to a defined population at risk. With growing concern about health services planning and evaluation, health care utilization rates have become important in epidemiologic studies.

Incidence and Prevalence

We deal with two basic kinds of rates—incidence and prevalence. An incidence rate for a given event is the number of new occurrences of the event in a specified time, as a ratio of the population at risk of experiencing the event during the specified time. Prevalence, strictly speaking, is not a rate but the ratio of the total number of all individuals who have an attribute or disease at a particular time (or during a particular period) to the population at risk of having the attribute or disease. It is important to distinguish between incidence and prevalence. Comparison or intermixing of data that are essentially incidence rates with data that are essentially prevalence ratios leads to erroneous results and conclusions. Incorrect labeling of incidence rates and prevalence ratios is common among those inexperienced or untrained in their use, with resulting errors in logic.

Essentially, an incidence rate is an expression of average frequency of occurrence of an event in a population. Incidence (attack, case) rates may allow for an individual being counted more than once as a case in a specified period, if the condition is one for which this is possible (e.g., accidents, colds).

Prevalence determinations are useful for measuring the frequency in a population of states that are either permanent or of long duration; thus they are useful in chronic disease. Calculation of prevalence ratios is simpler than calculation of incidence rates. The prevalence ratio is the number of persons with an attribute at a specified time, divided by the number of persons in the population or the number examined for the presence of the attribute. There is no time dimension for (point) prevalence.

The relationship among incidence, prevalence, and duration of a disease can be simply expressed, assuming that the population is stable and incidence and duration are unchanging:

$$\text{Prevalence} = \text{Incidence} \times \text{Mean duration}$$

when incidence is measured in the same terms as duration. For example, if incidence is at a constant level of 50 per 100,000 per year and mean duration is 6 years, the prevalence is 300 per 100,000 population. This relationship occasionally helps health planners predict future need for chronic care facilities, e.g., if the incidence of a certain type of birth defect such as spina bifida and mean survival time of children with this defect are known.

The relationship between incidence and prevalence is important in health resources planning. Here, "incidence" is the annual output of graduates from health professional training programs, and the mean duration in years is 30 or more; hence an increase in output to meet an apparent shortage leads rather quickly to a great increase in prevalence, or supply, which may become surplus to requirements. Had this been appreciated sooner by health planners, the surpluses of expensively trained professional personnel that have occurred in many nations could have been predicted and avoided. The situation is not, of course, unique to the health professions.

Certain rates used in infectious disease epidemiology and occasionally in other situations merit brief mention.

The **case-fatality rate** is useful in estimating the lethality of a condition. It has been used mainly in acute infectious disease and in studying the outcome of surgical procedures. It is simply the ratio of deaths to cases. This rate is meaningful only when calculated from cases that are actually followed until death or recovery. If it is estimated from the number of deaths certified in an area in relation to cases reported during a defined period of time, various biases in case reporting and in certifying cause of death make it less reliable. The **attack rate** is a cumulative incidence rate, often used for particular populations observed for a limited period, e.g., during an epidemic.

Rates and Risks

The probability of occurrence is another measure of risk of nonrecurrent events. When calculating probability, the number of events in the period is the numerator, and the population at risk at the beginning of the period is the denominator. Absence of in or out migration simplifies understanding and is assumed in the following example.

Consider mortality in an institution with 500 inmates; to simplify still further, there are no admissions or discharges between January 1 and December 31, during which time there are 18 deaths. If the deaths were evenly spaced, the average population during the year would be $500 - (18 \div 2) = 491$; the death rate is therefore 18 per 491, or 3.7 per 100 per annum. The probability (risk) of dying, however, is 18 per 500, or 0.036.

If we wished to measure the incidence of type A hepatitis in the same institution, given the same mortality figures and the occurrence of 28 cases during the year, we would eliminate the cases from the at-risk population as they occurred (since recovery from type A hepatitis confers good specific immunity), and again assuming that the cases were evenly spread throughout the year, the denominator for incidence rate becomes $500 - (18 + 28) \div 2$, i.e., 477; the incidence rate is therefore 28 per 477, or 5.9 per 100 per annum. For calculating the probability of contracting type A hepatitis, the denominator is $500 - (18 \div 2)$, i.e., 491, and the probability is 29 per 491, or 0.057.

► NOSOLOGY

Before we can count health-related events, we must name and classify them. Nosology is the classification of ill persons into groups, whatever the criteria for the classification, and agreement as to the boundaries between groups. A workable nosology is an essential prerequisite to meaningful health statistics. The names we give to health problems, and the ways we classify them, reflect our level of understanding of these problems. There were 83 rubrics in the 17th century Bills of Mortality that John Graunt discussed in *Natural and Political Observations*. The Ninth Revision of the International Classification of Diseases (ICD)[13] listed over 1000 rubrics. Many included a number of separate entities rather than synonyms for the same condition. This expansion of numbers and the changing names by which we identify diseases are eloquent testimony to the rapid advance of medical science, and a fascinating aspect of the history of ideas.[14] The classification of disease entities has changed little since 1855 when William Farr and Marc d'Espigne presented their ideas to the Second International Statistical Congress in Paris. Farr's principle of classifying disease primarily by anatomic site or body system, with a second level of classification according to pathophysiologic process, remains intact. Bertillon, the great French demographer and statistician, took procedural steps only when he modified the classification in a series of revisions beginning late in the 19th century and assigned code numbers to the rubrics. There is an orderly arrangement following morphologic, pathologic, or etiologic criteria; all conditions are assigned code numbers.

Until the ninth revision (ICD-9), the ICD remained largely unchanged from its structure early in the 20th century. The tenth revision, released in 1993 (ICD-10), has been renamed; it is now the *International Statistical Classification of Diseases and Related Health Problems*. ICD-10 added 4 chapters to the 17 of previous revisions by dividing diseases of the nervous system and sense organs into finer subdivisions and included a final Chapter XXI for factors influencing health status and contact with health services (Table 2–4). Altogether there are over 1200 rubrics in ICD-10. There are some significant renamed and rearranged disease entities. For example, there are rubrics for addiction, making it easier to certify that the underlying cause of death is tobacco addiction. The value of the additional chapters and rubrics is in their combination of specificity, flexibility, and utility both for primary care use and for use by specialized health care providers in an age of rapidly expanding medical knowledge and increasing specialization. Like its predecessor ICD-9, ICD-10 is the central element in a "Family of Classifications" (Fig. 2–1);

TABLE 2–4. The Chapters of the *International Statistical Classification of Diseases and Related Health Problems* (ICD-10)

I (A00–B99): Certain infections and parasitic diseases

II (C00–D97): Neoplasms

III (D50–D89): Diseases of the blood-forming organs and certain disorders involving the immune mechanism

IV (E00–E90): Endocrine, nutritional, and metabolic diseases

V (F00–F99): Mental and behavioral disorders

VI (G00–G99): Diseases of the nervous system

VII (H00–H59): Diseases of the eye and adnexa

VIII (H60–H95): Diseases of the ear and mastoid process

IX (I00–I99): Diseases of the circulatory system

X (J00–J99): Diseases of the respiratory system

XI (K00–K93): Diseases of the digestive system

XII (L00–L99): Diseases of the skin and subcutaneous tissue

XIII (M00–M99): Diseases of the musculoskeletal system and connective tissue

XIV (N00–N99): Diseases of the genitourinary system

XV (O00–O99): Pregnancy, childbirth, and the puerperium

XVI (P00–P96): Certain conditions originating in the perinatal period

XVII (Q00–Q99): Congenital malformations, deformations, and chromosomal abnormalities

XVIII (R00–R99): Symptoms, signs, and abnormal clinical and laboratory findings not elsewhere classified

XIX (S00–T98): Injury, poisoning, and certain other consequences of external causes

XX (V01–Y99): External causes of morbidity and mortality

XXI (Z00–Z99): Factors influencing health status and contact with health services

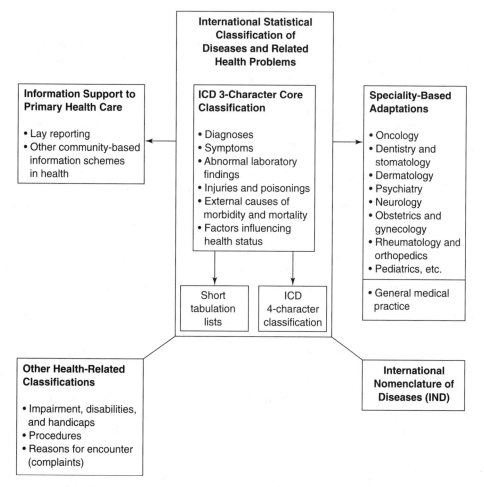

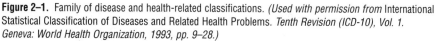

Figure 2–1. Family of disease and health-related classifications. *(Used with permission from* International Statistical Classification of Diseases and Related Health Problems. *Tenth Revision (ICD-10), Vol. 1. Geneva: World Health Organization, 1993, pp. 9–28.)*

another improvement is that the members of the family are more closely integrated with one another and with the ICD itself than previously.

It is useful for health workers to be aware of the overall architecture of classification systems; an understanding of how these work is an aid to orderly thought about the underlying conditions for which they are the labels.

► DIAGNOSIS, DISEASE TAXONOMIES, AND THE LOGIC OF MEDICINE

The central fact in epidemiologic study is usually the nature of the "health-related state or event" that we must identify and count. We often seek the highest possible degree of diagnostic precision. Alas! This can be the weakest link in the logical chain of the search for cause–effect relationships. A "diagnosis" can be anywhere on the continuum from a precisely defined disease entity, identified with 100 percent certainty by the best diagnostic tests available, through a range of possibilities suggested by the presenting symptoms and signs, to a guess based on pattern recognition ("I saw a case just like this once . . ."), or a shot in the dark. One of the ways medicine has improved in my lifetime is that we have moved along this continuum toward greater diagnostic precision. We have better diagnostic tools (imaging techniques, DNA typing, electrophoresis, polymerase chain reactions, etc.), and physicians now learn how to apply logic to the diagnostic process.[15]

Imprecise diagnoses raise doubts about the validity of vital statistics like secular trends and geographic differences in death rates from coronary heart disease and lung cancer. Even expert clinicians with the best available diagnostic tools can be wrong—reports of clinicopathologic conferences in the *New England Journal of Medicine* and other journals sometimes record necropsy findings indicative of different diseases from those identified while the same patients were alive.[16] National and cyclical fashions in diagnosis, the preferred diagnoses of male and female physicians, and of specialists in various fields further complicate matters. Women with lower back pain commonly receive "gynecologic" or "psychosomatic" diagnostic labels and treatment—especially from male physicians—whereas men with identical symptoms and signs are diagnosed "musculoskeletal."

How can we trust what we read in published papers reporting "statistically significant" associations between hypothesized causes and diseases when disease diagnoses are so unreliable? Obviously we must be reassured that the diagnostic labels are valid. Peer-reviewed medical journals now require investigators to state the evidence used to confirm diagnoses in case-control and cohort studies reporting on known or suspected causes of disease. In RCTs to test the efficacy of therapeutic regimens the same rules apply even more forcefully. Investigators must adhere to a protocol that begins with criteria on eligibility, i.e., states the way the diagnoses were made, then spells out exactly what was done at all subsequent steps from random allocation to completion of participation in the trial.[17]

When studying a particular condition the epidemiologist is often concerned with a different question: Which people in the population have the condition? The epidemiologist wants to identify all individuals who have the condition in any form—fatal, florid clinical, mild cases, subclinical cases, carriers, and premonitory and precursor states. A variety of criteria can be used to count the cases: registries and notifications, abstracts of clinical records, and surveys of the general population. Sometimes, a single test is used to identify presumptively all the people affected, as by tuberculin skin test or presence of parasitic ova in the stools. Another means is reporting of defects such as decayed, missing, and filled teeth or uncorrected errors of refraction, which may be detected at routine medical examinations of schoolchildren.

Another is statistical tables showing spells in hospitals by diagnostic category—which of course can lead to multiple counting if individuals have more than one spell during the period under study, so they can be used only for a limited range of conditions, and then only with reservations about their validity.

It is important to adopt and adhere to a definition of a case. How restrictive this definition should be depends on the purposes of study and the nature of the disease. Diagnosis usually depends on clinical features and results of laboratory procedures. It might seem that the definition of an acceptable case for epidemiologic purposes should be made on such exact criteria that there would be little chance of an erroneous diagnosis. This, however, can mean that cases that have been less well studied clinically are excluded. The adequacy of medical care is thereby introduced as one of the determinants of the disease, which is undesirable—and of course rapidly fatal cases also would be excluded if the patient died before diagnostic tests could be done.

Chronic diseases of unknown etiology present a problem, especially when there are no pathognomonic findings. Multiple sclerosis is an example. One expedient is to use a scoring system in which weights are assigned to various symptoms, signs, and laboratory findings, and a total score above a certain value is required for inclusion in the study. The validity of such a scoring system is influenced by the weighting factors employed, and excellent clinical judgment is required to establish a definition. The process of clinical diagnosis is similar to this process of arriving at a score, except that it is less formalized, more subjective, and is able to consider more factors than can be incorporated in the scoring system.

The concept of a disease state in an epidemiologic study is likely to differ from the clinician's in its concern with minor manifestations. Most diseases have a wide spectrum of severity. Many infectious agents produce inapparent infections more often than symptomatic disease. For example, hepatitis A virus infections lead to sickness only in one out of several hundred individuals from whom the infecting organism can be isolated.

Inapparent infections, subclinical cases of infectious disease, and carrier states can be identified by laboratory investigations, but no comparable procedures exist for diseases of unknown etiology. In chronic and degenerative diseases such as coronary heart disease, epidemiologic study has been hampered by inability to identify precisely the subclinical and precursor states.

▶ MORTALITY STATISTICS

Death is, for the epidemiologist, the least equivocal measure of health—although the significance of death rates as indicators of health status is increasingly disputed. In the United States and other nations at similar levels of development, a death certificate signed by a licensed physician is required before disposal of the dead and before next of kin can claim an estate, so for practical purposes, medical certification of the cause of death is universal. The facts in a death certificate (Fig. 2–2) therefore provide a basis for mortality statistics. In addition to the cause of death, these facts are place of residence and of death, sex, race, marital status, birth date, usual occupation, birthplace, service in armed forces, and Social Security number.

Death rates are computed and published for all causes and ages and in many combinations of place, race, and age and sex groups. The numerator for crude death rates is all deaths in a designated period, usually 1 year; and the denominator is the number of persons in the population in which the deaths occurred estimated to be living at the midperiod. Mortality rates are generally calculated for a political subdivision, since census population figures are available on this basis.

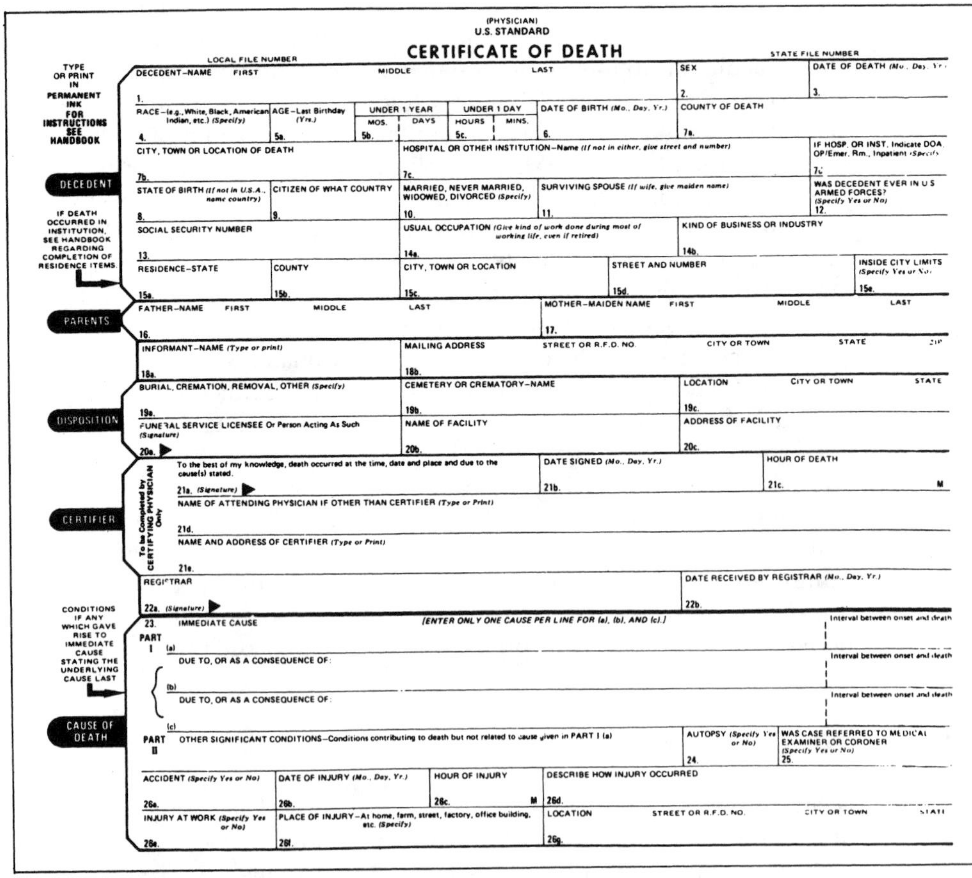

(PHYSICIAN)
U.S. STANDARD
CERTIFICATE OF DEATH

TYPE OR PRINT IN PERMANENT INK FOR INSTRUCTIONS SEE HANDBOOK

DECEDENT

IF DEATH OCCURRED IN INSTITUTION, SEE HANDBOOK REGARDING COMPLETION OF RESIDENCE ITEMS

PARENTS

DISPOSITION

CERTIFIER

CONDITIONS IF ANY WHICH GAVE RISE TO IMMEDIATE CAUSE STATING THE UNDERLYING CAUSE LAST

CAUSE OF DEATH

LOCAL FILE NUMBER — STATE FILE NUMBER

1. DECEDENT—NAME FIRST MIDDLE LAST / 2. SEX / 3. DATE OF DEATH (Mo., Day, Yr.)

4. RACE—(e.g., White, Black, American Indian, etc.) (Specify) / 5a. AGE—Last Birthday (Yrs.) / UNDER 1 YEAR 5b. MOS. DAYS / UNDER 1 DAY 5c. HOURS MINS. / 6. DATE OF BIRTH (Mo., Day, Yr.) / 7a. COUNTY OF DEATH

7b. CITY, TOWN OR LOCATION OF DEATH / 7c. HOSPITAL OR OTHER INSTITUTION—Name (If not in either, give street and number) / 7d. IF HOSP. OR INST. Indicate DOA OP/Emer. Rm., Inpatient (Specify)

8. STATE OF BIRTH (If not in U.S.A., name country) / 9. CITIZEN OF WHAT COUNTRY / 10. MARRIED, NEVER MARRIED, WIDOWED, DIVORCED (Specify) / 11. SURVIVING SPOUSE (If wife, give maiden name) / 12. WAS DECEDENT EVER IN U.S. ARMED FORCES? (Specify Yes or No)

13. SOCIAL SECURITY NUMBER / 14a. USUAL OCCUPATION (Give kind of work done during most of working life, even if retired) / 14b. KIND OF BUSINESS OR INDUSTRY

15a. RESIDENCE—STATE / 15b. COUNTY / 15c. CITY, TOWN OR LOCATION / 15d. STREET AND NUMBER / 15e. INSIDE CITY LIMITS (Specify Yes or No)

16. FATHER—NAME FIRST MIDDLE LAST / 17. MOTHER—MAIDEN NAME FIRST MIDDLE LAST

18a. INFORMANT—NAME (Type or print) / 18b. MAILING ADDRESS STREET OR R.F.D. NO. CITY OR TOWN STATE ZIP

19a. BURIAL, CREMATION, REMOVAL, OTHER (Specify) / 19b. CEMETERY OR CREMATORY—NAME / 19c. LOCATION CITY OR TOWN STATE

20a. FUNERAL SERVICE LICENSEE Or Person Acting As Such (Signature) / 20b. NAME OF FACILITY / 20c. ADDRESS OF FACILITY

21a. (Signature) To the best of my knowledge, death occurred at the time, date and place and due to the cause(s) stated. / 21b. DATE SIGNED (Mo., Day, Yr.) / 21c. HOUR OF DEATH M

21d. NAME OF ATTENDING PHYSICIAN IF OTHER THAN CERTIFIER (Type or Print)

21e. NAME AND ADDRESS OF CERTIFIER (Type or Print)

To be Completed by CERTIFYING PHYSICIAN Only

22a. REGISTRAR (Signature) / 22b. DATE RECEIVED BY REGISTRAR (Mo., Day, Yr.)

23. PART I IMMEDIATE CAUSE [ENTER ONLY ONE CAUSE PER LINE FOR (a), (b), AND (c).] / Interval between onset and death
(a)
DUE TO, OR AS A CONSEQUENCE OF: / Interval between onset and death
(b)
DUE TO, OR AS A CONSEQUENCE OF: / Interval between onset and death
(c)

PART II OTHER SIGNIFICANT CONDITIONS—Conditions contributing to death but not related to cause given in PART I (a) / 24. AUTOPSY (Specify Yes or No) / 25. WAS CASE REFERRED TO MEDICAL EXAMINER OR CORONER (Specify Yes or No)

26a. ACCIDENT (Specify Yes or No) / 26b. DATE OF INJURY (Mo., Day, Yr.) / 26c. HOUR OF INJURY M / 26d. DESCRIBE HOW INJURY OCCURRED

26e. INJURY AT WORK (Specify Yes or No) / 26f. PLACE OF INJURY—At home, farm, street, factory, office building, etc. (Specify) / 26g. LOCATION STREET OR R.F.D. NO. CITY OR TOWN STATE

Figure 2–2. The U.S. Standard Certificate of Death (Physician). *(From Department of Health, Education, and Welfare, Washington, DC: Public Health Service, National Center for Health Statistics, 1978 revision.)*

Cause-specific death rates have as their numerator the number of deaths for which the underlying cause, as given on the death certificate, is a particular condition, the denominator being the same as for all-cause rates.

Age-specific rates are derived from the number of deaths in the specific age range, with the population in that age range as the denominator. Age, sex, and cause-specific death rates are also used.

General, age-specific, and place-specific mortality rates are usually calculated on an annual basis. The midyear population is used as the denominator; this must be estimated in intercensal years by reference to census populations and use of an arithmetical approximation for estimating the changes in population. Mortality for those under 1 year of age is calculated with annual number of live births as the denominator.

Death Certification

The cause of death should be recorded in a particular way. The immediate cause is entered on the first line, two lines are reserved for conditions, if any, giving rise to the immediate cause, and the underlying cause is entered last. The underlying cause is coded and tabulated in all official publications of cause-specific mortality. The interval from onset of each stated condition to death is also entered. Part II of the death certificate identifies other significant conditions contributing to the death but not related to the terminal disease condition. Details are provided on deaths from accidents, suicide, or homicide.

Sources of Error in Mortality Statistics

Obviously, there are variations in the accuracy of these facts, and in some cases in their interpretation. Sex and age are recorded with close to 100 percent accuracy, but race, marital status, and occupation are not. In the United States, statistical tables commonly show deaths according to the usual place of residence, rather than place of occurrence.

The greatest inaccuracy arises in certification of the cause of death, a fact repeatedly confirmed in many studies. In general, broad groups of causes are more accurately certified than specific diseases. When someone dies suddenly and there is no suspicion of foul play, the physician may make a guess, or certify whatever is the currently most fashionable cause, usually heart disease, in order to spare the next of kin unnecessary distress that might be caused by requiring an autopsy. One problem in death certification concerns which disease is to be considered underlying. Consider persons who die from acute myocardial infarction or cerebral thrombosis and who also have diabetes. Should such deaths be attributed to the cardiovascular condition or, since diabetes is associated with an acceleration of such conditions, to the diabetes? There are coding rules to govern this and similar contingencies. Whatever cause the certifying physician may assign, the final published tables of causes of death, derived from the edited and coded death certificates, will follow these rules.

Another problem is the lack of recognition by many physicians of the importance of accurate certification in advancing medical knowledge.

Changing fashions, perceptions, and philosophies, as well as taxonomic revisions of the ICD codes for certain diseases, can undermine the validity of inferences about secular trends in mortality. For example, the nosology of heart disease was changed in 1948, making more difficult the direct comparison of death rates before and after that year. Further changes with each revision of ICD have had similar though mostly smaller effects on comparability of time series.

The international comparison of cause-specific mortality is hazardous. Not only does the availability of modern medical practice vary between and within countries, but there are habitual differences in diagnostic fashion and terminology. For example, the frequency with which induced abortions are reported and suicide is given as the cause of death may differ between primarily Catholic and non-Catholic countries.

Age-Related Features of Mortality

The burden of threats to health and life falls most heavily on the very young and those very old. As living conditions improve, the very young begin to benefit. We measure these changes in health experience by means of several vital statistical rates that focus on events in late pregnancy and early childhood. In populations that have high infant mortality rates, relatively small proportions of the population survive to age 65 years and over; in populations with low infant mortality rates, a higher proportion of the population reaches old age, where the causes of death are quite different.

Infant and Perinatal Mortality
The **infant mortality rate** is defined as:

$$\frac{\text{Number of deaths in a year of live-born infants less than 1 year of age}}{\text{Number of live births in the same year}} \times 1000$$

The infant mortality rate has two components, the **neonatal mortality rate,** in which the denominator is live births and the numerator is the number of deaths in a year of infants aged 0 to 28 days; and the **postneonatal mortality rate,** in which the numerator is the number of deaths in a year of infants aged 4 weeks to 1 year. The principal contributing causes to the neonatal mortality rate include birth defects, birth injuries, immaturity, and in some developing countries, certain infections such as neonatal tetanus. The principal contributing causes to the postneonatal mortality rate are respiratory and gastrointestinal infections; the burden of these is heaviest in the second 6 months of life, after weaning and the decline of passively acquired natural immunity to infections. The infant mortality rate is strikingly related to the living standards of the community or socioeconomic group in which it is recorded. Rates are consistently lowest in the most affluent, best educated, and best housed segments of the population.

The **perinatal mortality rate** has conventionally been defined as:

$$\frac{\text{Annual number of fetal deaths (28 weeks or more gestation) plus deaths in first week}}{\text{Number of fetal deaths plus live births in the same year}} \times 1000$$

The World Health Organization (WHO) has recommended that in developing countries where fetal deaths often are not recorded, live births only should be used as the denominator. Furthermore, there is sometimes uncertainty about the duration of gestation. A better biologic definition, recommended by WHO, is based on the size and weight of the fetus or infant. WHO recommends that perinatal statistics should include all fetuses and infants weighing 1000 g or more having a crown–heel length of 35 cm; these dimensions correspond to a gestational age of 28 weeks. Because of their biologic interest, fetuses weighing 500 to 1000 g or with a crown–heel length of 25 to 35 cm or both, corresponding to a gestational age of 22 to 28 weeks, are also included in perinatal statistics in some jurisdictions. These fetuses, though generally nonviable, may have readily visible anatomic abnormalities that make the diagnosis of birth defects feasible. Perinatal mortality reflects to a considerable extent the quality of care provided to women during pregnancy and childbirth. Incomplete registration and discrepancies in definition, however, may make it difficult to produce truly comparable perinatal mortality rates even between two or more advanced industrial nations.

The age curve of mortality has general features in common everywhere, with variations depending chiefly on environmental factors. Mortality is high during the first year of life (infancy), drops to its lowest level in childhood, and then gradually begins to climb during the third and fourth decades. After about the age of 35, the increase in mortality with age tends to be logarithmic for the remainder of the life span, i.e., the proportionate increase in mortality in each successive age class (of equal size) is about equal.

Figure 2–3 shows the decline in mortality since 1930 in the United States. The age-adjusted death rate for males has actually risen slightly since the late 1960s, while the female rate has continued to decline. This is due mainly to the effect of ischemic heart disease and cancer of the respiratory tract on male mortality rates.

▶ USE OF MORTALITY DATA IN EPIDEMIOLOGY

Mortality statistics reveal much about the health of the population; one derived statistic, life expectation at birth and at various subsequent ages, is often cited as an indicator of population health when comparisons are made over time or between nations. Changes in the frequency of disease or death

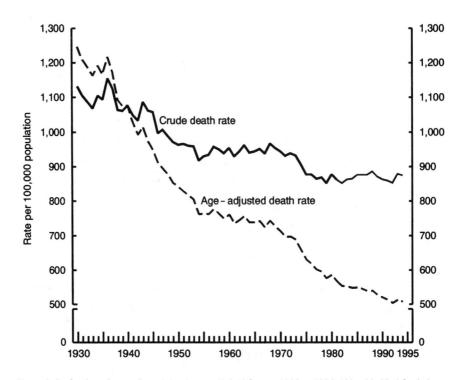

Figure 2–3. Crude and age-adjusted death rates: United States, 1930 to 1994. (*Monthly Vital Statistics Report. 45(3), September 30, 1996.*) Note: Crude death rates on an annual basis per 100,000 population; age-adjusted rates per 100,000 United States standard million population.

over time are sometimes difficult to interpret, however, and the reasons may be a matter for debate (Box 2–3).

Mortality Trends

Before concluding that an observed trend in mortality is genuine, we must consider other possibilities. Different proportions of the deaths may be inaccurately certified; there may have been changes in nomenclature or classification of disease, changes in the accuracy of diagnosis, or changes in the statistical classification or allocation of priorities; there may be uncertainty about the population at risk, changes in its age or in the racial composition in the registration area, or in the accuracy and completeness of census taking to define the population. It is also important to decide whether the observed change reflects a change in incidence, in case fatality (severity), or both. Some of these factors have been important in coronary heart disease. This condition was not even mentioned among the 189 specific causes of death in the U.S. mortality reports for 1920. In 1930 it constituted less than 1 percent of all deaths in the registration area, but by the mid-1960s the deaths certi-

---

BOX 2-3. Utility and Uses of Mortality Data

Comprehensive—Everybody dies eventually
A good (retrospective) measure of community health
Trends over time and regional variations tell us a lot
Proportional mortality
    Infant deaths
    Child deaths
    Male and female differences
    Proportion surviving to old age
Cohort analysis—Generation differences
Standardization for closer comparisons
Person-years of exposure
Life tables
Population pyramids

---

fied as caused by ischemic heart disease constituted about 40 percent of all male deaths in the United States. Since then, the age-adjusted mortality rate from ischemic heart disease has declined by over 40 percent, to reach the level that prevailed in the early 1950s.[18] Similar declines have been observed in some other nations, whereas in other countries, the rates have remained high or have risen further since the 1960s (see Chap. 7).

Time trends in mortality are presented graphically by plotting age-adjusted or age-specific death rates against time. Figure 2–3 shows such a secular trend in total mortality in the U.S. population. Figure 2–4 shows how mortality rates for lung cancer increased first in men, then in women, following in each sex about 20 to 25 years after cigarette smoking became a widespread habit among members of that sex. The recent rapid rise in female lung cancer death rates in the United States and other countries at similar levels of development reflects the increased prevalence of addiction to cigarettes among women and girls since World War II. The statistics on trends in cigarette smoking make it possible to predict with some confidence that the female lung cancer death rates will continue to rise until well into the 21st century, ultimately reaching levels close to those among men. Only a decline in the prevalence of addiction to cigarettes will change this for the better.

Refining Comparisons—Standardization of Rates

Age is an important determinant of most diseases, so mortality and incidence rates vary with the age composition of the population. Comparison of mortality and incidence rates is therefore confounded by differences in their age distributions. Consider two populations each of 5000, one with 45 deaths in

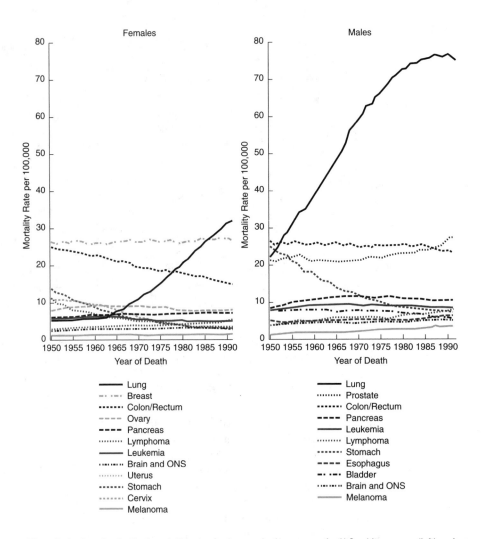

Figure 2–4. Age-standardized mortality rates for lung and other cancers for U.S. white women (left) and men (right) from the years 1950–1990. Rates are standardized on the U.S. population of 1950. *(Source: National Cancer Institute, 1996.)*

the year, the other with 29, giving crude death rates of 9.0 and 5.8 per 1000, respectively. We would be wrong to conclude that mortality has struck harder at the first than the second population, because their age distributions are very different (Table 2–5). We can compare communities by looking at their age-specific rates, but this produces lengthy columns of figures, which are difficult to assimilate, especially when we have to make many comparisons.

The usual procedure for comparing rates between populations with different age distributions is to adjust the rates for age, using an arithmetical procedure, direct or indirect standardization.

TABLE 2–5.   **Effects of Age Distribution on Mortality Incidence Rates**

Age	First Population			Second Population		
	No.	*Deaths*	*Rate*	*No.*	*Deaths*	*Rate*
0–14	1500	3	2.0	2000	4	2.0
15–44	2000	12	6.0	2500	15	6.0
45+	1500	30	20.0	500	10	20.0
Total	5000	45	9.0	5000	29	5.8

(From Last JM: Epidemiology and health information. In Last JM (ed): Maxcy-Rosenau Public Health and Preventive Medicine. 12th ed. E. Norwalk, CT: Appleton-Century-Crofts, 1986, p. 27.)

Age adjustment by direct standardization consists of applying to a standard population the age-specific rates that are observed in each of the populations being compared. The standard population can be Sweden in 1940, the United States in 1960, or any other arbitrarily chosen population for which the numbers in each age and sex class are known. For direct standardization, we must know the age-specific rates of the population in which the rates are to be age adjusted.

If we do not know the age-specific rates for the population in which we want to adjust the rates for age, or if numbers in some age classes are too small to produce stable rates, we can use indirect standardization. In this procedure, we project on the population in which age-adjusted rates are desired the age-specific rates that have been observed in a standard population.

These rates are then used to estimate the number of deaths (or events) that would be expected in the population under study if it had the same rates as the reference population. This estimate is used to compute the standardized mortality ratio (SMR) or standardized incidence ratio (SIR), i.e., the ratio of observed deaths or events to the number expected:

$$\text{SMR (SIR)} = \frac{\text{Number of deaths (events) observed in the population}}{\begin{array}{c}\text{Number of deaths (events) expected if each} \\ \text{age group had the same age-specific death} \\ \text{(incidence) rate as the reference population}\end{array}}$$

The arithmetic of these calculations is simple but tedious. Details are given in the reference books on vital statistical methods listed at the end of this chapter.

Person-Years

The **person-years method** can be used to measure risks over extended and variable periods.

Person-years can be calculated as follows. Suppose observations begin with 1000 persons. At the end of a calendar year, 950 remain under observation, the remainder having dropped out, been lost to follow-up, or died. Assuming that the losses occur evenly throughout the year, there were, on average, 975 persons observed during the year. At the end of the second year, 900 remain, and again assuming uniform rate of loss throughout the year, there were therefore on the average 925 persons observed. For the 2-year period the person-years of observation are therefore 975 + 925, that is, 1900. Age groups can be introduced into the calculation. If 10-year age groups are to be used, it can be assumed that one-tenth of the population in each 10-year age group will move into a higher age group each year, and a corresponding adjustment can be made to the person-years of observation in each 10-year group. Passenger-kilometers or passenger-hours may similarly be used as a denominator in estimating comparative risks of various forms of transport.

Life Tables, Life Expectancy, and Quality-Adjusted Life Years

A life table is the numerical way to express the death rates experienced by a particular population whose age-specific death rates are known. The life table begins with an arbitrary number of births, usually 100,000, sometimes 1000, and applies to this number the observed death rates in each year of life, thus arriving at numbers representing the survivors and the deaths, expressed conventionally by the symbols 1_x and d_x respectively (1_x is the number of survivors at age x, d_x is the number of deaths in the age group x years old). Further simple arithmetical calculation yields the probability of surviving each year of life (p_x) and the probability of dying before the next birthday (q_x). The final column of the life table, as it is conventionally published, is life expectancy ($\mathring{e}_x$), which is written with a subscribed number designating the year of life to which this life expectancy applies. Thus, $\mathring{e}_0$ is life expectancy at birth, $\mathring{e}_{40}$ is life expectancy at age 40, and so on. The details are given in textbooks of vital statistics. Table 2–6 is a sample life table.

Life expectancy at birth or at any other age is a statistical abstraction, like the gross national product; it is derived as stated earlier, by arithmetic calculation from the known age-specific death rates at a particular period and on the assumption that these rates will remain stable. Life expectancy at birth is heavily dependent on mortality in the first year of life and is reduced in communities with high infant mortality rates. The main reason for the recent impressive improvement in life expectancy in many developing countries is the sharp reduction in infant and early child mortality. For those who survive the first year, life expectancy is greater than it was for the population born alive, a seeming paradox explained by the fact that only age-specific death rates from the end of the first year of life are used in the calculation. We can calculate life expectancy at any age, using the age-specific death rates from that age onward.

TABLE 2–6. Abridged Life Table for the Total Population, United States, 1994

Age Interval Period of Life Between Two Exact Ages Stated in Years x to $x + n$	Proportion Dying Proportion of Persons Alive at Beginning of Age Interval Dying During Interval nq_x	Of 100,000 Born Alive		Average Remaining Lifetime Average Number of Years of Life Remaining at Beginning of Age Interval $\overset{\circ}{e}_x$	Life Expectancy, 1994, All Races	
		Number Living at Beginning of Age Interval l_x	Number Dying During Age Interval nd_x		Male	Female
0–1	0.00801	100,000	801	75.5	72.4	79.0
1–5	0.00169	99,199	168	75.3	72.0	78.5
5–10	0.00100	99,031	99	71.4	68.1	74.6
10–15	0.00124	98,932	123	66.5	63.2	69.7
15–20	0.00431	98,809	426	61.6	58.3	64.8
20–25	0.00544	98,383	535	56.8	53.6	59.9
25–30	0.00608	97,848	595	52.1	49.1	55.1
30–35	0.00807	97,253	785	47.4	44.5	50.2
35–40	0.01046	96,468	1009	42.8	40.0	45.4
40–45	0.01360	95,459	1298	38.2	35.5	40.7
45–50	0.01856	94,161	1748	33.7	31.2	36.0
50–55	0.02814	92,413	2601	29.3	26.9	31.5
55–60	0.04300	89,812	3862	25.1	22.8	27.1
60–65	0.06793	85,950	5839	21.1	18.9	22.9
65–70	0.09971	80,111	7988	17.4	15.5	19.0
70–75	0.14683	72,123	10,590	14.1	12.4	15.3
75–80	0.21249	61,533	13,075	11.0	9.6	12.0
80–85	0.32026	48,458	15,519	8.3	7.2	9.0
85 and over	1.00000	32,939	32,939	6.1	5.2	6.4

A refinement is quality-adjusted life years (QALY). This takes account of the prevalence of disabilities, activity limitation, and short- and long-stay hospital care (bed days); all the data are available from surveys such as the ongoing household interview surveys of the National Center for Health Statistics, from hospital statistics, and sometimes other sources. By applying rates of each of these, in each age–sex class, and perhaps in other categories such as socioeconomic status, QALYs, a more sensitive measure of community health status than life expectancy, can be derived.

Disability-Adjusted Life Years

Disability-adjusted life years (DALYs) are a refinement of national information on health status, developed by Murray and Lopez[19] and others for the

World Bank's 1993 annual report, *Investing in Health*. DALYs are a measure of the burden of disease on a defined population and the effectiveness of interventions. They are based on an adjustment of life expectancy to allow for long-term or permanent disability as estimated from available national statistics. Some forms of disability (such as blindness) can be counted quite well even in developing countries that lack comprehensive health information systems; others, however, cannot, and this is a weakness of the DALY approach. Moreover, the concept postulates a continuum from disease to disability to death that is not univerally accepted, especially among persons with disabilities. Despite these limitations, DALYs are being used increasingly both in developed nations with good health information systems and in less developed countries.

When constructing life tables, it is essential to obtain information about all cases in a series, especially if the life table analysis is to be used to evaluate the efficacy of a therapeutic regimen such as a method of treating cancer. All cases must be accounted for, including those of patients who have died of the disease of interest, of those who have died of all other causes, of those still alive, of those who have withdrawn from the study for any reason, and of those lost to follow-up. Only if an investigator states that all cases are accounted for in one of these ways can the life table be regarded as a valid statement of the outcome of the regimen under scrutiny (Box 2–4).

▶ MEASUREMENT OF MORBIDITY

Mortality statistics provide a comprehensive picture of the health of the public in the sense that sooner or later everyone becomes part of the statistics; but the picture reveals facets of health as it was or has been. To glimpse health as it is, we must use morbidity statistics, which are far from a complete record.

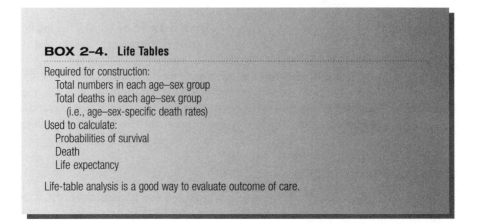

BOX 2–4. Life Tables

Required for construction:
    Total numbers in each age–sex group
    Total deaths in each age–sex group
       (i.e., age–sex-specific death rates)
Used to calculate:
    Probabilities of survival
    Death
    Life expectancy

Life-table analysis is a good way to evaluate outcome of care.

At any time, the population contains individuals who are in perfect health, as far as we can judge by the use of all available criteria, and individuals whose death is imminent; most of the people are scattered at all points along the continuum between these extremes. We have limited ability to identify and count those of epidemiologic and public health importance. Our sources of information are physicians and others in contact with the sick, the records maintained by the institutions that serve them, and the testimony of samples of the population.

Sources of health-related information used to calculate or estimate morbidity rates include notifications and registries of communicable and other diseases, e.g., cancer, records of spells in hospitals and attendance at ambulatory clinics, and health insurance claims. Surveys have been used to gather information on many kinds of physiologic measurements—e.g., blood pressure, respiratory function, hemoglobin concentration—and to ask questions about symptoms, disabilities, use of medical care, and many aspects of health-related behavior (Box 2–5).

BOX 2–5. Measurement of Morbidity

Notifiable (reportable) diseases
   Infectious diseases of public health importance
   Exotic infections
   Other conditions of interest
   Certain occupational diseases

Registries
   Cancer
   Substance abuse
   Birth defects

Hospital discharge statistics
   Numerator and denominator problems

Other health service utilization statistics, e.g., health insurance claims
   (often have problems with diagnosis, etc.)

Health surveys
   Total (census)
   Sample

Health status indicators

Notifiable Disease Statistics

For many years, we have required by statute the reporting to public health authorities of a number of communicable diseases (see Chap. 3). Partial information on some of these, mainly the major lethal epidemic diseases subject to international quarantine regulations, is also gathered in most developing countries.

Reporting is incomplete. The reasons include diagnostic inexactitude; the desire of patients and physicians to conceal the occurrence of conditions carrying a social stigma, e.g., sexually transmitted diseases (STDs); the reluctance of some countries to admit the occurrence of certain diseases that may hamper tourism (this can happen with cholera); and the indifference of physicians to the usefulness of information about such diseases as influenza. Yet notifications are very important. They furnish the starting point for local investigations into failure of preventive measures such as immunizations, for tracing sources of infection and routes of spread, for finding common vehicles of infection, for describing foci of infection and geographic clustering, for determining trends, and for evaluation of control measures.

Surveillance of Disease

Surveillance means the systematic regular ascertainment of incidence using methods distinguished by their practicability, uniformity, and frequently their rapidity, rather than by complete accuracy. Its main purpose is to detect changes in trend or distribution of disease in order to initiate investigative or control measures. Its elements are data-gathering mechanisms, central collection and analysis of the data, their publication and dissemination, and initiation of indicated action.

"Surveillance" suggests merely observation, but feedback is necessary— it encourages the cooperation of reporting agencies and informs them about the health status of the population. If practicing physicians report infectious disease, and local health departments consolidate the information and forward it promptly to a center, the assembled, analyzed, and interpreted information must be provided in return. It is the physicians in the community and the health officers who mainly have use for this information.

In the United States, reporting of notifiable diseases takes place weekly to the state health departments, which consolidate the information and forward it to the Centers for Disease Control and Prevention (CDC). CDC publishes the *Morbidity and Mortality Weekly Report* (MMWR), which also includes narrative reports of investigations of special significance. In 1995, MMWR published summaries by state of 24 diseases and 14 others of lower frequency when they occurred. WHO receives reports from all countries having reporting mechanisms, and publishes this information in a *Weekly Epidemiological Record* (WER) as well as the *World Health Statistics Quarterly*. Both MMWR and WER are readily available worldwide in the Internet. (See Appendix for URLs.)

Surveillance of Influenza

An outstanding example of epidemiologic surveillance is the collection of weekly mortality reports from large cities in order to detect influenza epidemics. This disease is almost the only cause of an abrupt rise in total mortality; other causes—such as severe heat wave, smog episode, or natural disaster—generally announce themselves. A system for regular signaling of the number of deaths from over 100 selected cities representing all geographic sections of the country has been operated by the U.S. Public Health Service for many years, and as a result the first week in which deaths are clearly in excess of the norm can be identified.

Influenza surveillance uses more sources of information than most conditions. In addition to these mortality reports, regular morbidity reports from schools, industries, and hospitals (including outpatient departments) have proved useful. None of these provide specific diagnoses; we rely on the rapid rise in acute febrile respiratory disease as an index of influenza. Reports of virus isolations and rising antibody titer in convalescent blood specimens establish the specific diagnosis and hence are vital to surveillance, but they are not by themselves sufficient for the purposes of surveillance.

Surveillance of Other Diseases

After the introduction of new control measures, such as vaccination, surveillance is important because it warns where and when the measures need intensification.

The raw data for surveillance programs are reports by physicians to health departments of cases of communicable diseases. These, however, are incomplete and variable. Supplementary and better sources of data for some diseases are reports from laboratories. Periodic reports from laboratories of total isolations of salmonella organisms have been useful gauges of salmonellosis, even though the reports include isolations from carriers as well as from clinical cases.

Surveillance and notifications of sexually transmitted diseases are enhanced if reporting of positive laboratory test results is routine, automatic, and mandatory. Physicians who attend patients with suspected STDs are more conscientious about notification if they know that the laboratory results are reported routinely to the health authorities. Since the main purpose of notification is to permit contact tracing and hence better control, this additional surveillance procedure is desirable. It has proved effective in the jurisdictions in the United States and Canada where laboratory reporting is required.

Surveillance of human immunodeficiency virus (HIV) infection has followed a different pathway: Most countries have adopted the WHO recommendation to use aliquots of maternal neonatal blood, stripped of personal identifiers. (See Chap. 10.)

After analysis of the data, periodic summary reports are sent to the agencies and people in the field who have made the reports possible as well as to all others with a need for the information. The surveillance reports published by the CDC on a number of diseases are excellent examples.

Surveillance is action oriented, having as its main goal the prompt initiation of steps to control a problem, particularly if such action is needed over a large area. It also helps us to understand the epidemiologic behavior of diseases.

Surveillance of occupational diseases would be valuable, but there are variations among jurisdictions as to what diseases are reportable and in the extent to which reporting is complete. Where there is a high standard of notification of occupational diseases, the reports can be a starting point for epidemiologic investigations, and the statistical tabulation of reported cases may be used to show trends in time and place. Unfortunately, information about reportable occupational diseases is seldom complete enough to be really useful. Its improvement is among the many measures that have been recommended to help promote better health for the American people.

Registries

Use of this term should be restricted to a registry of all cases in a defined region where the cases can be related to a population base, thus providing the ability to calculate incidence and prevalence rates as well as rates of progression, recovery, and mortality.

The oldest example of a disease for which population-based registries have been widely used is tuberculosis, but more effort now is directed to registries of cancer than any other condition. Attempts have been made to develop registries of high-risk infants, birth defects, mental disease cases, drug addicts, and some other conditions, but problems of definition and follow-up have proved difficult. Registries are usually either countrywide or statewide.

A cancer registry attempts to secure reports of all cancer patients as soon as possible after first diagnosis. Usually, skin cancer cases are omitted, as they are treated in physicians' offices and reporting is relatively poor. The main source of reports is hospitals, but a few cases are not reported until death. After initial notification, the registry attempts to follow patients, including collection of information on those who have moved out of the registry territory, date of last successful contact, and date of death. Where stage of disease or histologic type are provided, these are included in the patient's file. Further clinical details, such as therapy, presence of metastases, and progression or regression of disease, are sometimes included.

Incidence and prevalence rates disaggregate according to the usual demographic variables (sex, age, race, geography) and are the principal products of a register; life-table–based measurements of prognosis are another. Incidence trends may be the most valuable product of a register, insofar as they allow occurrence to be examined independently of changes in treatment that may confound mortality trends. Registries also have the practical use of permitting identification of lapsed cases that should be returned to treatment. They can also be used to forecast likely future trends and for many kinds of epidemiologic study.

Hospital Discharge Statistics

It is well over 100 years since Florence Nightingale remarked on the value of statistics that could be derived from the records of patients treated in hospitals.[20] Her advice is being followed in many countries: Hospital charts are being used to compile statistics. Charts from spells of inpatient care in hospitals are an important source of information despite their limitations, because they can be used for planning and evaluation of hospital services.

Medical charts contain several kinds of data (Box 2–6): clinical, e.g., diagnosis, procedures; demographic, e.g., age, sex; sociologic, e.g., occupation, family composition, region of residence; economic, e.g., method of payment (usually related to income); administrative, e.g., site of care, type of service; and behavioral, e.g., whether patients kept or broke appointments (which may be related to the patients' satisfaction with the care they received previously). All can be ingredients in an information system. The principal practical problem is to abstract the relevant information from many places in medical charts written by numerous health workers, few of whom have much interest in the eventual statistical analysis of these charts. Nevertheless, some efficient information systems have been functioning for many years, notably those which produce summary statistics about hospitalized patients. Computerized hospital discharge abstract systems, of which the Professional Activity Study (PAS) is the best known,[21] are essential to evaluate hospital care. Tabulations of length of stay by diagnosis, rates of removal of normal tissue at surgical operations, and other analyses of clinical activity are used in peer review. As Jick[22] has demonstrated, the diagnostic lists produced by PAS can be used to identify a series of cases of a condition with extremely low incidence, such as acute myocardial infarction in young women. The series can then be used in a case control study to test a causal hypothesis. Hospital discharge data, however, have limitations that preclude their use in most other types of

---

BOX 2–6.   Varieties of Data in Medical Records

Clinical	Diagnosis, procedures, etc.
Demographic	Age, sex, region of residence, etc.
Sociologic	Occupation, family composition, etc.
Economic	Method of payment (often reflects income)
Administrative	Site of care, type of service, etc.
Behavioral	Broken appointments (can reflect dissatisfaction)

epidemiology. They consist only of data from hospital charts; other relevant health-related events are not necessarily recorded. The population at risk is seldom well defined even if the system covers all hospitals in a state or region. Patients with conditions under study may die at home, move away, be lost to follow-up for other reasons, may not always be admitted to hospital, or may be counted more than once if readmitted to the same or a different hospital during the period under study.

Health Care Utilization Statistics

Every encounter between a patient and a provider of health care generates a record, which should often contain information of epidemiologic value. This source of data, however, has several limitations. First, an essential prerequisite, the denominator for rates, is missing because the provider of care—the hospital, clinic, or physician's office—seldom serves a defined population (although this is changing with the growth of capitation-based payment systems). Second, numerators are uncertain because the records relate to encounters, episodes of care, or spells in the hospital, not to the incidence of disease. Even for a condition that can occur only once in a lifetime and always requires hospitalization, such as acute appendicitis treated by surgical removal, a patient may have more than one spell in the hospital if there are complications requiring readmission, and the same discharge diagnosis, "acute appendicitis," may be recorded when the patient leaves the hospital after readmission. If the readmission is to a different hospital, it is very difficult to find out whether the numbers recorded in the statistical summaries from the different hospitals relate to the same individual. Multiple admissions of the same patient to the same or to different hospitals occur often for conditions such as unstable diabetes and chronic obstructive lung disease. Other conditions, such as peptic ulcer and coronary heart disease, may not lead to hospital admission, either because the disease is never severe enough to require it or because the patient dies before admission is possible. Hospital statistics therefore give a misleading impression of community-wide incidence or prevalence of such conditions. Finally, the records relate to a sample of patients that may be biased in various ways; some patients may not receive the service because they are not considered in need of it, are too remote from it, are ignorant of its existence, cannot afford it, are afraid of it, or are excluded for some administrative reason.

Records of ambulatory care have even greater limitations. They are scattered among innumerable physicians' offices and for practical purposes are mostly inaccessible, and they vary greatly in quality. At one extreme are meticulously detailed charts containing a lifetime medical history and at the other are cards with only the patient's name, the fee charged, and the date of service. Physicians whose records are in the former category have from time to time made valuable epidemiologic contributions. For example, Pickles, working in an isolated rural community, demonstrated the feasibility of his method of recording and its value in clarifying aspects of communicable disease epidemiology.[23]

A health insurance system that reimburses patients or physicians for each item of service and requires documented evidence of procedures or diagnoses provides an incentive to maintain complete records and to compile information in a systematic manner. Health insurance plans often serve defined populations, so denominators are known and rates can be calculated. Group Health Insurance, the Health Insurance Plan of Greater New York, the Kaiser Permanente Medical Group clinics, many HMOs, and the comprehensive health insurance plans of the Canadian provinces are among the organized systems of care from which it is possible to derive epidemiologic data.[24] Some promising results have been reported from several of these, mostly consisting of descriptive epidemiology and evaluations of medical care. In Britain, general practitioners in the National Health Service have defined "lists" of patients so they can calculate rates, but only enthusiastic volunteers maintain records of every encounter with their patients and compile a diagnostic list of the conditions from which their patients suffer. Such records have been used to generate several sets of "morbidity statistics"[25]—actually utilization statistics—which provide a perspective of disease that augments information about sickness experience available from other sources such as mortality statistics, hospital discharge statistics, and community health surveys. The general practitioners who have participated in the collection of these statistics come from all parts of the United Kingdom and their experience is probably representative of the country as a whole, but the fact that they are enthusiastic volunteers may have led to their selection by certain kinds of patients, so there could be some unknown biases in the distribution of morbidity in the population sample they constitute. Similarly, clients of prepaid group practices may differ sociologically, economically, and perhaps in patterns of disease from other people in the same community who select other forms of health care. Moreover, analysis of the morbidity statistics from British general practices has shown wide variations in the frequency of some diagnostic categories among the participating practices, suggesting that the individual physician's knowledge and attitudes may modify perceptions and diagnostic decisions, especially about emotional and personality disturbances.[26] This is a further source of possible bias, which applies to a varying extent to all collections of statistics from all forms of medical care. Despite these limitations, such types of health information have considerable value for planning purposes.

General practitioners who have maintained continuing records for many years[27,28] have been able to shed useful light on the long-term natural history of several conditions, e.g., recurrent respiratory infection in children.

Properly maintained medical records have many other uses in health care. For instance, it is possible to build into a record system a method for identifying persons in need of continuing care at intervals, such as chronic or convalescent patients who should return for assessment, mothers and their infants who require periodic health examinations, persons approaching retirement age, and persons at risk of certain disorders that may arise as a result of occupational exposures, past illnesses, etc. The use of microcomputers in office practice has facilitated record keeping with this aim. The same approach can be used in public health clinics; computerized record systems have long been used, for instance to provide a reminder service to parents that children's immunizations are due.[29]

Health Surveys

The National Center for Health Statistics (NCHS) has developed several ways to augment the supply of comprehensive information about the health of the American people and about manpower and resources to meet health needs.

In 1957, NCHS began conducting a nationwide household interview study (HIS). Area sampling ensures that all members of the civilian population not resident in institutions have a known chance of being selected for interview. Trained lay interviewers approach 40,000 households annually; diligent call-backs lead to a high response rate, generally over 95 percent. The details vary from year to year, but the facts collected include duration of long- and short-term disability, a broad classification of causes of disability, spells in hospitals, visits to physicians' offices, use of prescribed and nonprescribed medication, and smoking habits.[30]

The health examination survey (HES) began in 1959. Using similar sampling methods but a smaller sample size, this survey has concentrated on collecting sets of biologic measurements, e.g., height and weight, blood pressure, visual acuity, hemoglobin, blood sugar, first among adults and then among children. Apart from the light they shed on the health of Americans, HES reports are valuable sources of normal values for a wide range of biomedical variables, e.g., blood pressure, hemoglobin concentration, visual acuity.[31]

The national health and nutrition examination survey (NHANES) commenced in 1970; this survey gathers data on nutritional status and nutrient intake, together with some information on general health status and the need for medical care (Table 2–7).[32]

In addition to the sample surveys, NCHS is responsible for collecting and compiling several other sets of data. These are mostly derived from records of relevant agencies, sometimes augmented by survey. The health resources utilization statistics comprise the National Ambulatory Medical Care Survey, the Hospital Discharge Survey, the National Nursing Home Survey, and a reporting system for family planning services. Health manpower and facilities statistics include the master facilities inventory, the inventory of family planning clinics, and health manpower data systems—health manpower inventories and health manpower surveys.

There have been many smaller, localized health surveys, some resembling or modeled in those conducted by NCHS, others more specialized. An international survey provided useful cross-sectional data on use of health

TABLE 2–7.   Population Surveys of the National Center for Health Statistics (NCHS)

Survey	Purpose	Dates	Sample	Publications
Health Interview Survey (HIS)	National data on disease and impairments, extent of disability, use of health services, etc.	Continuous since 1957	40,000 households 120,000 persons per annum Response rate 96%	NCHS Vital and Health Statistics Series 1, 2, 3, and 10, NCHS Advance Data Reports
Health Examination Survey (HES)	Prevalence of certain chronic conditions, distribution of anthropometric and sensory characteristics	Cycle I 1959–1962 Cycle II 1963–1965 Cycle III 1966–1970	Ages 18–79, 6672 persons (86.5%) Ages 6–11, 7417 children (96%) Ages 12–17, 6768 youths (90%)	NCHS Vital and Health Statistics Series 1, 2, 11
National Health and Nutrition Examination Survey (NHANES)	Nutritional status, aspects of general health status, medical care needs	NHANES I 1970–1975 NHANES II 1976–1980	Ages 1–74, 20,769 (74%) Ages 6 mo–74 yr	NCHS Vital and Health Statistics Series 1, 2, 11, NCHS Advance Data Reports
National Health and Nutrition Examination Survey (NHANES)	Health status assessment (cardiovascular, respiratory, reproduction, etc.); Toxic exposures (lead, PCBs, etc.)	NHANES III 1988–1994	Ages 2 months and over Children, adolescents, older persons, women's health	NHANES III and Hispanic HANES also available on CD-ROM and Internet (http://www.nchs.gov)
Hispanic Health and Nutrition Examination Survey	Health status assessment (cardiovascular, respiratory, reproduction, etc.); Toxic exposures (lead, PCBs, etc.)	Hispanic HANES 1988–1990	Minority health Health care coverage	

care in relation to need for it in selected communities in several countries, demonstrating that for the most part the common health problems and the means people use to get help in solving them are the same everywhere, although there are some interesting exceptions, reflecting prevailing attitudes to certain symptoms and conditions in some cultures.[33]

Health Status Indices

Sometimes when we wish to compare the health of two or more populations, the numbers of deaths or cases of specific diseases are too small and the conventional indicators of health too insensitive to detect perceptible differences.

Increasing concern with the evaluation of alternative methods to provide primary care for chronic conditions such as arthritis and simply to define health more precisely has motivated development of sensitive indices to detect short-term fluctuations in the health of members of a small population.

The distinguishing characteristic of these indices is that they rely on subjective judgments provided by individuals in response to questions in an interview or in a self-completed questionnaire. The survey instrument usually consists of many questions, 20 or more being common, on such matters as physical function, emotional well-being, social interaction and adjustment, and satisfaction with life (or "quality of life"). Survey instruments designed to measure these aspects of health status often contain batteries of questions on several of the previously mentioned aspects. When the responses are analyzed, the scores obtained may be used as numerical indices of health status.

Most indices require the use of carefully composed rating scales, e.g., related to activities of daily living—feeding, washing, dressing, shopping, etc. Such sets have been useful in evaluating rehabilitation of patients suffering from chronic locomotor diseases and in assessing needs for care of the elderly.

While questions covering physical functioning normally refer to matters of fact, indices that deal with emotional well-being commonly record more subjective feelings and opinions. Most health status indices include numerical scoring procedures that enable the investigator to summarize levels of well-being in quantitative terms. Thus we can measure health, as well as the extent of departures from health.

Health status indices have provided a useful tool in epidemiologic studies, especially those intended to demonstrate the relative merits of alternative therapeutic regimens. There are many publications to which interested readers are referred for further information.[34,35]

▶ THE EPIDEMIOLOGIC APPROACH

There is nothing mysterious or arcane about epidemiology. At its best it is a synthesis of all the available biomedical, social, and behavioral information about a health problem: clinical information and laboratory-based studies, routinely collected health-related and other pertinent information (such as school performance, occupational records), and anything else that seems relevant. This information is gathered for all, or a representative sample, of the population and analyzed in various ways illustrated below with examples. The essence of epidemiology is to apply imagination and insight in studying and interpreting the facts that seem relevant to the problem.[36] Countless public health problems have been solved and control measures developed. For example, extrapolating hepatitis B epidemiology to aquired immunodeficiency syndrome (AIDS) disease epidemiology, and health education about "safer sex" among members of the gay community in San Francisco, began before the discovery of HIV—a modern reprise of John Snow's elucidation of cholera epidemiology.

Here are some more examples to illustrate the challenges. Consider "clusters" of childhood leukemia in communities adjacent to nuclear power plants in the United Kingdom. Epidemiologic studies showed what appeared to be significantly elevated incidence rates of childhood leukemia in relation to the father's employment in a nuclear power plant.[37] Martin Gardner, a medical statistician, postulated paternal chromosomal damage as the probable cause of the leukemia clusters.[38] Further study showed that the apparent increase was unrelated to the level of radiation exposure that the father had experienced (radiation exposure was never high anyway). It was first thought that some other unknown exposure, perhaps chemical rather than radiation-related, might be damaging the father's chromosomes. But no chromosomal abnormalities were found in the fathers. Then the incidence rates of childhood leukemia in communities adjacent to nuclear power plants were compared with incidence rates in other newly established communities to which families had moved from elsewhere, but where there were no environmental exposures to radiation or chemicals. Rates were found to be closely comparable in such communities. Review of all the assembled evidence suggests that if there is a true increase in leukemia incidence rates in new housing developments, it is related not to parental exposure to radiation or chemicals in the environment, but to some other factor such as an infectious agent that children encounter for the first time in such communities on moving there from elsewhere.[39] Thus, while the evidence failed to identify immediate environmental causes of childhood leukemia, it supports an earlier hypothesis, that an infectious agent is implicated in at least some cases of childhood leukemia.

Another example is the observation, replicated many times, that certain malignant conditions occur at higher than expected incidence rates among children living near high-voltage power cables and among occupational groups exposed to electromagnetic radiation.[40,41] Other studies have failed to find an association between exposure to electromagnetic radiation and cancers.[42] Is there a biologic explanation for these puzzling epidemiologic findings? A suggestion that high-voltage power cables emit radon gas, a known carcinogen, has not been confirmed, nor has any other credible explanation been forthcoming. An expert committee of the National Research Council reviewed all published studies and reported in 1996 that they found no convincing evidence of a causal relationship or biological explanation for the frequently replicated observation of the association.[43] Epidemiologic and animal studies continue in efforts to elucidate this mystery.

New challenges appear often. In Britain, in 1996, a variant form of Creutzfeld-Jakob disease (CJD), a fatal degenerative brain disease, was putatively linked to bovine spongiform encephalopathy (BSE) or "mad cow disease."[44] BSE first occurred in dairy cattle herds in Britain in the late 1970s; it is due to a prion, a protein-like substance at the border between living and nonliving things, often described as an "infectious protein" that causes disease by activating degenerative (spongiform) changes in the host's central nervous system. Kuru, another spongiform encephalopathy, affects a tribe of primitive aborigines in the highlands of New Guinea and is transmitted by eating the brains of tribe members who died of kuru. By analogy, supported by some experimental evidence, BSE appears to be transmitted by ingesting infected nerve tissue. Maternal–fetal transmission from cows to their calves has been demonstrated. BSE may have first occurred when carcasses or offal of sheep suffering from scrapie, another spongiform encephalopathy, were rendered down into meat-meal and fed to cattle to enhance growth and improve milk yield. The supposition is that the variant form of CJD identified in the United Kingdom early in 1996 may be due to ingestion of prions from affected beef cattle. If this is the sequence, it is an example of a commonly observed phenomenon, a "species jump" by an infectious agent—and it also suggests that feeding animal parts to herbivores was not a good idea. Another feature of this lamentable fiasco, the prevarication and deceit of elected government officials in the United Kingdom, has made matters worse by allowing bad animal husbandry practices to continue after the evidence suggested a need for change. Are the handful of cases of variant CJD so far confirmed the beginning, the middle, or the end of an epidemic? Are humans infected by eating meat from infected cattle? Or by milk or other dairy products? The implications are horrendous: The beef and dairy cattle economy of the United Kingdom has been devastated. If new variant CJD is confirmed as a prion disease originating in cattle, with an incubation period of many months or perhaps years, what will be the future course of the epidemic? These are questions of high public policy importance, with challenging implications for veterinary and human epidemiology. We urgently require answers, which may come from epidemiologic study combined with molecular biology (DNA typing, etc.). This may be the best and fastest way to control a deadly and mysterious threatened epidemic.

► EPIDEMIOLOGIC METHODS

Epidemiologic studies are based either on observations or on experiments. I will describe and comment on these study methods only briefly because many excellent textbooks (listed in the additional readings) give more detail than space allows here. I will offer my personal views on some of the highlights. Experiments clearly constitute research; observational studies also often deserve to be called research.

Observational methods are: (1) investigation of epidemics, both commonplace and unusual; (2) population-based surveys of health status, determinants of health, health-related behavior, etc.; (3) cross-sectional, case-control, and cohort studies that are aimed at identifying causes or defining risks of diseases such as cancer and coronary heart disease.

Epidemic Investigation[45]

An epidemic is defined as the occurrence of cases in excess of normal expectations. A single case of an infectious disease long absent from a community, such as a case of typhoid in a city with good sanitation, signals an epidemic threat. The occurrence of many cases of an acute respiratory or gastroenteric infection over a short period of time makes it obvious that an epidemic exists. Occurrence of four cases of hemangiosarcoma of the liver in 8 years among 500 workers in the same section of an industrial chemical plant manufacturing polyvinyl chloride[46] was an epidemic: it represented an incidence rate 5,000 times greater than in the general population. In all these and many other circumstances, epidemic investigation and control are of paramount importance.

Investigating epidemics is often a high-profile activity in epidemiology, a topic of TV documentaries and fictional dramas with heroic epidemiologists battling against time and bureaucracy to find the cause and protect the populace from being decimated by a deadly and mysterious disease. Epidemic investigation can really be a bit like this, but most of the time it is painstaking routine that adheres to tried and tested methods (Box 2–7).

The first step is to verify that the cases all have the same disease, perhaps variations along the continuum from subclinical through mild to severe, life threatening, and fatal; in short, accurate diagnosis is essential. This may be an easy clinical exercise requiring no more than careful history taking, physical examination, and confirmatory laboratory tests. Sometimes, e.g., with emerging infectious diseases (see Chap. 3), the task is more complex, and

BOX 2–7. **How to Investigate an Epidemic**

Make sure of diagnosis
Is occurrence outside normal expectations?
Identify feature(s) in common among cases
Delineate the case group
Epidemiologic history of all cases and sample of noncases
    Exposure(s)
    Ill and not ill
    Clinical and laboratory data
Laboratory and other investigations
Environmental and social conditions
Arrange, classify data
    Time (graph)
    Place (map)
    Persons
Compare and contrast cases, noncases
Write a report

perhaps also very urgent; it may require development of new methods or tests to identify cases precisely.

The numbers affected must be counted or estimated and a procedure established to determine whether new cases are occurring—is the epidemic curve rising, at a plateau, or declining? It is helpful to plot graphically the distribution of cases in time, place, or both. Figure 2–5 is a graph showing the course of an epidemic of measles in two high schools, and Figure 2–6 is part of the well-known spot map of cases of cholera, drawn by John Snow at the time of the epidemic in Soho in 1849. Snow's spot map was the first of its kind and has been a model for innumerable others ever since.

An epidemiologic history must be taken from every case, and from healthy individuals to allow classification into groups (ill and not ill, exposed and not exposed to the suspected agent). The cases should be oriented in time, place, and kinds of persons affected (the epidemiologic triad of "time, place, persons"). It is important to predict who is at risk of future attack and to take precautions to protect them. In many infectious disease epidemics this means isolating cases and contacts, immunizing susceptibles, etc.; in epidemics caused by chemical poisons and in "cancer clusters," protection and prevention may not be feasible until the underlying cause is established, perhaps only after lengthy investigation.

In epidemics of obscure origin, the investigation takes on a different character: It becomes a formal research project in which the investigators develop an explanatory hypothesis, test this against the established facts, and

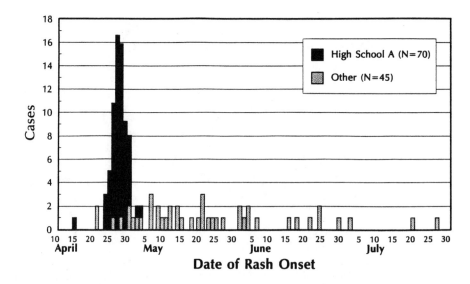

Figure 2–5. Reported measles cases by date of rash onset. Elgin, Illinois, April 15 to July 28, 1985. *(From Last JM, Wallace RB (eds): Maxcy-Rosenau-Last* Public Health and Preventive Medicine. *13 ed. E. Norwalk, CT: Appleton & Lange, 1992, p. 20.)*

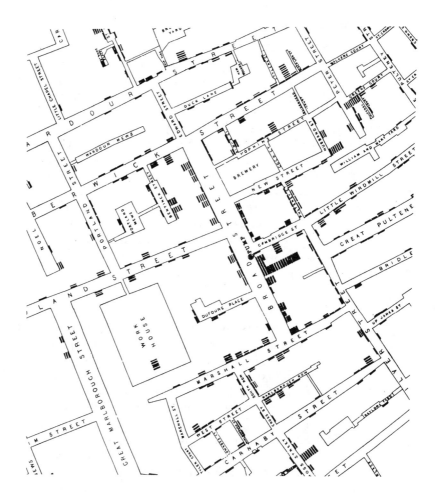

Figure 2–6. John Snow's spot map of cholera cases in Soho, London, 1849. Each case is represented by a short horizontal bar. *(From Snow J:* On the Mode of Communication of Cholera. *London: Churchill, 1855.)*

conduct systematic studies until all the questions raised by the epidemic can be answered and appropriate countermeasures can be put in place to protect the public from further epidemics of the same condition. In all epidemics, however trivial they may seem, a written report should be prepared. In major epidemics and outbreaks of new and emerging infections this is of highest importance. CDC publishes many reports of epidemics in *MMWR,* WHO in *WER,* and health departments in some other countries do the same. These reports are required reading for epidemiologists in public health departments. *MMWR* and *WER* are online on the Internet, so epidemiologists all over the world can obtain instantaneous notification of epidemics of public health importance.

Cross-Sectional Studies

Surveys are widely used to assess aspects of community health, notably by the NCHS as described previously; innumerable smaller and localized surveys are done, usually on random samples of a defined population, reinforced sometimes by physical examinations—e.g., of blood pressure, or vital capacity—or simple laboratory tests, e.g., of hemoglobin. If there is a distinction between a survey and a cross-sectional study, it is that the latter aims to be a hypothesis-testing research project. But cross-sectional studies are seldom a good way to conduct anything other than preliminary exploratory research. On the other hand, ongoing surveys like those done by NCHS yield much valuable information about health status and its changes over time, from place to place, and among people of differing socioeconomic, ethnic, and occupational backgrounds. These are often a starting point for scientific inferences that lead to hypothesis development, and from there to formal epidemiologic research projects.

Case-Control Studies

Observant physicians who take careful case histories are often able to make connections between present disease and past exposure. Percivall Pott described cancer of the scrotum in 1775 and observed that it occurred in chimney sweeps; he correctly deduced that it was associated with lodgement of coal tar in the rugae of the scrotal skin. In 1941, the Australian ophthalmic surgeon Norman Gregg saw many infants with congenital cataract and deduced correctly that this was related to an epidemic of rubella that had affected the mothers of these children during their pregnancies.

The case-control study is a carefully designed extension of clinical history taking. Individuals, commonly patients with a disease or condition of interest (cases) are identified and their past history of exposure to a suspected risk factor is compared to the past history of exposure to the same risk factor among other people who resemble them in as many ways as possible but do not have the disease or condition of interest (controls).

Case-control studies produced the first convincing evidence to link smoking to lung cancer,[47] and have repeatedly demonstrated their value ever since. Some methodologic flaws limit their validity,[48] but this is nevertheless an excellent method of investigation in a clinical setting, particularly when specialization leads to rapid accumulation of large numbers of cases of a condition that is rare in the general population. It is usually inexpensive, and results are obtained quickly. When a case-control study demonstrates that cases have been exposed to a presumed risk factor significantly more often than controls, it is possible to estimate approximately the relative risk associated with exposure. If the method of inquiry is to ask many detailed questions about known and suspected risk factors and also about seemingly unrelated factors, it is possible to investigate several risk factors simultaneously and sometimes to discover previously unsuspected associations by serendipity. With a large series of cases and controls, it is possible to stratify the population investigated in the analysis and so to estimate the approximate importance of each known risk factor, e.g., smoking and occupation in relation to bladder cancer.

Many conditions have been the subject of case-control studies—infections such as tuberculosis; malignant, inflammatory, and degenerative disease; birth defects. When it has been possible to conduct a cohort study to test the same hypothesis, the results of the case-control and cohort studies have usually been consistent. Thus, the value of the method is established (Box 2–8).

A good illustration of the value of the case-control method is the epidemiologic study of eight cases of clear-cell cancer of the vagina, a very rare cancer that affected young women in Boston in the early 1970s.[49] In seven of the eight cases the mothers of these girls and young women had been given stilbestrol during pregnancy because this drug was believed to reduce the risk of miscarriage. This history of maternal use of estrogens was compared with the history of matched controls (Table 2–8).

Subsequently there were other reports not only of vaginal cancers but also of other genital dysplasias in offspring of both sexes with a history of maternal use of estrogens. This episode is particularly tragic—and hard to forgive—because evidence that estrogens were useless in preventing threatened miscarriage had been reported about the time this regimen came into vogue in the 1950s.[50] Unfortunately the report was not heeded and many women were given stilbestrol over the next 20 years (an estimated 3 million in the United States alone); their offspring are the victims of this, one of the worst modern tragedies attributable to a medical mistake.

Case-control studies have been accused of being scientifically unsound, producing results that cannot be trusted. The principal reason for this is that sometimes investigators have ignored or made insufficient allowance for possible sources of bias and confounding, which can invalidate their results. If due care is taken in the design to minimize sources of bias and confounding, case-control studies are scientifically acceptable. For some important investigations, case-control study is the only feasible approach.

Bias can arise in several different ways. If the cases are hospital patients, they may be unrepresentative: Other people with the condition may have been excluded from the series because they died before admission to hospital, were not sick enough to require admission, or failed to be admitted because they could not afford it or lived too far away. Hospital patients with one disease may be more likely also to have another disease—a factor that may apply as well to controls, if these are also hospital patients, but could affect cases and controls differently. It is often convenient to use hospital patients as controls. This has the advantage of allowing for circumstances such as anxiety, which might be expected to have an equal effect on the memory of cases and controls regarding recall of past events to help determine the amount of

BOX 2–8. Strengths and Weakness of Case-Control and Cohort[a] Studies

Case Control

Advantages
Excellent way to study rare diseases and diseases with long latency
Relatively quick
Relatively cheap
Requires few study subjects (usually)
Can often use existing records
Can study many possible causes of a disease

Disadvantages
Relies on recall or existing records for information about past exposures
May be difficult or impossible to validate data
Control of extraneous factors may be incomplete
May be difficult to select suitable comparison group
Cannot calculate rates (no denominators)
Cannot study mechanism of disease

Cohort

Advantages
Provides complete data on cases, stages
Allows study of more than one effect of exposure
Can calculate, compare rates in exposed, unexposed
Choice of factors available for study
Quality control of data
Can accommodate a "nested" case-control study

Disadvantages
Need to study large numbers
May take many years
Circumstances may change during study
Expensive
Control of extraneous factors may be incomplete
Rarely possible to study mechanism of disease

[a] *(Modified from Schlesselman.[52])*

exposure to the presumed risk factor. However, patients who know they have a particular condition such as breast cancer may more accurately recall past events such as breast trauma than controls with other conditions. Thus, knowledge of the condition from which they suffer may lead to bias because of its different effects on cases and controls. The best controls in some circumstances might be a random sample of the general population, matched

TABLE 2–8.   Carcinoma of the Vagina in Young Women in Relation to Prenatal Use of Estrogens (Diethylstillbestrol) by Their Mothers

	History of Maternal Use of Estrogens	No History of Maternal Use of Estrogens
Cases of vaginal cancer	7	1
Matched controls	0	32

$P < 0.00001$
(From Herbst AL, Ulfelder H, Poskanzer DC, 1971.[49])

with the cases for age and sex and for such other variables as the investigator wants to control in order to avoid their possible confounding effect; for example, if occupation is a known risk factor, the investigator would want to match controls for age, sex, and occupation. Such a complex matching procedure on a sample from the general population is troublesome and expensive, so it is rarely used. Other tactics to achieve matching include asking siblings, neighborhood acquaintances, healthy friends, and working colleagues to volunteer as controls. Only incident cases should be used in case-control studies. Prevalent cases may be unrepresentative because they include a higher proportion of longer duration, the survivors, whose exposure history and biologic reaction may be atypical.

The effect of confounding variables can sometimes be controlled by stratifying the analysis of results. For example, lung cancer is known to be associated with smoking and with certain occupational exposures. The possible effect of urban atmospheric pollution can be determined by stratifying smokers and nonsmokers and those occupationally exposed and not exposed, so the variable of interest, atmospheric pollution, can be examined separately from the other factors. Obviously, this can be done with greatest confidence when numbers are large.

Cohort Studies

In a cohort study, healthy individuals with differing levels of exposure to a risk factor are identified and observed over a period, commonly years rather than weeks or months, and the rates of occurrence of the condition of interest are observed, measured, and compared in relation to exposure levels. This is a more robust scientific method than case-control study to test a hypothesis about causes, and as cohort studies generate rates, they can also measure levels of risk; but it requires prolonged study of large numbers, often for many years. It is therefore costly in money as well as time. Usually it involves no direct intervention (other than perhaps x-rays or laboratory tests). A famous example is Doll's and Hill's study of mortality in British doctors, in relation to their smoking habits. This began in 1951. I registered to practice medicine in the United Kingdom earlier in 1951, so I was among the 40,000 doctors recruited to this study. Each of us received a postcard that

TABLE 2–9.   Features of Cohort and Case-Control Studies

Cohort Study Population	Case-Control Study		
	Cases (Disease Present)	Controls (Disease Absent)	
Risk factor present	a	b	a + b
Risk fact or absent	c	d	c + d
	a + c	b + d	a + b + c + d

Reading from left to right shows the procedure of a cohort study, which begins by identifying persons in a population who are exposed to various levels of the risk factor of interest. Reading from top to bottom shows the procedure of a case-control study.

In cohort studies, the total population (a + b + c + d) and the numbers in all cells of the table (a, b, c, d) are known. Incidence rates and the relative risk of persons exposed to risk can therefore be calculated. In case-control studies, only a, b, c, d are known.

asked about our smoking habits (I smoked about 20 cigarettes a day at that time); a covering letter told us the investigators would examine our death certificates in due course, to test their hypothesis that smoking and lung cancer were related. The modest amount of information requested—a few questions on a postcard—contributed to a high response rate. The evidence published at the 5-year follow-up[54] (Table 2–10) was enough to convince me, and many other doctors, to quit smoking. Incidentally, the fact that so many doctors quit smoking provided Doll and Hill with a "natural experiment," an opportunity to study the effect of quitting smoking, as well as the effect of smoking, on lung and other respiratory cancers and other smoking-related diseases. The results at the 10-year[55] and at the 20-year follow-up[56] (Table 2–11) show this well.

Table 2–11 shows very clearly the dose–response relationship of smoking to respiratory and some other cancers; it shows that smoking adds to the risk of cancer in many other organs and that smoking increases the risk of death from ischemic heart disease. As ischemic heart disease is much commoner than lung cancer, this adverse effect of smoking kills more people than die of lung or other respiratory cancers. Smoking appears to confer a protective effect against Parkinson's disease and perhaps malignant disease of the hemopoietic system.

Cohort studies have obvious advantages over case-control studies but they also have disadvantages (Box 2–8). The long time needed to yield results and the high costs are drawbacks that can be overcome if pertinent data on exposure to risk of individuals in a large population at some time in the past are available and can be analyzed.

This is a **historical cohort study.** MacMahon used this design to assess the risk of childhood cancer among offspring of women who had had diagnostic x-rays during pregnancy.[57] Alice Stewart and others[58] had done a case-control study suggesting that even a single diagnostic x-ray exposure increased the risk of childhood cancer (Table 2–12). That study was criticized because it relied on mothers' memories of events during the relevant preg-

TABLE 2–10. Annual Death Rates of Male British Doctors from Carcinoma of the Lung According to Cigarette Smoking Habits; 5-Year Follow-up

Smokers	Deaths/100,000 Person-Years
Nonsmokers	7
Light smokers	47
Moderate smokers	86
Heavy smokers	166

(From Doll and Hill.[54])

nancy. This is an example of recall bias: Mothers whose children subsequently died were more likely than mothers of healthy children to remember details of events during pregnancy that might have led to their child's death. MacMahon used records from most maternity hospitals in the New England states to assemble a cohort of 734,243 live births and counted the deaths from leukemia and other childhood cancers in this population. He demonstrated an increased risk of about 40 percent among children exposed to diagnostic doses of x-ray (Table 2–13). Childhood cancer is rare, so large numbers are needed to demonstrate an increased risk.

Calculation and Estimation of Relative Risk
A cohort study yields the data needed to calculate incidence rates. These are then used to measure the risk that an individual will get the condition of interest. Relative risk is the ratio of incidence rate in the exposed to incidence rate in the unexposed groups (Table 2–9):

$$\text{Relative risk} = \frac{a \div (a + b)}{c \div (c + d)}$$

Estimates of Risk in Case-Control Studies
If the condition is rare, the total number exposed $(a + b)$ is close to the number of healthy exposed (b); and the total number not exposed $(c + d)$ is close to the number of healthy nonexposed (d). Therefore, we can estimate the relative risk as:

$$\frac{a \div (a + b)}{c \div (c + d)} \approx \frac{a \div b}{c \div d} \text{ or } \frac{a \times d}{b \times c}$$

This approximation is useful in a case-control study, when a, b, c, and d, are known but the populations at risk are not known.

The aim of case-control studies is to demonstrate whether a significant association exists between the condition and a presumed risk factor. Unlike a cohort study, which yields incidence rates in exposed and unexposed groups,

TABLE 2–11. Death Rate by Cause of Death and Smoking Habits When Last Asked[a]

		Annual Death Rate per 100,000 Men, Standardized for Age							
Cause of Death	No. of deaths	Non-Smokers	Current or Ex-smokers	Ex-smokers	Current Smokers, Any Tobacco (g/day) 1–14	15–24	25	Non-smokers and Others	Trend
Cancer									
Lung	441	10	83	43	52	106	224	41.98	197.04
Esophagus	65	3	12	5	12	13	30	3.94	14.94
Other respiratory sites	46	1	9	4	6	9	27	3.31	21.68
Stomach	163	23	28	21	28	38	32	—	—
Colon	195	27	34	34	35	33	31	—	—
Rectum	78	6	14	14	10	14	27	2.81	10.76
Pancreas	92	14	16	12	14	18	27	—	3.98
Prostate	186	39	30	31	28	31	38	—	—
Kidney	46	3	8	9	8	9	9	—	—
Bladder	80	9	14	11	16	16	12	—	—
Marrow and reticuloendothelial system	152	33	24	26	27	22	19	—	(3.51)
Unknown site	64	12	11	9	10	13	14	—	—
Other site	151	25	26	29	19	24	35	—	—
Respiratory disease									
Respiratory tuberculosis	57	3	11	11	8	7	21	3.83	10.51
Asthma	40	4	7	12	5	7	0	—	—
Pneumonia	345	54	59	62	47	62	91	—	6.94
Chronic bronchitis and emphysema	254	3	48	44	38	50	88	25.58	47.23
Other respiratory disease	121	16	21	24	20	14	26	—	—
Pulmonary heart disease									
Pulmonary heart disease	50	0	9	7	9	10	19	4.72	8.37
Cardiac and vascular disease									
Rheumatic heart disease	77	14	13	12	14	16	5	—	—
Ischemic heart disease	3191	413	554	533	501	598	677	22.59	53.56
Myocardial degeneration	615	67	108	98	111	111	160	9.58	13.92
Hypertension	239	37	41	41	33	43	58	—	4.67
Arteriosclerosis	117	21	20	17	17	21	46	—	4.85
Aortic aneurysm (nonsyphilitic)	121	5	22	16	18	28	45	8.40	25.60
Venous thromboembolism	48	9	8	8	8	5	14	—	—
Cerebral thrombosis	616	86	106	105	92	123	131	—	9.54
Other cerebrovascular disease	692	107	118	122	112	114	128	—	—
Other cardiovascular disease	267	53	44	49	37	42	52	—	—
Other diseases									
Parkinsonism	51	14	8	13	8	1	4	—	(9.10)
Peptic ulcer	79	8	14	12	10	20	23	—	8.26
Cirrhosis of liver, alcoholism	80	7	14	10	10	10	40	—	22.53
Hernia	16	0	3	2	3	4	7	—	4.16
Other digestive disease	144	20	25	27	18	33	26	—	3.25
Nephritis	79	10	14	10	15	14	21	—	—
Other genitourinary disease	136	19	23	24	22	24	26	—	—
Other disease	391	59	67	73	65	58	73	—	—
Violence									
Suicide	173	21	31	27	30	28	46	—	6.26
Poisoning	74	9	13	6	12	14	26	—	6.86
Trauma	240	46	39	36	47	25	56	—	—
All causes	10,072	1317	1748	1652	1581	1829	2452	68.47	244.16
(No. of deaths)		(940)	(9132)	(3114)	(2707)	(1986)	(1325)		

[a] Figures are given whenever the value was greater than 2.71 ($P < 0.1$); figures in parentheses indicate a decreasing trend from nonsmokers to heavy smokers; others indicate an increasing trend.

(Source: Doll and Peto.[56])

TABLE 2–12. **Number of Mothers Reporting X-ray Examination of the Abdomen and Other Sites in Three Periods; Ratio of Case Mothers to Control Mothers**

	X-ray Examination		
Period	*Abdominal*	*Other*	*Any*
Before marriage	44/26 = 1:69	335/275 = 1:22	361/296 = 1:22
Between marriage and relevant conception	109/121 = 0:90	213/184 = 1:16	304/285 = 1:07
During relevant pregnancy	178/93 = 1:91	117/100 = 1:17	273/184 = 1:48
Any period	296/215 = 1:38	531/456 = 1:16	692/593 = 1:17

The case:control ratio of 1:91 for abdominal x-ray exposures during relevant pregnancy
(1) differs from the "expected" ratio (1:00) at level of $P < 10^{-7}$;
(2) differs from the contemporary ratio for other x-ray exposures (1:17) at the level $P \approx 0.011$ and from the ratio for other x-ray exposures in any period (1:16) at the level $P < 0.001$;
(3) differs from the ratio for abdominal x-ray exposures in any period (1:38) at the level $P \approx 0.012$.
(From Stewart A, et al.[58])

a case-control study does not provide data from which to calculate incidence rates. Instead, the case-control study yields the **odds ratio.** This is the exposure ratio in the cases, divided by the exposure ratio in the controls (Table 2–9). If the condition is uncommon, the odds ratio is a close approximation to the relative risk. The mathematical theory underlying this statement was discussed by Mantel and Haenszel[51] and, more recently, by Schlesselman[52] and others.[53]

Attributable Risk

It is useful to estimate how much of the risk of suffering or dying from a condition should be attributable to exposure to several known risk factors, for instance how much of the risk should be attributed to cigarette smoking and to occupational exposure in cases of respiratory or bladder cancer. The term **attributable risk** is used to describe this but has been defined in different ways by various writers on the subject, thus causing some confusion. It is therefore preferable to use the term **attributable fraction,** qualifying this according to whether the exposed group or the whole population is being considered.

The attributable fraction (exposed) is the proportion of cases among the exposed that can be attributed to exposure to the risk factor of interest. It is defined as:

$$AF_e = \frac{I_e - I_u}{I_e}$$

where I_e is the incidence rate among the exposed and I_u is the incidence rate among the unexposed members of the population.

TABLE 2–13. Observed and Expected Number of Children Dying from Leukemia and Other Childhood Malignant Diseases Who Were Exposed to Prenatal Diagnostic Irradiation, by Age at Death

Age	Leukemia			Cancer of Nervous System and Other Sites			Total of All Malignant Diseases		
	Observed	Expected	Ratio	Observed	Expected	Ratio	Observed	Expected	Ratio
0–2	9	8.1	1:1	15	10.0	1:5	24	18.1	1:3
3–4	17	11.1	1:5	9	7.3	1:2	26	18.4	1:4
5–7	21	10.4	2:0	12	6.3	1:9	33	16.7	2:0
8+	0	2.9	—	2	2.9	0:7	2	5.8	0:3
Total	47	32.5	1:4	38	26.5	1:4	85	59.0	1:44

The ratio of observed to expected can also be expressed as a percentage risk. Thus the ratio of observed cases of all malignant diseases at all ages to the expected number is 1:44 (bottom row, last column in the table); this means that the excess risk of malignant disease following fetal irradiation is 44 percent.
(From MacMahon B.[57])

The attributable fraction (population), also called the population-attributable risk or Levin's attributable risk, is the proportion of the disease that can be attributed to exposure to the risk factor. It is defined as:

$$AF_p = \frac{I_p - I_u}{I_p}$$

where I_p is the incidence rate in the population and I_u is the incidence rate among the unexposed. Note that incidence rates are used in these calculations. Attributable fraction cannot be estimated from prevalence data nor from the distribution of risk ratios obtained in case-control studies but must always be calculated from data obtained in cohort studies.

Association and Causation

These examples illustrate how epidemiologic studies can be used to show statistically significant differences among groups exposed to different levels of risk. Dose–response relationships are apparent in some case-control as well as cohort studies. The observed effect (disease, death) follows the putative cause. The putative cause is biologically plausible: For example, we have known since 1915 that tobacco contains carcinogens, and ionizing radiation has been known to cause cancer for almost as long. Different research methods have yielded consistent results, and in studies of smoking and lung cancer, the association is very strong. It has also been demonstrated experimentally in dogs that exposure to inhaled tobacco smoke in concentrations comparable to those of cigarette smokers will produce lung cancer. Precancerous lesions comparable to those observed in dogs have been observed in human smokers. These criteria of causation were offered by the British medical statistician Austin Bradford Hill (1897–1991).[59] If all

BOX 2–9. Hill's Criteria of Causation

Strength of association	Frequency of occurrence of factor with (and without) disease High relative risk
Consistency	Association found by different methods in different populations
Dose–response relationship	Greater exposure → greater risk
Chronologic relationship	Exposure must occur before disease
Specificity	The factor alone (as well as in combination with other factors) can induce the disease
Biologic plausibility	The association accords with previous knowledge (but the observation may still be valid, perhaps the first evidence of a previously unknown biologic phenomenon)
Coherence	The evidence fits related facts
Analogy	For example, chemical compounds resembling known carcinogens or teratogens can be expected to have similar effects
Experiment	Though it is unethical to do experiments to induce disease, it is ethical, even desirable, to do experiments (e.g., RCTs) aimed at reducing suspected risk factors

of Hill's criteria (Box 2–9) are demonstrated, we have a powerful array of evidence. But it is circumstantial evidence; it cannot provide absolute proof that the putative cause produces disease in humans. Can epidemiologic evidence alone ever prove a cause–effect relationship? The question has been much debated.[60] Susser[61] affirmed the importance of clinical credibility as well as the capability of the epidemiologic evidence to persuade skeptics. Rothman[62] drew attention to the problem of dissecting actual causes in individuals and groups from multiple causal factors that might operate in populations generally. I think this debate will continue indefinitely: We will never obtain absolute epidemiologic proof of many associations between risk factors and resulting disease, because experiments on human subjects that would have disease or premature death as the outcome are unethical. But it is sometimes ethical, indeed essential, to do experiments on human subjects, as I discuss in the following section.

Epidemiologic Experiments

An experiment is research in which an investigator intentionally alters one or more factors under controlled circumstances in order to study the effects of doing so. The experimental method in epidemiology is the RCT in which people—human subjects—are randomly allocated to receive an experimental or a "control" regimen. Human subjects are therefore "experimental animals," so informed consent and other ethical requirements must always be satisfied in epidemiologic research (see Chap. 10).

RCTs came into vogue soon after World War II when new and costly antibiotics became available to treat tuberculosis and other previously untreatable diseases. It was imperative to determine as rapidly as possible which drug or combination of drugs worked best.[63] The same approach was used to determine the efficacy of vaccines for polio and measles, and over the years since then it has become generally accepted that all innovative preventive and therapeutic regimens (and some long established ones, too) should be tested in RCTs to establish beyond doubt what is the "best" regimen. Before RCTs were invented, decisions about therapeutic regimens were arbitrary; many forms of treatment were established on the basis of the opinions of leading figures in medical teaching and practice. If the president of the medical association or the professor of medicine said rhubarb was the best treatment for constipation, every physician for miles around prescribed rhubarb until the next president or professor pronounced that senna pods were better than rhubarb. Patients sometimes influenced treatment choices if, for example, family members or friends knew of or had been treated with apparent success using a particular medical or surgical regimen. RCTs remove the elements of bias and personal preference from treatment decisions, putting in place instead a decision about choice of regimen for a particular patient that is determined by chance alone. At first glance this looks callous or brutal, but when we are uncertain about the relative merits of two or more alternative courses of action, the only way we can ever know for sure which is the best is to conduct an experiment in which every person has an equal chance of receiving any of the alternatives that are offered. Of course as soon as the results demonstrate unequivocally that one way is better than all others, the RCT is stopped and the demonstrably best method is adopted.

Like cohort and case-control studies, RCTs have methodologic problems that it is inappropriate to describe and discuss in this brief account[64]; they also have well-defined ethical features that were established during the trials of the Nazi war criminals at Nürnberg after World War II. Medical experiments on humans, including children, were among the heinous crimes of the Nazis; the Nürnberg Code[65] was the first clear statement of what is acceptable (as well as what is totally unacceptable) procedure for research involving human subjects. The voluntary consent of human subjects is absolutely essential. Much has been written since 1947 on this and other ethical aspects of RCTs. If you have time to read only one short book on this, read Silverman's.[66]

As Silverman and others have emphasized, when there is genuine doubt about the efficacy of a particular preventive or therapeutic regimen, we have an ethical obligation to conduct a rigorous test to discover what is the best regimen. This is particularly necessary when a therapeutic regimen is dangerous, painful, or merely distressing. For many years surgeons and radiotherapists argued fiercely about the relative merits of radical surgery or minimal surgical intervention plus radiation or chemotherapy for breast cancer. This is far from a simple question because the anatomy and pathology of breast lesions is so variable. But it is now accepted that the best way to resolve the uncertainty is a trial in which as far as possible women with comparable lesions are randomly allocated to each of the alternative regimens. Results as of 1992[67] suggest that minimal surgery and chemotherapy (or sometimes radiotherapy) is best.

When an undesirable treatment regimen has become established and customary practice, it can be difficult to persuade people to change. Silverman's example of this is the resistance of neonatal intensive care nurses to giving up the practice of administering supplemental oxygen to premature and very-low-birth-weight babies. An association of supplemental oxygen with retrolental fibroplasia, a cause of irremediable blindness, had already been empirically observed. It was imperative to discover as rapidly as possible whether this observation was due to chance or to a pathologic process. It was difficult to prove the association because nurses surreptitiously continued using oxygen despite orders not to do so.

Epidemiologic versus Legal Evidence

Epidemiologic evidence and its interpretation may not be acceptable in law. Epidemiologic evidence applies to populations, is concerned with the probability that an association between variables is statistically significant, and that an association is or may be causal. There are few absolute certainties, however; only probabilities. We customarily accept 95 percent confidence limits. Courts of law, on the other hand, may accept an argument based on a 50.1 percent probability, or they may require 100 percent certainty. Courts of law, moreover, can be swayed by emotion or rhetoric. Above all, most decisions made in courts of law apply to individuals rather than to entire populations. The weight of epidemiologic evidence overwhelmingly supports the belief that mesothelioma of the pleura is caused by exposure to asbestos; the evidence is based upon studies of exposed populations. But a court of law, faced with the arguments from two opposing attorneys, may have difficulty deciding that a particular person's mesothelioma is due to a particular occupational exposure. This situation is a variation on the old theme of the ecologic fallacy—we cannot extrapolate risks based upon studies of populations to determine the risks faced by a particular individual. Hoffman[68] and others[69] have reviewed the use of epidemiologic data in courts in the United States.

Evidence-Based Medicine: The Cochrane Collaboration

Evidence-based medicine is the process of determining the best way to treat each individual patient. The process begins by searching pertinent published (and sometimes unpublished) work and applying a few simple rules of science and common sense to the evidence from these sources, in order to assess the truth, validity, and relevance of this evidence to the problem at hand. Much, often virtually all, the valid evidence comes from RCTs. Sometimes the evidence from multiple sources, e.g., multiple RCTs, is assembled and analyzed collectively in a meta-analysis.[70] When this is done it is more necessary than ever to scrutinize the evidence most rigorously for reliability and validity.[71]

There is a hierarchy of evidence (Box 2–10) developed by the Canadian Task Force on the Periodic Health Examination[72] and refined by the U.S. Preventive Services Task Force.[73] This was developed for evaluating evidence on screening procedures and preventive interventions, but it is equally applicable in other settings including clinical medicine. Indeed, it has had its apotheosis in clinical epidemiology.

The **Cochrane collaboration** is named in honor of A.L. ("Archie") Cochrane (1909–1988), who developed to a fine art the use of RCTs. It is an international network of clinicians, epidemiologists, and others committed to preparing, maintaining, and disseminating systematic reviews of the effects or outcomes of medical care. The *Cochrane Reviews* are prepared by collaborating authors (a Cochrane Review Group) using explicitly defined methods, mainly RCTs, to minimize the effects of bias. The aim is to identify

---

BOX 2-10. **The Hierarchy of Evidence**

I   Evidence from at least one properly designed randomized controlled trial

II-1 Evidence from a well-designed trial without randomization

II-2 Evidence from well-designed cohort or case-control analytic studies, preferably from more than one center or research group

II-3 Evidence obtained from multiple time series, with or without the preventive or therapeutic intervention; dramatic results in uncontrolled experiments (e.g., the first use of penicillin)

III   Opinions of respected authorities, based on clinical experience, descriptive studies, or reports of expert committees (e.g., NIH Consensus Conferences)

(Source: Canadian Task Force on the Periodic Health Examination; U.S. Preventive Services Task Force)

optimum preventive and therapeutic methods. The findings of Cochrane Review Groups appear in *Evidence-Based Medicine*.[74]

Record Linkage

Some events can happen to a person only once; birth and death are the obvious examples. Other events can occur many times to the same person; admission to the hospital or visits to a doctor for treatment of a chronic or continuing disease like diabetes, coronary heart disease, or cancer and repeated minor accidents at work are examples. It is helpful for many purposes to be able to count the actual persons rather than their repeated hospital admissions, encounters with a doctor, or episodes of a chronic recurring illness. It can be useful and very enlightening to relate events or experiences at one time in a person's life to other events, including their death, perhaps many years later. A record linkage system enables us to do this.[75]

A record linkage system requires a reliable method to identify individuals precisely, even if they change their names. The sequence of digits of an individual's date of birth is the starting point; mine, for instance, is 19260922. We add another digit, 1 for a male, 2 for a female; and a further sequence of several digits (or letters of the alphabet) for the place of birth. By now the probability of repeating the same sequence for two individuals has become quite small. The final steps are a sequence of alphabet letters for the individual's own name and for the individual's mother's maiden name. A record linkage system with these properties has been in place in parts of the United Kingdom and Canada since the 1960s. In Canada it can be linked to a very large mortality database, comprising all deaths since 1954.[76] Names and other identifying information and certified causes of death are preserved on microfiche. The United States has had a similar National Death Index since 1979. Linking causes of death to past occupational experience, e.g., in a dangerous trade like asbestos mining and refining, or to past medical history, e.g., exposure to diagnostic doses of x-rays, can generate very large numbers, measurable in the millions, for historical cohort studies.

▶ EPIDEMIOLOGY IN IMPERFECT CIRCUMSTANCES

Much of the foregoing discussion relates to epidemiology under ideal conditions; but three-quarters of the human race live in developing countries where ideal conditions are an impossible dream—and epidemiology is a powerful aid to upgrading health conditions in these regions. Some concessions must be made to recognize this reality. Several useful guides to the problems and methods are available.[77]

The Minimum Data Set

In rural villages in developing countries, epidemiologic studies cannot be based on precise diagnostic labels. A minimum data set and short list of causes of death and disease has been developed,[78] making it possible to sort disease categories into several relevant classes: perinatal deaths, deaths following diarrhea, acute respiratory disease, alternating chills and fever characteristic of malaria, etc. This information can be gathered by a village headman or tribal healer even in the most primitive setting, to compile a profile of the main causes of premature death and disabling diseases (Box 2–11). A "verbal autopsy" in which field epidemiologists ask questions to reduce the range of diagnostic possibilities can refine the information further.[79]

Epidemiology Without Denominators: Capture–Recapture Methods

Some health problems are difficult to study not only in developing but also in developed countries, because the affected populations are elusive. Examples include STDs, HIV disease, and other conditions in prostitutes; drug abusing teenagers; and homeless "street people" (who may suffer from burnt-out schizophrenia, chronic alcoholism, and other mental disorders). A useful approach is the capture–recapture method. This was adapted from wildlife biology and veterinary epidemiology, where observers have no way to count numbers precisely. It is possible to estimate not only the numbers of cases but also the population at risk. Two or more independent overlapping sample frames are compared. If two frames are used, the population at risk is calculated by multiplying the two and dividing by the number caught in both "captures"; denominators are calculated the same way. With larger numbers of "captures" the mathematics become more difficult but the reliability and validity of the method increases. Interested readers should consult the sources I cite for more details.[80, 81]

► SCREENING

Screening is the examination by a single test or procedure of a population of apparently well people for the purpose of detecting those with a particular unrecognized disease or defect. Prescriptive screening is aimed at early detection of disease in presumptively healthy people that can be better controlled if detected early in its natural history. Multiple or multiphasic screening is the examination of people by a battery of tests during a single visit to a screening center or clinic. A screening test should be capable of identifying all the people in the population who have a high probability of being affected by the disease or defect and capable of excluding the majority of those not affected. A screening test should be inexpensive, easily and quickly done, and free from hazard. The aim of a screening test is not to diagnose disease but to sort the population into those who are and are not suspected to suffer from the disease or defect of interest.

BOX 2–11. Minimal Mortality List for Lay Reporting of Health Information

Description	Possible diagnosis
1 Fever with skin eruptions	Measles, chickenpox, smallpox
2 Fever with neck rigidity, vomiting, skin rash	Meningitis
3 High fever, intermittent, with chills and prostration	Malaria
4 Fever, unqualified	
5 Diarrhea, unqualified	
6 Abdominal pain, rigidity of abdominal wall	Acute abdomen
7 Chronic cough with loss of weight, blood in sputum, slight fever	Tuberculosis
8 Acute cough, fever, chest pain, shortness of breath	Pneumonia
9 Breathing difficulty, shortness of breath, chest pain, swollen ankles	Heart disease
10 Cessation of urination	Renal shutdown
11 Fear of drinking water, convulsions, history of animal bite	Rabies
12 Locked jaw, muscle spasms, history of open wound or childbirth	Tetanus
13 Sudden paralysis and unconsciousness	Stroke
14 Pregnancy with complications	Complicated pregnancy
15 Abortion	Abortion
16 Childbirth with complications	Complicated childbirth
17 Puerperium with complications	Complicated puerperium
18 Impaired physical or psychological function due to old age	Senility
19 Sudden death, cause unknown	
20 Injuries	
21 Other unspecified causes of death	
22 Cause unknown	

External cause of injury:

23 Bites or stings of venomous animals
24 Burns
25 Drowning
26 Falls
27 Poisoning
28 Transport (traffic) accidents
29 Suicide, homicide
30 Other violence

(From: WHO[78])

Terminology

When discussing epidemiologic aspects of screening, it is important to use certain terms correctly (Box 2–12). **Validity** is an expression of the frequency with which the result of the screening test is later confirmed by other diagnostic procedures. The components of validity are sensitivity and specificity. **Sensitivity** is the ability to identify correctly those who have the disease. **Specificity** is the ability to identify correctly those who do not have the disease. These similar sounding words and the concepts they describe are often confused. For this reason, the terms "false positive" and "false negative" are preferable.

False positives are those whose test is positive who do not have the disease, and **false negatives** are those who have the disease but in whom the test gives a negative result. When large populations are being screened, it would be undesirable to have large numbers of individuals with false-positive results, but it could be disastrous for diseased individuals to be falsely labeled negative when in fact they have a condition for which early detection might make an important difference to prognosis. The **predictive values** of the result of a screening test are the proportions of people correctly labeled diseased and nondiseased by the test.

Table 2–14 shows the relationship between these properties of screening tests. The properties become important in different ways depending on the frequency of the condition in a population and the type of population in which the screening procedure is conducted. In practice, the decision to use the screening test is based upon existing knowledge of its sensitivity and specificity. This knowledge is often derived from clinical and laboratory study. Other elements in the decision to use a screening test include the importance of the health problem and the potential for benefit as a result of early detection and the evidence, preferably obtained as a result of RCTs, that the test is effective and efficient.

Ideally, a screening test and a diagnostic test would have the same properties. Each would be capable of detecting with 100 percent accuracy all diseased individuals and capable also of correctly identifying all nondiseased individu-

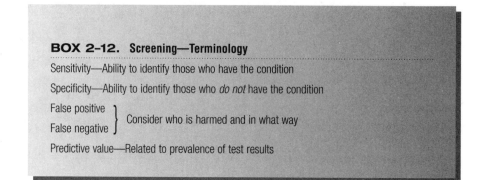

BOX 2–12. Screening—Terminology

Sensitivity—Ability to identify those who have the condition

Specificity—Ability to identify those who *do not* have the condition

False positive
False negative } Consider who is harmed and in what way

Predictive value—Related to prevalence of test results

TABLE 2–14. Properties and Relationships in Screening

Test Result	"True" Diagnosis		
	Disease Present	Disease Absent	
Positive	a	b	a + b
Negative	c	d	c + d
a + c	b + d		

Sensitivity $= \dfrac{a}{a+c}$

Specificity $= \dfrac{d}{a+d}$

Predictive value of positive test $= \dfrac{a}{a+b}$

Predictive value of negative test $= \dfrac{d}{c+d}$

als. This might be possible if the biologic variables generally used to measure the presence or absence of the disease had a bimodal distribution in the population, such that all diseased individuals had values within a certain range and all nondiseased individuals had values in an entirely different range. In reality, most biologic variables used to measure the extent to which disease is present or absent have a distribution in the population that is either normal or skew (Fig. 2–7). This being so, we are forced to select some arbitrary level of measurement beyond which we say that disease is probably present. For example, in screening for hypertension, this may be a resting diastolic blood pressure

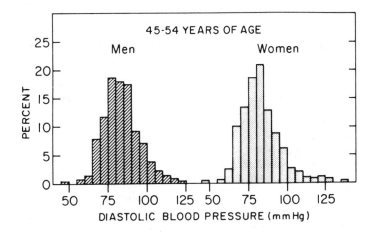

Figure 2–7. Distribution of diastolic blood pressure in men and women aged 45 to 54. In a screening survey of the population, all subjects with a resting diastolic blood pressure above a certain arbitrarily chosen level (generally 95 mm Hg) would be selected for further investigation. *(Based on data from the U.S. National Health Survey.)*

over 95 mm Hg. Under these circumstances the sensitivity and specificity of a screening test become important. For example, consider a screening test with 90 percent specificity and 95 percent sensitivity, which is applied to a population of 10,000 people to detect cases of a condition with a prevalence of 1 percent (Table 2–15, column A). In this situation, the predictive value of a negative screening test is close to 100 percent, while the predictive value of a positive test is 8.7 percent. Now consider the situation where the prevalence of the condition is 10 percent. Here, the predictive value of a negative test remains close to 100 percent, but the predictive value of a positive test has risen to 51.3 percent (Table 2–15, column B). This relationship provides the rationale for applying certain screening tests primarily in populations where a high prevalence of the disease of interest is expected, e.g., screening multiparous and sexually active women for preinvasive cancer of the cervix. Sensitivity, specificity, predictive value, and prevalence are interrelated. With conditions of very low prevalence, a test with very high specificity is required in order to ensure that the number of false negatives is minimized, but as a rule, the cost of using such a test is a high proportion of false positives.

Surveys to detect more than one disease (multiphasic screening) were first undertaken on a large scale at the end of World War II. Some have included many different measurements and examinations—e.g., height and weight, blood pressure, chest x-ray, vision testing, audiometry, dental inspection, urinalysis, and blood sugar determinations after ingesting a standard amount of glucose. The main purpose of such surveys has generally been case finding, in order to provide an early diagnosis and prompt medical care. There has been much debate over their value, which is limited when the chosen screening tests are inappropriate or improperly performed so that sensitivity and specificity are low. Public and personal funds may be wasted in the effort to confirm false-positive findings, the patient unnecessarily alarmed, and clinicians in the community overburdened and alienated. A false-negative report, on the other hand, engenders a feeling of security, which may

TABLE 2–15. Predictive Values of a Screening Test at 1 Percent and 10 Percent Prevalence of a Condition

| Screening Test | (A) Prevalence 1 Percent | | (B) Prevalence 10 Percent | |
	Not Diseased	Diseased	Not Diseased	Diseased
+	95	990	950	900
−	5	8910	50	8100
Total	100	9900	1000	9000

$$\text{Predictive value of positive} = \frac{95}{95 + 990} = 8.7\% \qquad \text{Predictive value of positive} = \frac{950}{950 + 900} = 51.3\%$$

$$\text{Predictive value of negative} = \frac{8910}{8910 + 5} = 99.9\% \qquad \text{Predictive value of negative} = \frac{8100}{8100 + 50} = 99.3\%$$

cause a delay in diagnosis. Yet all screening procedures do produce both false-positive and false-negative reports. The task is to minimize these, putting the premium on whichever quality—sensitivity or specificity—is more important in the particular disease. Thus, a high sensitivity in a cervical cytology screening program is desired, even at the cost of rather low specificity, since the penalty for missing a case may be severe. In diabetes screening, on the other hand, because the benefits of early diagnosis are uncertain, more sensitivity may properly be sacrificed, if necessary, to ensure an acceptably low number of false-positive results.

▶ PROBLEMS OF MEASUREMENT AND CLASSIFICATION IN EPIDEMIOLOGY

The important properties of a measurement are validity, accuracy, precision, and reproducibility. Errors can arise because of faults in any of these (Box 2–13).

Validity is an expression of the degree to which a measurement measures what it purports to measure. For example, forced expiratory volume in one second (FEV_1) is a valid measure of respiratory function. Subscapular skinfold thickness is not, by itself, a valid measure of obesity, although in combination with other measurements it can be used to assess how fat or lean someone is.

Accuracy is the extent to which a measurement conforms to or agrees with the true value. A measurement can be precise but inaccurate; for example, if a faulty thermometer records the body temperature to be 36.56°C when it is actually 37.10°C.

BOX 2–13. Problems of Measurement and Classification

Validity—Does it measure what it purports to?
Accuracy—Does it agree with true value?
Precision—How clearly defined is it?
Reproducibility—Same result every time
Instrumental error
Digit preference
Observer variation—Between observers; within observers
Variation in individual response
Biologic (gaussian, log-normal, etc.)
Bias—Many varieties!
Confounding

Precision is the quality of being sharply defined. It can be expressed numerically, e.g., when a measurement is stated to two decimal places or a person's height is stated to the nearest millimeter.

The quality of the measuring instrument is the principal ingredient of precision, but the circumstances under which the measurement is made, the presence of faulty reagents or impurities, and sources of error attributable to the individual making the measurement are also important. These sources, called observational errors, include simple varieties such as parallax, digit preference, and the important class known as observer variation.

Reproducibility or **reliability** is the degree of stability exhibited when a measurement is repeated under closely similar conditions. Lack of reproducibility may arise from faults in the instrument, the observer, or in standardization of circumstances under which the measurements are made. Reproducibility should not be confused with ability to replicate, which means obtaining the same results when conducting an experiment or test in strict accordance with a defined protocol.

Instrumental error includes all the sources of variation inherent in the test itself. We can evaluate instrumental error by doing the same test twice or more independently, on each of a series of subjects. Independence implies that the second test is performed and the result recorded without knowledge of the first result. For example, in doing a chemical determination on blood serum, each specimen can be divided into two aliquots, which are separately analyzed. This permits determination of a laboratory's instrumental error.

Even the simplest measurements exhibit errors. No study should be undertaken without determining the amount of error existing under the test conditions. Procedures can sometimes be adopted to reduce the test error.

Digit preference is an idiosyncrasy of the person making the measurement that leads to a predilection for rounding off the measurement to the nearest whole number, even number, or multiple of 5 or 10.

Observer Variation

Observer variation is particularly troublesome when complex clinical qualities are being assessed.[82] For example, if several radiologists examine a large series of chest x-rays, they will not agree 100 percent on the interpretation, or even on which are normal or not, let alone on the nature and extent of abnormality. The same is true of many other clinical characteristics, for example, electrocardiograms; the size, shape, and texture of a lump in the breast or a mass in the abdomen; the appearance of abnormal cells in a cervical smear; and the assessment of personality. Interobserver variation may be as high as 20 percent. Intraobserver error also occurs: the same observer, viewing for the second time a chest x-ray, electrocardiogram, or histopathologic specimen, may assess and grade it differently; the frequency of intraobserver variation can be as high as 10 percent.

Whatever is being measured, the criteria should be as objective as possible and efforts made to avoid having the measurements influenced by extraneous factors. If, for example, two different skin test antigens are to be applied to each of a series of subjects for comparative purposes, the same test should not always be applied on the same site, as the reader would then know which antigen produced the reaction under study.

The same principle applies to the use of a questionnaire to elicit a history of disease, the presence of symptoms, or some host or environmental attribute. There can be large variations in information thus elicited. The design and wording of a questionnaire, as well as the training of the interviewers, their supervision, the rules they follow, and their approach to the subjects all influence the reliability. This is of special importance where results of one survey are to be compared with those of another done by a different research team, as in international comparisons of chronic bronchitis prevalence in relation to smoking history. Valuable experience on these issues has been acquired in sociologic studies.

Individual Variation

Biologic variables do not have a precise value but a range, which has a Gaussian (normal) or log-normal (skew) distribution in the population (Fig. 2–8).

Many biologic variables also vary within the same individual, depending upon circumstances such as the phase of certain body rhythms and the presence or absence of emotional stress. If reliance is to be placed upon such measurements, whether in clinical medicine or in epidemiology, the circumstances under which the measurement is made must as far as possible be standardized. For example, blood pressure recording can be standardized by always measuring it in the same arm with the same sized cuff, with the subject sitting, after 5 minutes' rest.

Bias

Bias is defined as any effect at any stage of investigation or inference tending to produce results that depart systematically from the true value. Bias must be distinguished from random error, which is discussed later. Any kind of bias will invalidate comparisons of rates and proportions between groups that are the subject of epidemiologic study. Many varieties of bias have been described[83]; only the most important of these are discussed here.

Selection Bias

This is a common cause of erroneous results and conclusions. It is due to systematic differences between those selected and those not selected for study. It occurs if nonrandom methods are used to select subjects for study. Unless the sampling method ensures that all members of the "universe" or reference population have a known chance of selection into the sample, bias is likely to occur. The best way to ensure a known chance of selection for all is to use a

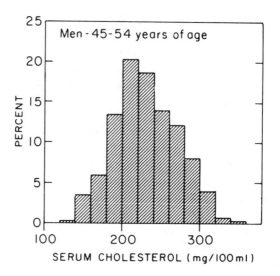

Figure 2–8. Distribution of a biologic variable: serum cholestrol in U.S. men aged 45 to 54. The distribution is distinctly skewed. Other biologic variables show varying degrees of skewness and some (e.g., body weight at a given height) are very close to a normal distribution (see also Fig. 2–10). *(Based on data from the U.S. National Health Survey.)*

probability sampling method, such as a table of random numbers. Sampling methods that lead to selection of individuals whose names begin with certain letters of the alphabet, who are enrolled on lists of voters, who have a listed telephone number, and various other methods that are sometimes used are all subject to certain kinds and degrees of bias.

Investigators frequently select for study those members of a population whom it is convenient to study, e.g., a consecutive series of patients attending a clinic, or persons whose names are listed in a health insurance plan. If only cases admitted to hospitals or cases under the care of a physician are studied, those who die before admission or before receiving care, those not sick enough to require hospital admission or care, and those excluded by distance, cost, or other factors will not be included in the investigation; conclusions based on this biased group can be misleading. Selection bias also invalidates generalizable conclusions from a survey of blood pressure or glycosuria at a shopping center or county fair. Only those fit enough to attend will be included—and only volunteers among them.

In case-control studies, the validity of results is based upon the assumption that the cases are a random sample of all the cases that have arisen in a defined period, and the controls are a random sample of all the noncases at risk during the same period. Yet this assumption hardly ever holds true. Usually the cases are a convenient sample, most often newly diagnosed cases at a hospital or other health facility; and the controls are often a sample of patients with other conditions who happen also to be attending the same institution. As Berkson[84] pointed out, this gives rise to a particular kind of bias—hospital patients are likely to suffer from more than one disease; biologically speaking, they are quite unrepresentative of the population and probably should not be selected for comparison purposes.

Response Bias

Volunteers and those who willingly comply with requests to participate in a study are often different from those who do not. For example, those who did not readily come forward for chest x-ray at the time of a mass radiography survey were often found to include high proportions of unusual individuals—alcoholics, criminals, vagrants, the mentally retarded, and so forth; the prevalence of tuberculosis was usually higher among these than in the general population. In any survey, there are always some who decline to participate, and it is desirable to find out as much as possible about these individuals in other ways, e.g., their demographic and cultural characteristics, in order to identify similarities and differences between responders and nonresponders.

Observer Bias

Interviewers and others who collect data in epidemiologic investigations may subconsciously or even consciously gather only such data as they want to in order to prove their point. Strategies to overcome this source of bias include random allocation of interviews among all the interviewers who are collecting data for a survey, and keeping the data gatherers as far as possible in ignorance of the nature of the individuals about whom they are gathering data—e.g., not revealing whether subjects belong to study or control groups in a randomized trial.

A variation of observer bias is recall bias. When subjects of a case-control study are asked about their past medical or occupational history, those who have the disease of interest may more completely recall the pertinent details than healthy controls who are asked the same questions. For instance, women with breast cancer may more completely recall past breast trauma than women without breast cancer.

Detection Bias

This term is applied to the form of bias that can arise if persons with a condition are detected because of circumstances related to some special prior experience that might distinguish them from other persons who have the same condition. Those who have had the special prior experience might be subject to closer surveillance because of this. For instance, women who have anomalous vaginal bleeding around the time of menopause may be more likely both to have a diagnostic curettage on one or more occasions and to be given estrogens to control menopausal symptoms. It is argued that if these women develop endometrial cancer, early detection of this cancer is more likely than in women who have a menopause without anomalous bleeding.

Confounding

This term describes the situation in which the effects of two processes are not separated. The distortion of the apparent effect of an exposure to risk is thus brought about by the association of another factor that can influence the outcome. The factor that distorts the apparent magnitude of the effect of a study factor is called a confounding variable. It is a determinant of the outcome that is being studied, and it is unequally distributed among exposed and unexposed groups that are being compared. Age can be a confounding variable when the age distribution of two populations being compared is very different; age standardization is used to remove the confounding effect of age differences. There are many other commonly encountered confounding variables. For example, in studies of the effects of occupational exposure upon respiratory disease, smoking would be a confounding variable unless allowance were duly made, which can be done by stratifying between smokers and nonsmokers in the analysis of results.

Further Sources of Error

Data Processing

Most epidemiologic studies generate large quantities of data, which are usually collected on survey forms, coded, keypunched, and then machine sorted or entered in a computer file for electronic data processing. Error can arise at several stages during these steps in an epidemiologic investigation. Errors of transcription and coding are minimized but never entirely eliminated by double-checking, every step being verified by a second clerical worker; this should be standard practice when data are keypunched or entered directly into the computer memory. When the data are tabulated, however, errors almost invariably occur—they are revealed by appearance in the tables of numbers that make no sense, such as women who have had a prostatectomy and men who have had a hysterectomy. The frequency of such errors is generally small, and most are easily detected, but occasionally large errors of this nature go undetected.

Interpretation and Logic

Finally, no account of sources of error in epidemiology would be complete without mention of the errors of interpretation that can result from faulty logic on the part of the investigator. It is easy to reach false conclusions about the explanation for associations between variables. An example from 19th-century epidemiology is Farr's suggestion that cholera mortality rates, which were highest at low altitudes, could be explained by the theory that a poisonous miasma from swamps and marshes was the cause of the disease. There are many contemporary parallels, often vigorously debated. For example, there was argument for some years about the epidemiologic evidence on distribution of blood pressure in populations. Was it bimodal or unimodal? If bimodal, a genetic basis for essential hypertension could be and was inferred by those who held this view of the evidence. More careful and larger epidemiologic studies ultimately showed no evidence of bimodal distribution of blood pressure in populations. This led to a reappraisal of the simple genetic hypothesis for the cause of essential hypertension. All too often, otherwise capable scientists have forced the facts (often incomplete facts) to fit a theory.

It is always easy to derive a false theory that appears to explain the known or apparent facts. For example, it was once believed that pellagra was infectious. Supposed causal organisms were confidently demonstrated by several investigators early in the 20th century, and the theory of infectious origin appeared to fit the then known epidemiologic and clinical evidence. Goldberger's work[85] dispelled this theory forever.

Statistical Concepts Relevant in Epidemiology

Samples and Sampling Error

Much of the time, epidemiologists study samples of the population, and even when they do not, every event of interest, e.g., deaths, births, new cases of specific diseases, affects a sample rather than all of the population.

Every rate, ratio, or average measurement is subject to sampling variation—an expression of the amount of variation to be expected from the operation of chance. Assumptions about the shape of the distribution, that it is normal rather than skew, and about the randomness of the sample are implicit in the calculation of sampling variation. Estimation of the sampling variation permits determination of the confidence interval within which the true value of measurement is likely to lie. Furthermore, the probability that two or more rates or means of measurement really differ from one another, i.e., that they are drawn from different populations, may be calculated by taking into consideration the sampling variation of each value.

Sampling error is a complex subject. It is dangerous to assume that a simple set of equations suffices to test the reality of all apparent differences. The whole subject of statistical significance, methods to test for it, and its meaning under various circumstances is properly treated in textbooks of medical statistics, such as those listed at the end of this chapter.

Type I and Type II Error

Sample size and types of error in randomized trials have received much attention.[86] If the experimental and control groups do not in reality have different outcomes, an apparent difference may nevertheless be observed by chance—a phenomenon known as type I error. Another possibility is that real differences do exist between experimental and control regimens, but by chance these differences are not detected on statistical analysis—type II error. The relationship of type I and type II errors is a function of sample size. In many RCTs, it is desirable to keep to a minimum the number of people who are subjected to the experimental regimen, which may be expensive or potentially hazardous. This aim must be balanced against the likelihood that the results will be invalidated by type II error. Type I and type II errors can occur in any study in which inferences are made on a sample, e.g., in case-control studies. Type I error is sometimes called an alpha and type II a beta error.

Normal and Skew Distributions

When there are many observations of a given biologic variable such as heights or weights of 10-year-old boys, blood pressure of 45-year-old men, or hemoglobin concentrations of healthy adult males, a range of values is recorded; this range is either symmetric about a mean or central value, as with heart rate (Fig. 2–9) or somewhat asymmetric, as with serum cholesterol (Fig. 2–8). A symmetric distribution is known as normal or gaussian, and the mean or central value is also the median and the mode. An asymmetric distribution is described as skew or log-normal when logarithmic transformation of the data convert it to a normal or symmetric distribution. In a skew distribution, the mode or most frequently occurring value is different from the mean, and so is the median or middle value in the sequence from highest to lowest.

Statistical Tests in Epidemiology

In epidemiology as in other biomedical sciences, we must often decide whether a difference between observations is statistically significant. Two questions arise: What is meant by "statistically significant?" How can we test for statistical significance? A complete answer to these questions demands a

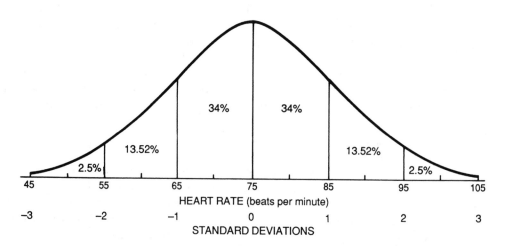

Figure 2–9. Normal distribution for heart rates. *(From Rimm AA, et al.:* Basic Biostatistics in Medicine and Epidemiology. *New York: Appleton-Century-Crofts, 1980, p 52.)*

thorough understanding of statistics, which can be acquired in courses and textbooks on the subject. The following discussion is all that space permits in such a book as this; I must assume familiarity with the terms and concepts of elementary statistics.

The Meaning of Statistical Significance

When data have normal or gaussian distribution, 5 percent of observations lie more than two standard deviations from the mean or central value. This fact leads to the rather arbitrary decision that the 5 percent level is a suitable point to set for observed differences to be described as statistically significant. In the conventional notation, the probability of an observation falling in this range is less than 5 percent, or $p < 0.05$. This level of statistical significance is suitable for many purposes in epidemiology, but sometimes we are justified in insisting on higher levels, e.g., a difference that could occur by chance less often than once in 100 times, i.e., $p < 0.01$, or less often than once in 1000, i.e., $p < 0.001$. When we set a 5 percent level, i.e., $p < 0.05$, one observed difference in 20 can be expected to be "statistically significant" just by chance; the type I error described previously illustrates this phenomenon. It must be remembered when many comparisons are being made in sets of data, e.g., in multivariate analysis, when on the average 1 in 20 of the correlations will be "statistically significant" by chance alone.

Significance Tests

The most widely used tests of statistical significance in epidemiology are the χ^2 (chi-squared) and t-test, correlation coefficient and analysis of variance. A detailed description of ways to perform these tests and their underlying mathematical theory can be found in the reference books listed at the end of this chapter; here is a brief and necessarily oversimplified account of the circumstances under which each should be used.

The chi-squared test is used to determine whether two or more series of proportions or frequencies are significantly different from one another or whether a single series of proportions differs from a theoretically expected distribution. There are a number of variations on the chi-squared test, e.g., the Mantel–Haenszel test, widely used in epidemiology to test for statistically significant differences in two-by-two tables when confounding variables are present.

The t-test is used when we want to compare the means of two or more populations or groups of data in which the standard deviation is not known, which is often the case when dealing with small numbers. The t-test is based on the assumption that the data are normally distributed; in many biomedical data sets, the distribution is skew rather than normal, but if the skewness is not extreme, the assumption of normal distribution is considered approximately valid.

The correlation coefficient is used to detect a trend in the relationship of two variables, e.g., heights and weights of a sample of schoolchildren, national per capita consumption of dietary fats, and mortality rates from coronary heart disease or cancer of the large bowel. These relationships are often represented visually as scatter diagrams, which reveal how two variables are related but do not fully describe the nature of the statistical relationship, which is provided by calculating the correlation coefficient.

If we know the means of two or more distributions, we can use analysis of variance to compare these and detect statistical differences or similarities. When we use analysis of variance, we could search for close similarity or parallelism of trends. In interpreting the results of these tests, it must be remembered that observed parallelism of trends does not necessarily imply a causal relationship. For example, the death rate from coronary heart disease in the United States rose in the period from the 1940s to the mid-1960s at about the same rate as the number of licensed automobiles per thousand population; but this does not mean, of course, that automobile use causes coronary heart disease. There are many such "nonsense correlations." Common sense as well as logic must be brought to bear in interpreting data and the statistical significance tests that are applied to the data.

Confidence Intervals

Results of hypothesis-testing studies have conventionally been expressed in terms of probabilities that the distributions observed are due to chance. This assumes that the populations in the study groups are truly representative of the "universe," and that the data have a normal or other known distribution. Often, neither assumption is true and, more important, undue attention has been focused upon statistical, rather than clinical or epidemiologic, significance. For instance, in an early case-control study of cigarette smoking and occurrence of lung cancer, Doll and Hill[87] observed the distribution of cigarette smoking in the cases and controls cited in Table 2–16 (male patients only). The probability of this distribution occurring by chance, according to Fisher's exact test, was given as 0.00000064. But this seemingly impressive level of statistical significance means much less than the confidence intervals derived from an estimate of relative risk. Using the odds ratio method of estimation, the relative risk of lung cancer among smokers compared to nonsmokers is 14, i.e., smokers had about 14 times higher risk of lung cancer than nonsmokers. This figure is consistent with the relative risks derived from distributions observed in later, more carefully conducted case-control

TABLE 2–16.   Case Contol Study of Lung Cancer and Past History of Smoking

History of Smoking	Cases	Controls
Yes	647	622
No	2	27
Total	649	649

studies (and also with the risks calculated from cohort studies). The confidence intervals, however, are wide and therefore these results must be interpreted with caution. Confidence intervals are related to sample size, as Table 2–17 clearly shows.

Several authorities have argued cogently that scientific papers must show the confidence intervals rather than, or in addition to, the p values derived from statistical significance testing.[88,89] As from 1986, a number of important journals are insisting that confidence intervals be included in the results intended for publication. A confidence interval is defined as the range of possible values for the attribute that is being measured or assessed, constructed so that this range has a specified probability, usually greater than 95 percent, of including the true value. Methods of calculating confidence intervals vary according to the nature and quality of the data and are a branch of applied biostatistics beyond the scope of this book. Details are given in some of the references cited at the end of this chapter. Anyone who has to calculate confidence intervals should be able to use the appropriate statistical methods and, if unable to do so, should consult a statistician.

Sampling Methods

Almost the only kind of epidemiology that can be done with the total population is analysis of vital statistics and other official records. While useful for many purposes, these have many flaws, as mentioned earlier; the most serious is the lack of diagnostic precision that raises questions about their validity. Many epidemiologic studies must be done using a sample of the population, and as a rule we want this sample to resemble as closely as possible the total population of the country or region. To ensure this, we rely on probability sampling methods, which can ensure that all members of the "universe" population have a known chance of being selected for study. The chance may not be equal if we elect to stratify the sample in some way, for instance by age, sex, or occupational grouping; but the chance of selection must be known

TABLE 2–17. Infant Mortality Rate: Sample Size and Confidence Interval

Sample Size: Number of Persons	Number of Births Observed	Number of Infant Deaths Observed	95% Confidence Interval for the Infant Mortality Rate
1000	40	4	4-196
5000	200	20	58-142
10,000	400	40	70-130
50,000	2000	200	87-113
100,000	4000	400	91-109
250,000	10,000	1000	94-106
500,000	20,000	2000	96-104

(Adapted from Development of Indicators for Monitoring Progress towards Health for All by the Year 2000. Geneva: WHO, 1981.)

and it must be based on a probabilistic method. This is called a random sample. A widely used random sampling method is to work from a suitable list that is reckoned to be representative of the population as a whole, such as a voters' list or the telephone directory; but neither is truly representative since not everyone is registered to vote nor does everyone have a telephone—and some who do have unlisted numbers. The U.S. National Health Survey and similar important field studies often use a cluster sampling method in which geographic regions are sampled, and households within the sampled regions are then sampled. Details of this and other sampling methods can be found in the sources cited at the end of this chapter.

► REFERENCES

1. Lloyd GR (ed): *Hippocratic Writings.* Harmondsworth, England: Penguin, 1978.
2. Graunt J: *Natural and Political Observations, Mentioned in a Following Index, and Made Upon the Bills of Mortality.* London: T Roycroft for J Martin, J Allestry, and T Dicas, 1662.
3. Snow J: *On the Mode of Communication of Cholera,* 2nd ed. London: Churchill, 1855. Reprint with annotations by Wade Hampton Frost, New York: Commonwealth Fund, 1936; reprint New York: Hafner, 1965.
4. Humphries N (ed): *Vital Statistics: A Memorial Volume of Selections from the Reports and Writings of William Farr.* London: Stanford, 1885. Reprint, Susser MW, Adelstein A (eds). New York Academy of Medicine, 1975.
5. Lilienfeld AM, Lilienfeld D: A century of case-control studies: Progress. *J Chronic Dis* 32:5–13, 1979.
6. Laporte RE, Akazawa S, Hellmonds P, et al.: Global public health and the information superhighway. *Br Med J* 308:1651–1652, 1994.
7. Last JM (ed): *A Dictionary of Epidemiology.* 3rd ed. New York: Oxford University Press, 1995.
8. Morris JN: Uses of epidemiology. *Br Med J* 2:305–401, 1955.
9. Last JM: The iceberg: "Completing the clinical picture" in general practice. *Lancet* 2:28–31, 1963.
10. Paul JR: Clinical epidemiology. *J Clin Invest* 17:539–541, 1938.
11. Shapiro S: Evidence on screening for breast cancer from a randomized trial. *Cancer* 39:2772–2782, 1977.
12. McDowell IW, Newell C: *Health Measurement Scales.* 2nd ed. New York: Oxford University Press, 1996.
13. World Health Organization: *International Classification of Disease.* 9th revision (ICD-9). Geneva, 1975.
14. Last JM: Nosography: Conceptual, epidemiological and statistical implications. In Kupka K (ed): *Health Statistics for the Year 2000.* Budapest: Statistical Publishing House (for WHO), 1984, pp. 34–48.
15. Murphy EA: *The Logic of Medicine.* Baltimore: Johns Hopkins University Press, 1976.
16. Heasman MA: Accuracy of death certification. *Proc Roy Soc Med* 55:733–736, 1962.
17. Begg C, Cho M, Eastwood S, et al.: Improving the quality of reporting of randomized trials; the CONSORT statement. *JAMA* 276:637–639, 1996.

18. Feinlieb M, Havlik RJ, Thom TJ: The changing pattern of ischemic heart disease. *J Cardiovasc Med* 7:139–148, 1982.

19. Murray CJL, Lopez AD (eds): *Global Comparative Assessments in the Health Sector: Disease Burden, Expenditures, and Intervention Packages.* Geneva: WHO, 1994.

20. Nightingale F: *Notes on Hospitals.* London: J.W. Parker, 1859.

21. *Length of Stay in PAS Hospitals.* Ann Arbor, MI.: Commission on Professional and Hospital Activities (published annually).

22. Jick H: The Commission on Professional and Hospital Activities—Professional activity study. A national resource for the study of rare illnesses. *Am J Epidemiol* 109:625–627, 1979.

23. Pickles WN: *Epidemiology in Country Practice.* Bristol, England: Wright Brothers, 1939.

24. Avnet HG: *Physician Service Patterns and Sickness Rates.* Chicago: Group Health Insurance Institute, 1967.

25. Logan WPD, Cushion AA: *Studies on Medical and Population Subjects, No. 14: Morbidity Statistics from General Practice.* Vol. 1. (General). London: General Register Office, HMSO, 1958.

26. Logan WPD, Cushion AA: *Studies on Medical and Population Subjects, No. 14: Morbidity Statistics from General Practice.* Vol. 3. (General). London: General Register Office, HMSO, 1963.

27. Fry J: *Profiles of Disease.* Edinburgh: Churchill-Livingstone, 1966.

28. Hodgkin G: *Towards Earlier Diagnosis.* 2nd ed. Edinburgh: Churchill-Livingstone, 1973.

29. Galloway TM: Computers: Their use in local health administration. *Roy Soc Health J* 86:213–216, 1966.

30. National Center for Health Statistics: *Vital and Health Statistics.* Series 1, 2, 3, 10. Washington, DC: U.S. DHHS.

31. National Center for Health Statistics: *Vital and Health Statistics.* Series 1, 2, 11. Washington, DC: U.S. DHHS/NCHS.

32. National Center for Health Statistics: *Vital and Health Statistics.* Series 1, 2, 11. Washington, DC: U.S. DHHS.

33. Kohn R, White KL: *Health Care: An International Study.* New York: Oxford University Press, 1976.

34. Clearinghouse on Health Indices: *Cumulated Annotations 1976.* Washington DC: U.S. Department of HEW Publications No. (PHS) 78–1225, 1978.

35. McDowell IW, Newell C: *Measuring Health.* 2nd ed. New York: Oxford University Press, 1996.

36. Ashton J (ed): *The Epidemiological Imagination.* Buckingham, England: Open University Press, 1994.

37. Gardner MJ, Snee MP, Hall AJ, et al.: Results of case-control study of leukaemia and lymphoma among young people near Sellafield nuclear plant in West Cumbria. *Br Med J* 300:423–429, 1990.

38. Inskip H: Introduction to Gardner's paper. In Ashton J (ed): *The Epidemiological Imagination.* Buckingham, England: Open University Press, 1994, p. 65.

39. Doll R, Evans HJ, Darby SC: Paternal exposure not to blame. *Nature* 367: 678–680, 1994.

40. Wertheimer N, Leeper E: Electrical wiring configurations and childhood cancer. *Am J Epidemiol* 109:273–284, 1979.

41. Armstrong B, Thériault G, Gunel P, et al.: Association between exposure to pulsed electromagnetic fields and cancer in electrical utility workers in Quebec, Canada, and France. *Am J Epidemiol* 140:805–820, 1994.

42. Poole C: Invited commentary: Evolution of epidemiologic evidence on magnetic fields and childhood cancers. *Am J Epidemiol* 143:129–132, 1996; see also accompanying original articles in the same journal.

43. National Research Council: *Possible Health Effects of Residential Electric and Magnetic Fields.* Washington, DC: National Academy Press, 1996.

44. Will RG, Ironside JW, Zeidler M, et al.: A new variant of Creutzfeld-Jakob disease. *Lancet* 347:921–925, 1996.

45. Gregg MB (ed): *Field Epidemiology.* New York: Oxford University Press, 1996.

46. Creech JL Jr, Johnson MN: Angiosarcoma of the liver in the manufacture of polyvinyl chloride. *J Occup Med* 16:150, 1974.

47. Doll R, Hill AB: Smoking and carcinoma of the lung; preliminary report. *Br Med J* 2:739–748, 1950; see also Wynder EL, Graham EA: Tobacco smoking as a possible etiologic factor in bronchogenic carcinoma. A study of six hundred and eighty-four proved cases. *JAMA* 143:4:329–336, 1950.

48. Schlesselman JJ: *Case-Control Studies—Design, Conduct, Analysis.* New York: Oxford University Press, 1982; see also Wacholder S, McLaughlin JK, Silverman DT, Mandel JS: Selection of controls in case-control studies. *Am J Epidemiol* 135:1019–1050, 1992.

49. Herbst AL, Ulfelder H, Poskanzer DC: Association of maternal stilbestrol therapy with tumor appearance in young women. *N Engl J Med* 284:878–881, 1971.

50. Dieckmann WJ, Davis ME, Rynkiewicz LM, et al.: Does the administration of diethylstilbestrol during pregnancy have therapeutic value? *Am J Obstet Gynecol* 66:1062–1068, 1953.

51. Mantel H, Haenszel W: Statistical aspects of the analysis of data from retrospective studies of disease. *J Natl Cancer Inst* 22:719–748, 1959.

52. Schlesselman JJ: *Case-Control Studies—Design, Conduct, Analysis.* New York: Oxford University Press, 1982.

53. Breslow NE, Day NE: *Statistical Methods in Cancer Research.* Vol. 1. The Analysis of Case-Control Studies. Lyon, France: WHO/IARC Scientific Publications No. 32, 1980.

54. Doll R, Hill AB: Lung cancer and other causes of death in relation to smoking: A second report on the mortality of British doctors. *Br Med J* 2:1071–1082, 1956.

55. Doll R, Hill AB: Mortality in relation to smoking: ten years' observations of British doctors. *Br Med J* 1:1399–1410; 1460–1467, 1964.

56. Doll R, Peto R: Mortality in relation to smoking: 20 years' observations on male British doctors. *Br Med J* 2:1525–1536, 1976.

57. MacMahon B: Prenatal x-ray exposure and childhood cancer. *J Natl Cancer Inst* 28:1173–1191, 1962.

58. Stewart A, Webb J, Hewitt D: A survey of childhood malignancies. *Br Med J* 1:1495–1508, 1958.

59. Hill AB: The environment and disease; association or causation? *Proc Roy Soc Med* 58:295–300, 1965.

60. Susser MW: *Causal Thinking in the Health Sciences.* New York: Oxford University Press, 1973. [This book is a classic that all aspiring epidemiologists should read.]

61. Susser MW: Judgment and causal inference: Criteria in epidemiologic studies. *Am J Epidemiol* 105:1–15, 1977; see also Susser MW: What is a cause and how do we know one? A grammar for pragmatic epidemiology. *Am J Epidemiol* 133:635–648, 1991.
62. Rothman KJ: Causes. *Am J Epidemiol* 104:587–594, 1976.
63. Witts LJ (ed): *Medical Surveys and Clinical Trials.* Oxford: Oxford Medical Publications, 1959.
64. Meinert CL, Tonascia S: *Clinical Trials: Design, Conduct, and Analysis.* New York: Oxford University Press, 1986.
65. *Trials of War Criminals before the Nürnberg Military Tribunals under Control Council Law No. 10.* Vols. 1, 2. The Medical Case (Military Tribunal I, 1947). Washington, DC: U.S. Government Printing Office, 1948–49.
66. Silverman WA: *Human Experimentation. A Guided Step into the Unknown.* Oxford: Oxford Medical Publications, 1985.
67. Early Breast Cancer Trialists' Collaborative Group: Systematic treatment of early breast cancer by hormonal, cytotoxic, or immune therapy. *Lancet* 339:1–15, 71–85, 1992.
68. Hoffman RE: The use of epidemiologic data in the courts. *Am J Epidemiol* 120:190–202, 1984.
69. Lilienfeld DE, Black B: The epidemiologist in court: Some comments. *Am J Epidemiol* 123:961–964, 1986.
70. Dickerson K, Berlin JA: Meta-analysis: State of the science. *Epidemiol Rev* 14:154–176, 1992.
71. Petitti D: *Meta-Analysis, Decision Analysis and Cost-Effectiveness Analysis: Methods for Quantitative Synthesis in Medicine.* New York: Oxford University Press, 1994.
72. Canadian Task Force on the Periodic Health Examination: Task Force report. *Can Med Assoc J* 121:1193–1254, 1979.
73. U.S. Preventive Services Task Force: *Guide to Clinical Preventive Services.* Baltimore: Williams & Wilkins, 1989.
74. *Evidence-Based Medicine.* 1:1 (Nov/Dec), 1995. (Published bi-monthly by BMA Publishing Group.) Tavistock Square, London WC1H9JR, UK.
75. Acheson ED: *Medical Record Linkage.* New York: Oxford University Press, 1967.
76. Newcombe HB, Kennedy JM, Axford SJ, et al.: Automatic linkage of vital and health records. *Science* 130:954, 1959; see also Smith ME, Newcombe HB: Use of the Canadian mortality data base for epidemiological follow-up. *Can J Public Health* 73:39–46, 1982; and Newcombe HB: *Handbook of Record Linkage.* Oxford: Oxford Medical Publications, 1988.
77. Beaglehole R, Bonita R, Kjellström T: *Basic Epidemiology.* Geneva: WHO 1993.
78. Lay reporting of health information. Geneva: WHO 1978; see also Murnaghan J: Health indicators and information systems for the year 2000. *Annu Rev Public Health* 2:299–361, 1981.
79. Chandramohan D, Maude GH, Rodriques LC, et al. Verbal autopsies for adult deaths; issues in their development and validation. *Int J Epidemiol* 23:213–230, 1994.
80. Wittes JT, Colton T, Sidel VW: Capture-recapture methods for assessing the completeness of ascertainment when using multiple information. *J Chron Dis* 27:25–36, 1974.
81. Laporte RE, Tull ES, McCarty D: Monitoring the incidence of myocardial infarctions; applications of capture-mark-recapture technology. *Int J Epidemiol* 21:258–262, 1992.

82. Abercrombie MLJ: *The Anatomy of Judgment.* London: Hutchinson, 1960.
83. Last JM (ed): *A Dictionary of Epidemiology.* New York: Oxford University Press, 1983.
84. Berkson J: Limitations of the application of fourfold table analysis to hospital data. *Biometrics Bull* 2:47–53, 1946.
85. Terris M (ed): *Goldberger on Pellagra.* Baton Rouge: Louisiana State University Press, 1964.
86. Freiman JA, Chalmers TC, Smith H, et al.: Importance of beta, the type II error and sample size in the design and interpretation of the randomized control trial. *N Engl J Med* 299:290–294, 1978.
87. Doll R, Hill AB: Smoking and carcinoma of the lung. *Br Med J* 2:739–748, 1950.
88. Gardner, MJ, Altman DG: Confidence intervals rather than P values: Estimation rather than hypothesis-testing. *Br Med J* 292:746–750, 1986.
89. Poole C, Lanes S, Rothman KJ: Analyzing data from ordered categories. *N Engl J Med* 311:1382, 1984.

▶ ADDITIONAL READINGS

Epidemiology and Biostatistics

Colton T: *Statistics in Medicine.* Boston: Little, Brown, 1974.
Evans RS: *Causation and Disease: A Chronological Journey.* New York: Plenum, 1993.
Fletcher RH, Fletcher SW, Wagner EH: *Clinical Epidemiology.* 3rd ed. Baltimore: Williams & Wilkins, 1990.
Gregg MB (ed): *Field Epidemiology.* New York: Oxford University Press, 1996.
Hennekens CH, Buring JE: *Epidemiology in Medicine.* Boston: Little, Brown, 1987.
Hill AB: *Principles of Medical Statistics,* 12th ed. New York: Oxford University Press, 1996.
Kelsey JL, Thompson WD, Evans AS: *Methods in Observational—Epidemiology.* 2nd ed. New York: Oxford University Press, 1996.
Kleinbaum DG, Kupper LL, Morgenstern H: *Epidemiology—Principles and Quantitative Methods.* Belmont: Lifetime Learning Publications, 1982.
Lilienfeld DE, Stolley PD: *Foundations of Epidemiology.* 3rd ed. New York: Oxford University Press, 1994.
Morris JN: *Uses of Epidemiology,* 3rd ed. London: Churchill-Livingstone, 1975.
Schlesselman JJ: *Case-Control Studies—Design, Conduct, Analysis.* New York: Oxford University Press, 1982.
Susser MW: *Causal Thinking in the Health Sciences.* New York: Oxford University Press, 1973.

Historical Background

Farr W: *Vital Statistics: A Memorial Volume of Selections from the Reports and Writings of William Farr.* Intro. by Susser MW, Aldelstein A, Metuchen, NJ: Scarecrow Press, 1975.
Frost WH: *Collected Papers.* Maxcy KF (ed). New York: The Commonwealth Fund, 1941.

Greenwood M: *Medical Statistics from Graunt to Farr.* Cambridge, Cambridge University Press, 1935.

Lilienfeld AM (ed): *Times, Places and Persons: Aspects of the History of Epidemiology.* Baltimore: Johns Hopkins University Press, 1980.

Panum PL: *Observations Made During the Epidemic of Measles on the Faroe Islands in the Year 1846.* Hatcher AS (trans): New York: American Public Health Association, 1940.

Snow J: *The Mode of Communication of Cholera (1855).* (Reprinted) New York: The Commonwealth Fund, 1936.

Terris M: *Goldberger on Pellagra.* Baton Rouge: Louisiana State University Press, 1964.

Infectious Disease

Centers for Disease Control and Prevention, United States Public Health Service: *Morbidity and Mortality Weekly Reports.*

Centers for Disease Control and Prevention, United States Public Health Service: *Surveillance Reports* on selected diseases (published periodically).

Evans AS: *Viral Infections of Humans: Epidemiology and Control.* New York: Plenum, 1976.

3

Ecology and Control of Communicable Diseases

A communicable disease develops after transmission of a specific infectious agent or its toxic products from an infected person, animal, or reservoir to a susceptible host, either directly or indirectly through an intermediate plant or animal host, vector, or the inanimate environment. Infection is usually—but by no means always—accompanied by overt manifestations of disease in the human host.

Communicable diseases can occur as sporadic cases or in epidemics; sometimes they are always present at a relatively low level in the population, or endemic. Rarely, they occur on a massive international, even worldwide scale, as pandemics. The last great pandemic of influenza in 1918–19 killed more people than had died in combat in World War I. Since the early 1980s, the world has been hit by a pandemic of aquired immunodeficiency syndrome (AIDS) that is no nearer control now than when it was first identified.

Control of communicable diseases requires that the chain of transmission be broken. Epidemiology, which originally meant the scientific study of epidemics, has played its most important role in finding causes and associated risk factors, and thus it has led to the successful control of many communicable diseases.

Most of the great epidemic diseases of the past are under control but infectious and parasitic diseases still cause almost a third of all the deaths in the world every year, many of them in infancy and childhood. Smallpox has been eradicated by a World Health Organization (WHO)-coordinated international effort; plague and epidemic louse-borne typhus are rare; but cholera still occurs in many parts of the world, even occasionally in affluent industrial nations; yellow fever has flared up again in equatorial Africa and in Brazil.[1] We have no reliable long-term vaccine defense against epidemic influenza. Many sexually transmitted diseases (STDs) are largely uncontrolled. In tropical and subtropical regions of developing nations, malaria, schistosomiasis, filariasis, trypanosomiasis, leishmaniasis, and leprosy, although all the target of intensified research, are often poorly controlled and are out of control in some places.

In rich industrial nations, many formerly common and often fatal infectious diseases are rare or have disappeared entirely. These include diphtheria, typhoid, whooping cough, measles, the gastrointestinal diseases of infancy and early childhood, and poliomyelitis. In developing nations, many of these diseases and others, e.g., malaria and several parasitic infections, are serious and widespread. In much of the former Soviet Union, public health infrastructure has broken down: Diphtheria has reemerged as a serious problem with high mortality and morbidity rates. In the first 6 months of 1996 there were 125,000 cases and 4000 deaths from diphtheria in Russia and other former Soviet republics.[2] Acute respiratory infections remain as common as ever all over the world. Tuberculosis, which had virtually died out in affluent industrial nations by the mid-1960s, is common among homeless and indigent people in large cities, its virulence potentiated by human immunodeficiency virus (HIV) infection. The common cold defies preventive efforts. Several "new" or emerging infectious diseases, notably HIV/AIDS, present formidable challenges.

In the 1940s and early 1950s, when I was a medical student and hospital resident, optimism and "can-do" attitudes toward all infections were the prevailing mood. We used penicillin and streptomycin to cure innumerable patients with serious infections whose outlook had been hopeless a decade earlier. This followed soon after the triumphs of vaccines and sera that could prevent a wide range of previously lethal or dangerous infectious diseases. We believed that human ingenuity would soon find magic bullets to conquer all other diseases caused by microorganisms and many other incurable and fatal conditions like cancer and multiple sclerosis. How wrong we were! We had overlooked a fundamental biologic reality: The brief generation time of microorganisms led to selective survival and breeding of antibiotic-resistant pathogens. By the early 1960s antibiotic-resistant staphylococci, gonococci, and many other pathogens were taxing our ingenuity to find ways to treat the infections they caused. Microorganisms not previously identified as causes of infection, such as *Proteus* and *Pseudomonas* species, became a serious problem in hospitals, causing obstinate nosocomial infections. This was just the beginning. We began to see and recognize new kinds of infection: legionnaires' disease, Lyme disease, deadly exotic infections out of Africa—Lassa fever, Marburg and Ebola virus infections—and others. In 1981, the first cases of AIDS were identified, and we soon realized that we were confronted by one of the most dangerous epidemic diseases ever to challenge us.

In this brief account I will discuss principles rather than details. Details are available in *Control of Communicable Diseases Manual*[3] (CCDM), now in its 16th edition, published by the American Public Health Association. This is an indispensable desk reference for practicing physicians and public health workers.

► CLASSIFICATION

The most practical way to arrange communicable diseases is according to the principal mode by which they are transmitted and gain entry to the human host: person-to-person, by insect or other vectors, from animals to man, etc. But some important infectious diseases do not fit this simple system: They may be transmitted and invade the host in several different ways. CCDM simply lists them all in alphabetical order. Another way to arrange them is according to the type of infecting organism: virus, bacterium, protozoon, multicellular parasite, and some infectious agents that lie outside this list. Many textbooks use a classification that combines the method of transmission and the nature of the infecting organism. This is flexible enough to include conditions that, strictly speaking, are not communicable such as those caused by contamination of food by toxic chemicals, which often behave epidemiologically like infectious processes.

► EPIDEMIC THEORY

Ronald Ross (1857–1932), who discovered the malaria parasite, followed William Farr in using mathematical formulae to explain his field observations of malaria. Hamer,[4] Soper, Greenwood,[5] and other epidemiologists expanded on this approach, which Bailey explored in a famous monograph[6] on the mathematical theory of epidemics. The mathematical models were tested in field studies or in "experimental epidemiology"—observations on the spread of infection among captive colonies of animals such as rats, mice, and guinea pigs. Hamer developed the fundamental principle of infectious disease epidemiology, the **mass action principle:** The course of an epidemic depends on the rate of contact between susceptibles and infectious individuals.[7] With the decline of epidemic infectious diseases in rich industrial nations, epidemic theory fell into disuse, although it remained valuable in control programs for malaria and other infectious diseases in developing and tropical regions. With the resurgence of antibiotic-resistant infectious diseases and emergence of new diseases, particularly HIV/AIDS, epidemic theory has undergone a renaissance.[8] Application of the mathematical theory of epidemics can help to predict epidemics, to plan effective control measures, and to evaluate the success of the plan after it has been implemented.

Infectivity

Persons harboring infectious organisms can transmit them at various stages of the infection, depending on the organism and its effects on the host.

Some common infectious diseases are most infectious in the prodromal or incubation periods, before they declare themselves by causing symptoms or sickness. Measles and many varieties of the common cold are spread in this manner. Once acquired, some conditions remain infective to others more or less indefinitely, as with some STDs. Some remain infectious after the host has become apparently well again, the convalescent carrier state, as with many cases of typhoid. Some important infectious diseases do not incapacitate the host, who can remain at large in the community to infect others; this commonly occurs with tuberculosis and many STDs. Many infectious diseases manifest varying degrees of severity, including subclinical cases that can lead to serious infection when transmitted to other people.

Gradient of Infection

An important feature of many kinds of infection is variation in individual response, graphically presented in Figure 3–1. The response to invading pathogenic organisms can range from an overwhelming and rapidly lethal disease with profound toxemia to a completely symptomless invasion, in which the only detectable evidence of infection is a rise in titer of antibodies, indicating that the individual has been infected. From the point of view of the infectious organism, inapparent infection is most likely to ensure its survival and

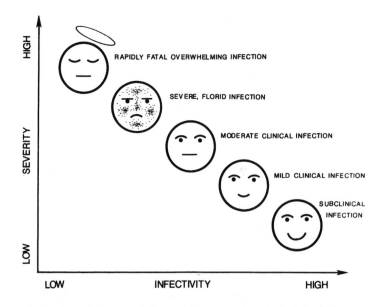

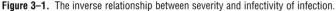

Figure 3–1. The inverse relationship between severity and infectivity of infection.

further propagation; if the infected individual remains apparently well and continues normal activities, especially remaining in contact with others who may be susceptible to infection, the organism is more likely to be passed on—and thus infect others, not all of whom will escape unscathed. Many infections produce clinical signs and symptoms in only a minority of those who are invaded by the infectious agent, but many of those who have no signs or symptoms are infectious to others for short or sometimes prolonged periods, i.e., they have subclinical infections—but they are carriers of pathogens that are capable of infecting others. Epidemiologically, subclinical cases and carriers are the most significant among all who become infected. The more serious the symptoms and signs of infection, the more likely it is that infected persons will be confined to bed or to the house, in contact with relatively small numbers, and therefore less likely to infect others.

Evolutionary biology has enlightened us about the complex interactions among infectious pathogens, host susceptibility and resistance, and myriad environmental and behavioral factors that influence the ecology of infectious diseases.[9] We are beginning to appreciate the nature of some of these interactions. We can never eradicate most pathogens as we eradicated smallpox. Instead, we should try to live in harmony among the microorganisms that in sheer biomass outweigh us, just as they outnumber us by many orders of magnitude. We can best do this by enhancing immunity.

Herd Immunity

This means the collective immunity of a group or community. The resistance of a group to invasion and spread of an infectious agent is a product of the number susceptible to infection and the probability that those who are susceptible will encounter a source of infection. This essentially mathematical concept can be calculated empirically for many common infections. Its utility is its capacity to define the **herd immunity threshold,** i.e., the proportion of the total population that has to be immunized in order to reduce to near vanishing point the probability of a susceptible person encountering a source of infection. The herd immunity threshold is $1 - 1/R_0$, where R_0 is the rate at which new infections are produced in a susceptible population in the early stages of an epidemic when all or almost all members of the population are susceptible. Other variables include the characteristics of the organism, its mode of transmission and period of infectivity, the incubation time, the duration of artificial and postinfection immunity, the involvement of vectors, and the size of the population. The herd immunity threshold varies; for instance, for diphtheria the incidence of infection declines sharply when 50 to 60 percent of the population has been vaccinated, whereas for measles the herd immunity threshold is much higher, in the range of 80 to 95 percent. Herd immunity was comprehensively reviewed in 1993.[10]

Immunization campaigns, by raising the level of herd immunity, protect not only individuals but entire populations. If nearly all infants and children in the population are immunized against the common communicable diseases, i.e., if the number of susceptibles is close to zero, there is little likelihood of epidemic spread because the propagation of an infectious disease requires that there be a large enough pool of susceptibles among whom the condition can spread.

Seroepidemiology, the use of serologic tests to assess antibody titer and thereby identify infections, is a valuable way to determine the distribution of susceptibility and resistence to infection in populations and to observe how this changes over time and in response to occurrence of infection, which may be acquired by far higher proportions of the people than those with symptoms or signs. Seroepidemiology measures the immune status of the population, irrespective of whether the immunity is naturally or artificially acquired.

Molecular epidemiology offers more.[11] The techniques of molecular biology allow us to determine precisely the origin and passage through successive hosts of a specific strain of an organism, using DNA markers. Thus, we can identify who was the source of an outbreak of an infection such as tuberculosis or an STD (raising ethical questions about disclosure and stigmatizing, discussed in Chap. 10). Once identified, this source, the nidus of infection, is the logical place to begin preventive efforts such as chemoprophylaxis.

► **CONTROL**

A good reason for classifying communicable diseases is to aid our application of ways to control them; therefore, as I mentioned previously, a good way to classify communicable diseases is according to the principal method of control. This classification is imperfect because some important communicable diseases can only be controlled by applying several methods together. For example, typhoid is best controlled by a combination of personal hygiene, environmental sanitation, purifying water, and hygienic methods of preparing, preserving, and serving pathogen-free foods, and when all of these cannot be guaranteed, immunization; identifying and treating symptomless carriers is also important. On the other hand, there is only one way—good food hygiene—to prevent staphylococcal food poisoning, and only one way—mass immunization—to prevent epidemics of diphtheria, measles, and poliomyelitis.

Box 3–1 is a summary of control measures for some important varieties of communicable diseases. The family physician and pediatrician are most often concerned with providing immunization or vaccination for infants and children. There is a well-defined schedule for this (Table 3–1).

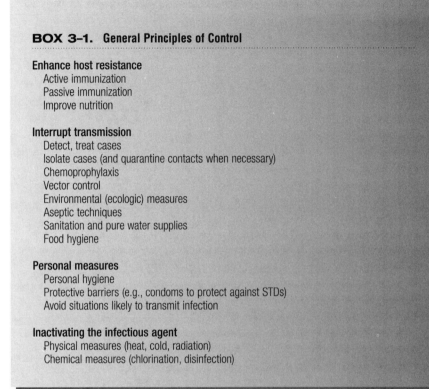

BOX 3–1.   **General Principles of Control**

Enhance host resistance
  Active immunization
  Passive immunization
  Improve nutrition

Interrupt transmission
  Detect, treat cases
  Isolate cases (and quarantine contacts when necessary)
  Chemoprophylaxis
  Vector control
  Environmental (ecologic) measures
  Aseptic techniques
  Sanitation and pure water supplies
  Food hygiene

Personal measures
  Personal hygiene
  Protective barriers (e.g., condoms to protect against STDs)
  Avoid situations likely to transmit infection

Inactivating the infectious agent
  Physical measures (heat, cold, radiation)
  Chemical measures (chlorination, disinfection)

▶ MODES OF TRANSMISSION OF INFECTION

Infection can be transmitted in several ways (Box 3–2):

1. **Person-to-person spread.** This may be by direct contact, as with the STDs, or indirect, as by droplet spread or through utensils, articles of clothing, etc. that are contaminated with infectious microorganisms, to which the term *fomites* is applied. The STDs generally require quite intimate contact of mucous membranes. Some other conditions that require direct body contact, e.g., scabies and fungus infections of the skin (athlete's foot, ringworm, etc.), and body and head lice are spread from infected (infested) skin surfaces rather than by mucous membrane contact.

Even the most fastidious people can become infested with lice when they are unable to maintain personal hygiene. Anne Frank described in her diary[12] how she and her family kept clean while hiding from the Nazis in wartime Amsterdam. She and her sister, Margot, died of epidemic louse-

TABLE 3–1.   Recommended Childhood Immunization Schedule[a]—United States, January 1995

Vaccine	Birth	2 Months	4 Months	6 Months	12[b] Months	15 Months	18 Months	4–6 Years	11–12 Years	14–16 Years
Hepatitis B[c]	HB-1									
		HB-2		HB-3						
Diptheria-Tetanus-Pertussis (DTP)[d]		DTP	DTP	DTP	DTP or DTaP at ≥ 15 months			DTP or DTaP	Td	
Haemophilus influenza type b[e]		Hib	Hib	Hib	Hib					
Poliovirus		OPV	OPV	OPV				OPV		
Measles-Mumps-Rubella[f]					MMR			MMR or	MMR	

[a] Recommended vaccines are listed under the routinely recommended ages. Shaded bars indicate range of acceptable ages for vaccination.

[b] Vaccines recommended for administration at 12–15 months of age may be administered at either one or two visits.

[c] Infants born to hepatitis B surface antigen (HBsAg)-negative mothers should receive the second dose of hepatitis B vaccine between 1 and 4 months of age, provided at least 1 month has elapsed since receipt of the first dose. The third dose is recommended between 6 and 18 months of age. Infants born to HBsAg-positive mothers should receive immunoprophylaxis for hepatitis B with 0.5 mL hepatitis B immune globin (HBIG) within 12 hours of birth, and 5 μg of either Merck & Co., Inc. (West Point, Pennsylvania) vaccine (Recombivax HB) or 10 μg of SmithKline Beecham Pharmaceuticals (Philadelphia) vaccine (Engerix-B) at a separate site. For these infants, the second dose of vaccine is recommended at 1 month of age and the third dose at 6 months of age. All pregnant women should be screened for HBsAg during an early prenatal visit.

[d] The fourth dose of DTP may be administered as early as 12 months of age, provided at least 6 months have elapsed since the third dose of DTP. Combined DTP-Hib products may be used when these two vaccines are administered simultaneously. Diphtheria and tetanus toxoids and acellular pertusis vaccine (DTaP) are licensed for use for the fourth and/or fifth dose of DTP in children ≥ 15 months of age and may be preferred for these doses in children in this age group.

[e] Three *H. influenza* type b conjugate vaccines are available for use in infants: (1) oligosaccharide conjugate Hib vaccine (HbOC) (HibTITER, manufactured by Lederle, [Wayne, New Jersey]); (2) polyribosylribitol phosphate-tetanus toxoid conjugate (PRP-T) (ActHIB, manufactured by Pasteur Mérieux Sérums & Vaccins, S.A. [Lyon, France] and distributed by Connaught Laboratories, Inc. [Swiftwater, Pennsylvania], and OmniHIB, manufactured by Pasteur Mérieux Sérums & Vaccins, S.A. and distributed by SmithKline Beecham Pharmaceuticals [Philadelphia]); and (3) *Haemophilus* b conjugate vaccine (meningococcal protein conjugate) (PRP-OMP) (PedvaxHIB, manufactured by Merck & Co., Inc.). Children who have received PRP-OMP at 2 and 4 months of age do not require a dose at 6 months of age. After the primary infant Hib conjugate vaccine series is completed, any licensed Hib conjugate vaccine may be administered as a booster dose at age 12–15 months.

[f] The second dose of MMR vaccine should be administered *either* at 4–6 years of age *or* at 11–12 years of age.

(Advisory Committee on Immunization Practices, American Academy of Pediatrics, and American Academy of Family Physicians.)

borne typhus in Bergen-Belsen concentration camp in February or March of 1945, only weeks before this death camp was liberated. It is easy to visualize the appalling conditions of crowding in cattle trucks and the total absence of facilities to preserve personal cleanliness that precipitated this deadly epidemic and killed so many innocent people. All uprooted and refugee populations are at risk of such person-to-person epidemic diseases when their personal hygiene cannot be maintained. Provision of facilities for maintenance of personal hygiene is an important part of refugee community health care.

Droplet spread is an important means for transmitting many infectious fevers of childhood. Coughing, sneezing, and even speaking lead to ejection from the mouth or nose of aerosol particles containing infectious microorganisms. These can enter the body of susceptible persons by being inhaled or ingested, lodging in the mucous membranes of the mouth, nose, or conjunctiva. Some infectious agents remain viable in desiccated droplets, micro-

BOX 3-2. Modes of Transmission of Infection

Person-to-person spread
Direct
    Sexually transmitted
    Other
Indirect
    Droplet spread
    Fomites
    Airborne desiccated droplets

Common vehicle spread
Water
Food and milk
Air
Biologic products (blood, serum, etc.)

Vectorborne
Biologic life cycle transfer
Passenger transfer

Zoonoses

Other (soil saprophytes, etc.)

scopic particles that remain suspended in the atmosphere or form part of the accumulated dust in households or public buildings, e.g., hospitals. Tuberculosis can be spread this way.

2. **Common vehicle spread** is the mode of transmission of many foodborne diseases and waterborne diseases and of infection transmitted in biologic products such as sera, vaccines, blood, and blood products. Air can also be a common vehicle for the spread of some organisms, e.g., the legionellae that cause legionnaires' disease.

From the viewpoint of the causative organism, common vehicle spread is an efficient means to ensure its survival and sometimes widespread dissemination. Typhoid can be widely spread by common vehicles such as polluted drinking water, milk, or improperly canned foods, perhaps consumed far from where they were prepared. An epidemic that caused many cases and some deaths in Aberdeen, Scotland, in 1964 was traced to a can of beef, contaminated via a tiny hole when the can was cooled in a river adjacent to the canning works after being packed in Argentina.

Waterborne diseases can affect very large numbers. In Milwaukee, in 1994, an outbreak of waterborne cryptosporidiosis caused over 403,000 people to become ill and led to deaths among the immunocompromised persons in the city. A similar outbreak occurred about the same time in Las Vegas.[13] In neither Milwaukee nor Las Vegas was the waterborne nature of the outbreak recognized for a time (not until after the epidemic ended in Las Vegas). Other waterborne outbreaks during the same reporting period in the United States were caused by *Campylobacter jejuni, Shigella sonnei,* and *S. flexneri,* non-O1 *Vibrio cholerae,* and *Salmonella typhimurium.* Fortunately, these other outbreaks affected only small numbers of people.

3. **Vectorborne spread** is transmission by a living organism, commonly an arthropod. Frequently the infectious microorganism undergoes part of its development in the insect vector, as with malaria and rickettsial diseases; in other instances, the vector is merely a means of transport for the infectious agent, as when houseflies transmit shigellae and other agents that cause gastrointestinal infections.

4. A fourth form of transmission is of infections that primarily affect animals but for which humans may be alternate hosts; these are called **zoonoses.** Examples include bubonic plague, rabies, brucellosis, and some parasitic worms.

5. Finally, there are some important diseases caused by invading microorganisms or their toxins that are not spread by any of the previous means. An example is tetanus, transmitted by the spores of *Clostridium tetani,* which can invade the body as a result of a laceration and which normally are saprophytic in soil, etc.

► SURVEILLANCE

Surveillance involves the collection, analysis, and dissemination of all data pertinent to the control of a disease. Reporting or notification of certain infectious diseases is one form of data collection, but there are others (Chap. 2).

Some communicable diseases are so dangerous that precise and timely information about their impact on populations is required. This information is provided by notification to the public health authorities of all cases as they occur. Table 3–2 lists the notifiable diseases in the United States, on which statistical summaries regularly appear in *Morbidity and Mortality Weekly Reports* (*MMWR*), published by the Centers for Disease Control and Prevention (CDC) and accessible on the Internet.

Complete notification is seldom achieved, except in the event of cases of rare and exotic diseases imported from another part of the world or of formerly commonplace but now rare conditions such as poliomyelitis or diphtheria. Most diagnosed active cases of pulmonary tuberculosis are also likely to be reported, as are most cases of STDs treated in public clinics or in juris-

TABLE 3–2.   Notifiable Diseases—Summary of Reported Cases, United States, 1993–1995

Disease	1993	1994	1995
Acquired immunodeficiency syndrome (AIDS)	103,533	78,279	71,547[a]
Amebiasis	2,970	2,983	[b]
Anthrax	—	—	—
Aseptic meningitis	12,848	8,932	[b]
Botulism, total (including wound and unsp.)	97	143	97
Foodborne	27	50	24
Infant	65	85	54
Brucellosis	120	119	98
Chancroid	1,399	773	606[c]
Chlamydia[d]			477,638[c]
Cholera	18	39	23
Diphtheria	—	2	—
Encephalitis, primary	919	717	[b]
Postinfectious	170	143	[b]
Escherichia coli O157:H7		1,420	2,139
Gonorrhea	439,673	418,068	392,848[c]
Granuloma inguinale	19	3	[b]
Haemophilus influenza, invasive	1,419	1,174	1,180
Hansen's disease (leprosy)	187	136	144
Hepatitis A	24,238	29,796	31,582
Hepatitis B	13,361	12,517	10,805
Hepatitis C/non-A, non-B[e]	4,786	4,470	4,576
Hepatitis, unspecified	627	444	[b]
Legionellosis	1,280	1,615	1,241
Leptospirosis	51	38	[b]
Lyme disease	8,257	13,043	11,700
Lymphogranuloma venereum	285	235	[b]
Malaria	1,411	1,229	1,419
Measles (rubeola)	312	963	281
Meningococcal disease	2,637	2,886	3,243
Mumps	1,692	1,537	906
Murine typhus fever	25		[b]
Pertussis (whooping cough)	6,586	4,617	5,137
Plague	10	17	9
Poliomyelitis, paralitic[f]	4	5	2
Psittacosis	60	38	64
Rabies, animal	9,377	8,147	7,811
Rabies, human	3	6	5
Rheumatic fever, acute	112	112	[b]

(continued)

TABLE 3–2. *(continued)*

Disease	1993	1994	1995
Rocky Mountain spotted fever	456	465	590
Rubella (German measles)	192	227	128
Rubella, congenital syndrome	5	7	6
Salmonellosis, excluding typhoid fever	41,641	43,323	45,970
Shigellosis	32,198	29,769	32,080
Syphilis, primary and secondary	26,498	20,627	16,500[c]
Total, all stages	101,259	81,696	68,953[c]
Tetanus	48	51	41
Toxic-shock syndrome	212	192	191
Trichinosis	16	32	29
Tuberculosis	25,313	24,361	22,860[g]
Tularemia	132	96	[b]
Typhoid fever	440	441	369
Varicella (chickenpox)[i]	134,722	151,219	120,624
Yellow fever	Last indigenous case reported in 1911; last imported case, 1924		

[a] The total number of AIDS cases includes all cases reported to the Division of HIV/AIDS Prevention, National Center for HIV, STD, and TB Prevention (NCHSTP) through December 31, 1995.
[b] No longer nationally notifiable.
[c] Cases were updated through the Division of Sexually Transmitted Diseases Prevention, NCHSTP, as of March 1, 1996.
[d] Chalmydia refers to genital infections caused by *C. trachomatis*.
[e] Anti-HCV antibody test available May 1990.
[f] Numbers may not reflect changes based on retrospective case evaluations or late reports (see MMWR 1986;35:180-2). Seven additional suspected cases of paralytic poliomyelitis were reported in 1995.
[g] Cases were updated through the Division of Tuberculosis Elimination, NCHSTP, as of May 29, 1996.
[h] Varicella was taken off the nationally notifiable disease list in 1991. Many states continue to report these cases to CDC.

dictions where positive laboratory test results as well as physicians' clinical diagnoses are reported in a routine mandatory procedure. The notification to authorities of some other diseases of public health importance, such as hepatitis A, is quite incomplete. In any event, notification of hepatitis A only provides partial information because subclinical or anicteric cases are usually missed. Seroepidemiology can reveal the true extent of community infection with hepatitis A virus.

Communicable disease surveillance serves several purposes. The most important is to facilitate control. A second purpose is to evaluate control programs. A third purpose is to learn more about emerging problems, as has been done by surveillance of HIV infection. Regular routine reports enable us to detect when an epidemic occurs. Reports of some diseases, e.g., epidemic influenza and paralytic poliomyelitis, are transmitted to WHO. One of the most valuable uses of the Internet is to allow instantaneous worldwide notification of infectious outbreaks of international public health importance.

▶ **GENERAL PRINCIPLES OF CONTROL**

The cycle of transmission of infectious diseases can be broken at several places (Box 3–3).

The infectious agent can be killed or inactivated or its reproduction can be inhibited. Infectious agents in food, water, or milk can be killed by heat sterilization, pasteurization, or cooking. Their reproduction can be inhibited by freezing or drying (although this does not necessarily kill pathogens). Infectious organisms that have invaded a human host who might transmit the infection can be rendered safe by killing the organisms with a specific antibiotic or chemotherapeutic agent; this procedure is called chemoprophylaxis. Simple isolation or quarantine of the infected person reduces or removes the possibility that the infection can be transmitted to others.

Without actually isolating people who may be capable of transmitting in-

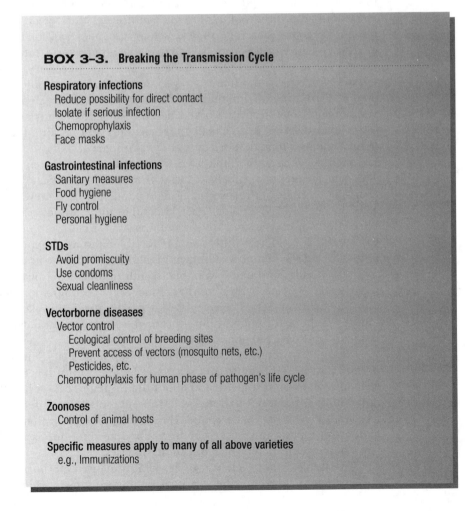

BOX 3–3. Breaking the Transmission Cycle

Respiratory infections
  Reduce possibility for direct contact
  Isolate if serious infection
  Chemoprophylaxis
  Face masks

Gastrointestinal infections
  Sanitary measures
  Food hygiene
  Fly control
  Personal hygiene

STDs
  Avoid promiscuity
  Use condoms
  Sexual cleanliness

Vectorborne diseases
  Vector control
    Ecological control of breeding sites
    Prevent access of vectors (mosquito nets, etc.)
    Pesticides, etc.
  Chemoprophylaxis for human phase of pathogen's life cycle

Zoonoses
  Control of animal hosts

Specific measures apply to many of all above varieties
  e.g., Immunizations

fection, it is possible to reduce the risk of transmission by imposing barriers between them and susceptible hosts. An example is the use of condoms to reduce the risk of transmission of gonorrhea and HIV disease. Face masks, as used by staff in hospital operating rooms and more widely by public officials and others in Japan and China, are alleged to help impede the transmission of pathogens, and modern types of properly fitted face masks may actually do this, but most conventional masks generally do not.

The resistance (immunity) of vulnerable hosts can be enhanced by immunizing them against many infectious agents of disease, as discussed previously. The eradication of smallpox made use of a different strategy, which was worked out in part using principles of theoretical epidemiology. This was the strategy of containment, suggested by Fred L. Soper[14] in 1949 and formally proposed to the World Health Assembly by the Soviet delegates in 1958. Smallpox was almost always a clinically unmistakable disease; if, therefore, all those in immediate contact with an identified case of smallpox were vaccinated before they could develop the disease, they would neither get it nor be able to transmit it to others, such as susceptibles in the neighborhood or district who had not been vaccinated—in other words, total coverage of the population by smallpox vaccination was not necessary. This strategy worked very well in the final stages of the smallpox eradication campaigns, despite disruptive civil and military disturbances in the affected areas, Eritrea and Somalia. This strategy worked because smallpox is not as infectious as some other diseases (e.g., chickenpox, measles) and because the incubation period is longer than that of other viral exanthemata.

It has been suggested that similar strategies and tactics could be used to eliminate measles and rubella, at least from the United States and Canada; complete coverage of the susceptible child population is, however, generally regarded as more likely to be efficacious, and as there are fewer dangerous adverse effects of measles and rubella immunization than there were with smallpox vaccination, there is little support for the alternative approach. Greater infectivity and shorter incubation periods also would militate against success.

WHO and some national public health authorities aspire to eradicate poliomyelitis, but probably a more realistic target is elimination, meaning reduction of the incidence below a level at which infection is likely to be transmitted to others; for poliomyelitis, this might occur with an incidence rate of less than 1 per 100,000 population.

Education about the risks of transmitting infectious agents plays an important part in reducing these risks. Food handlers must be educated about elementary personal hygiene and about the hygiene of food handling in order to minimize the risk that they will transmit food-borne infections to those for whom they are preparing food. Community-wide education, especially of mothers of infants and young children, is required to emphasize the importance of immunization against infectious diseases.

The transmission cycle can be broken in many vectorborne diseases by environmental control of the vectors. Draining swamps in which mosquitoes breed and reducing or eliminating other breeding places has played an important part in control of malaria and other mosquito-borne diseases such as yellow fever and filariasis. This is often combined with use of knock-down pesticide sprays inside houses to kill mosquitoes there, too.

This combination successfully eliminated malaria from some parts of the world where it was previously a serious public health problem. Unfortunately this method of control has broken down in regions where mosquitoes have been difficult to eradicate or have become resistant to pesticides. Other mosquito-borne diseases, Japanese B encephalitis and dengue, both transmitted by culicine mosquitoes, have been controlled in Singapore by a rigorous policy of eliminating breeding sites for mosquito larvae: Householders are heavily fined if breeding sites are found on their property. Few other places could sustain such a strict control program, and ecologic and environmental conditions rule out this approach in other regions such as Bangladesh.

It is more difficult to control the snail vectors of schistosomiasis by environmental or ecologic methods. In China, with abundant labor, some success has been achieved by cutting vertical walls on canals and ponds; the snails copulate at the water's edge on the sloping banks of ponds and canals and cannot find places to copulate when the banks are vertical. A similar strategy would not work with African schistosomiasis because of the snail vectors' different breeding habits.

General environmental measures, not specifically intended to improve health, did much to reduce mortality from some infectious diseases in the period from the early 19th to the mid-20th centuries in industrial nations. The reduction of tuberculosis, diphtheria, and other lethal respiratory infections of childhood and of gastrointestinal diseases such as typhoid, salmonella, and shigella infections is attributable to improved housing, better nutrition, and the provision of sanitary services and pure piped water supplies. The most spectacular declines in mortality from these diseases took place before significant advances in medical science that contributed to their control (Fig. 3–2). Future ecologic changes could increase the lethal impact of infectious diseases; for instance, if orderly social conditions and cleanliness are disrupted by wars or by the decay of essential public health infrastructure. This has happened, as noted earlier, in the former Soviet Union and could happen in some U.S. cities if tax revolts lead to decay of public health infrastructure.

▶ SPECIFIC INFECTIOUS DISEASES

The previously mentioned general principles can be illustrated by examples from important common infectious diseases. I will briefly discuss acute respiratory infections, tuberculosis, STDs, nosocomial infections, viral hepatitis, food poisoning, infectious diseases of children, malaria and other tropical vectorborne and parasitic diseases, and important emerging and reemerging diseases, notably HIV/AIDS. I will also mention the interaction of infections and changing regional ecology and human settlement patterns.

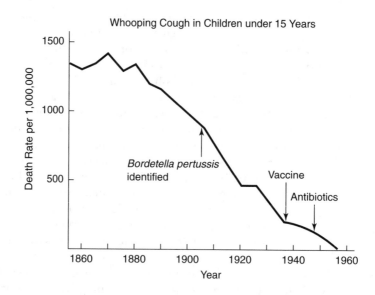

Figure 3–2. Mean annual death rates from whooping cough in England and Wales from 1860 to 1960. *(From Winikoff B:* Nutrition and National Policy. *Cambridge, MA: MIT Press, 1978, pp. 444–445.)*

Acute Respiratory Disease

This is the most difficult of all infections to control. It is caused by several kinds of viruses and by other organisms such as bacteria and mycoplasma. Some of these organisms readily mutate, altering their immunologic structure sufficiently to render susceptible even persons who have recently recovered from infection with closely similar organisms and who should therefore still have some immunity to it. Moreover, acquired immunity is often short-lived. Control is difficult because most people regard a cold as trivial, so they continue their usual activities and spread the infection.

Influenza is a more serious respiratory infection. The influenza virus more often penetrates deeply into the respiratory system, more often causes pneumonia or prepares the way for secondary bacterial pneumonia. Often there is a severe toxemia, especially among infants, the elderly, and those already in poor health from other causes. Several varieties of the influenza virus cause serious disease; these are mostly type A viruses. At least one influenza A virus type, perhaps more than one, occurs from time to time in pandemic form, sweeping across the world, causing many millions of cases and heavy mortality. The most recent pandemics were in 1919, 1957, and 1968, but epidemics of milder, less lethal strains of influenza affecting much of the world's population have occurred more often.[15] There has not been a worldwide influenza epidemic since 1968–69, though there have been both false alarms and several extensive epidemics. Many authorities believe that another pandemic is overdue. Table 3–3 lists the pandemic and epidemic outbreaks of influenza in recent history.

An effective vaccine against influenza can be prepared rapidly when an epidemic strain of the virus has been isolated. The logistics of immunizing large populations rapidly enough to prevent epidemic spread can be formidable. In the 1957 pandemic, few communities were able to deploy enough doses of vaccine in time. In 1976, the threat of an epidemic of pandemic proportions led the U.S. government to initiate a mass immunization campaign. The speedy development and distribution of the "swine influenza" vaccine were impressive. About 40 million doses were given; but no epidemic occurred, and some cases of Guillain-Barré syndrome (GBS) were attributed to the vaccine.[16] This episode was widely perceived as a fiasco, that could inhibit national action to control future epidemics. However, reappraisal of the evidence suggests that the number of cases of GBS was no greater among the immunized than the general population, i.e., that the cases of GBS were not attributable to the influenza vaccine.[17] Ultimately, the decision to launch a mass vaccination campaign is political rather than epidemiologic, so next time there is a credible threat of an epidemic or pandemic of influenza, epidemiologists and public health policy makers will have to weigh the evidence and political costs of action versus inaction very carefully.

Tuberculosis

Tuberculosis, the "Captain of all these men of death,"[18] the "white plague,"[19] cut a swath through several generations in the industrial world in the 18th and 19th centuries. It shortened the lives of millions, including many great writers and artists—John Keats, the Brontë sisters, Frederick Chopin, and

TABLE 3–3. Influenza Pandemics

1732–1733	Worldwide pandemic; overall death rate two to three times above usual levels in many European cities
1781–1782	Pandemic in Europe, North America, China, India; up to two-thirds of population affected, high mortality; may have started in China
1830–1833	Worldwide pandemic, affected half or more of population in many places; began in China
1847–1848	Widespread influenza epidemics in Europe, North and South America; probably started in Russia
1857–1858	Epidemics in North, Central, and South America, spread to Europe; probably started in Panama
1889–1890	"Asiatic influenza" pandemic, probably started in Russia, spread worldwide; very high attack rate, moderate to high mortality
1918–1919	The great pandemic of "Spanish" influenza; three waves; attack rate 20 to 40 percent, exceptionally high death rate among young adults; overall death rate about 0.5 percent in United States; total deaths worldwide estimated to be 15 to 25 million; first wave may have started in China
1957–1958	"Asian" influenza pandemic, began in Southeast Asia; high morbidity, moderate mortality
1968–1969	"Hong Kong" influenza; similar to 1957 "Asian," but lower mortality rate; first epidemic in which vaccines may have been efficacious

some of the characters they created; provided poignant opera plots: Who has watched *La Bohème* without tears? Wade Hampton Frost[20] analyzed mortality rates from tuberculosis and showed what appeared to be susceptible birth cohorts, followed by generations that were less vulnerable. The same phenomenon was observed in other countries. Probably the main factors responsible for the reduced impact of tuberculosis on generations born after the late 19th century were improved living conditions, better nutrition, housing, and education. Tuberculosis is not caused by the tubercle bacillus alone, but by a combination of the tubercle bacillus and poverty, overcrowding, ignorance, and poor nutrition, all of which declined in industrial countries from early in the 20th century. By the time effective antituberculosis drugs were developed in the 1950s, the epidemic was already waning; by the early 1960s it was over (Fig. 3–3).

A very different state of affairs has prevailed in almost all the rest of the world, notably in much of Africa, the Indian subcontinent, elsewhere in East and South Asia, and parts of Latin America. Tuberculosis never retreated in those regions. Moreover, in the 1990s it has reemerged in industrial nations among an urban underclass of homeless people and all over the world in immunocompromised populations afflicted with HIV/AIDS. It is now estimated to affect about 1.7 billion people, about a third of the world's population.[21] It will not be controlled until we eradicate its causes: poverty, overcrowding, ignorance, and poor nutrition. In an overcrowded world full of people who can barely eke out a living, of refugees and displaced, often malnourished

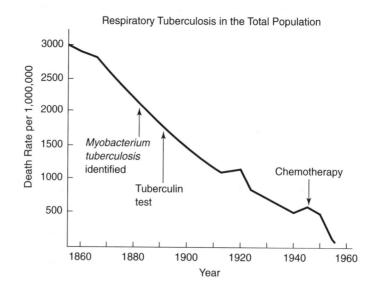

Figure 3–3. Mean annual death rates from tuberculosis in England and Wales from 1860 to 1960. *(From Winikoff B:* Nutrition and National Policy. *Cambridge, MA: MIT Press, 1978, pp. 444–445.)*

populations, of immunocompromised populations devastated by HIV/AIDS, it may be a long time before we succeed. HIV disease has confounded case-finding procedures too, because tuberculin skin tests do not work among the immunocompromised.

Sexually Transmitted Diseases (STDs)

At least 25 diseases can be transmitted by sexual contact, i.e., contact between mucosal surfaces of an infected person or carrier and mucosal surfaces of a susceptible person (Table 3–4). Numerically, the most important STDs are gonorrhea and chlamydia. Clinically, syphilis used to be the most important because of its prolonged course, devastating late effects on the nervous and cardiovascular systems, and its social stigma. However, *Treponema pallidum*, the cause of syphilis, is a delicate organism that is very sensitive to antibiotics, and these have for the most part successfully controlled syphilis. It remains refractory among promiscuous homosexual and heterosexual groups. Also, it has a synergistic relationship to HIV and occurs in a highly virulent and perhaps more easily transmissable form in the presence of HIV infection. Thus, after two decades of slipping into obscurity, it has again become a serious public health problem.

Gonorrhea is highly infectious. Control is difficult for several reasons. Sexual promiscuity is widespread, especially among young people; the use of the contraceptive pill increases the risk of transmission because there is no mechanical barrier to the gonococcus, as there is when a condom is used. Moreover, the vaginal mucosa may be more hospitable to the gonococcus when it is influenced by the hormonal changes produced by the pill. Finally, in women the symptoms and signs are often insignificant enough to escape notice. Gonorrhea has reached near pandemic proportions in many countries since the mid-1970s. Antibiotic-resistant organisms, particularly the penicillinase-producing *Neisseria gonorrhoeae* (PPNG), and patients who default from treatment and are reluctant to identify contacts add to the difficulty of control.

Sex education plays an important role in control, but there is resistance to this in some communities in the United States, on the grounds that it implies approval of promiscuous sexual behavior. But the evidence on the relationship between sex education and sexual behavior indicates precisely the opposite: that education about human sexuality and STDs reduces the prevalence of promiscuous sexual activity.[22]

Other important STDs include herpes, chlamydial infections, and non-gonococcal urethritis. The herpes II virus not only causes cutaneous herpes but may also cause cancer of the cervix.

The HIV epidemic may be having some impact on patterns of sexual activity. Media publicity—even without explicit details about unprotected sexual intercourse as the most important mode of transmission—has led to fear of AIDS, and this may act as a deterrent to sexual promiscuity; this could

TABLE 3–4. Sexually Transmitted Pathogens and the Diseases They Cause

Agent	Disease or Syndrome
Bacteria	
Neisseria gonorrhoeae	Urethritis, epididymitis, proctitis, cervicitis, endometritis, salpingitis, perihepatitis, bartholinitis, pharyngitis, conjunctivitis, prepubertal vaginitis, ?prostatitis, accessory gland infection, amniotic infection syndrome, disseminated gonococcal infection, chorioamnionitis, premature rupture of membranes, premature delivery
Chlamydia trachomatis	Urethritis, epididymitis, proctitis, cervicitis, endometritis, salpingitis, perihepatitis, bartholinitis, prepubertal vaginitis, otitis media in infants, inclusion conjunctivitis, infant pneumonia, trachoma, lymphogranuloma venereum, ?rhinitis, ?pharyngitis, ?chorioamnionitis, ?premature rupture of membranes, ?premature delivery
Mycoplasma hominis	Postpartum fever, ?salpingitis
Ureaplasma ureolyticum	?Nongonococcal urethritis, ?chorioamnionitis, ?premature delivery
Treponema pallidum	Syphilis
Gardnerella vaginalis	Bacterial ("nonspecific") vaginosis (in conjunction with *M. hominis* and vaginal anaerobes, such as *Mobiluncus* spp.)
Haemophilus ducreyi	Chancroids
Calymmatobacterium granulomatis	Donovanosis (granuloma inguinale)
Shigella spp.	Shigellosis in homosexual men
Campylobacter spp.	Enteritis, proctocolitis
Group B streptococcus	Neonatal sepsis, neonatal meningitis
Viruses	
Herpes simplex virus	Initial and recurrent genital herpes, aseptic meningitis, neonatal herpes, cervical dysplasia and carcinoma, ?vulvar carcinoma
Human papillomavirus	Condylomata acuminata, laryngeal papilloma, cervical intraepithelial neoplasia and carcinoma, vaginal carcinoma, anal carcinoma, vulvar carcinoma, penile carcinoma
Hepatitis B virus	Acute hepatitis B, chronic active hepatitis, persistent (unresolved) hepatitis, polyarteritis nodosa, chronic membranous glomerulonephritis, ?mixed cryoglobulinemia, ?polymyalgia rheumatica, hepatocellular carcinoma
Hepatitis A virus	Acute hepatitis A (anal–oral transmission)
Cytomegalovirus	Heterophil-negative infectious mononucleosis, congenital infection, gross birth defects and infant mortality, cognitive impairment (e.g., mental retardation, sensorineural deafness), ?cervicitis, protean manifestations in the immunosuppressed host
Molluscum contagiosum virus	Genital molluscum contagiosum
Human immunodeficiency virus (HIV)	AIDS
Human T-lymphotrophic retrovirus, type I	Adult T-cell leukemia/lymphoma
Protozoa	
Trichomonas vaginalis	Trichomonal vaginitis, ?salpingitis
Entamoeba histolytica	Amebiasis in homosexual men
Giardia lamblia	Giardiasis in homosexual men
Fungi	
Candida albicans	Vulvovaginitis, balanitis
Ectoparasites	
Phthirus pubis	Pubic lice infestation
Sarcoptes scabiei	Scabies

(From Cates W, Holmes K: Diseases transmitted from person to person. In Last JM (ed): Maxcy-Rosenau Public Health and Preventive Medicine, 12th ed. East Norwalk, CT: Appleton-Century-Crofts, 1986, p. 259.)

prove to be more effective than any previous forms of sex education in controlling STDs.

Nosocomial Infections

Until the late 19th century (before the era of antisepsis) hospital-acquired, or nosocomial, infections killed huge numbers of patients and made hospitals places to dread. Mortality was especially high among women after childbirth and among soldiers wounded in warfare. The connection between exposure to sepsis and childbed fever was made by Oliver Wendell Holmes in Boston in 1843 and by Ignaz Semmelweiss in Vienna in 1847. The antiseptic conduct of childbirth since that time has saved innumerable women from an untimely death. In the American Civil War, more than half of the approximately 1 million deaths were caused by infected wounds. The infections included streptococcal and staphylococcal septicemia, gas gangrene, and tetanus. By the time of World War II, vaccination against tetanus and gas gangrene eliminated these as causes of death from war wounds, and antibiotics reduced deaths from staphylococcal and streptococcal infections to insignificant levels.

But the problem of nosocomial infection has not been solved by the development of antisepsis, immunizations, and antibiotics. In the industrial nations, the nosocomial infection rate remains about 5 to 6 percent of all hospital patients; in the United States alone this means some 2 million infections annually, accounting for about 6 million excess days of hospital stay. About 1 percent of patients with nosocomial infections die as a result, and infection is a contributing cause of death for an additional 2 to 3 percent.[23] Nosocomial infection rates are probably higher in developing countries, but information is scanty.

Debilitated patients, patients with tissue devitalized by injury or operation, or patients who have an instrumental procedure on mucocutaneous tissue such as the urogenital tract are at high risk of nosocomial infection. The urinary tract is particularly vulnerable, accounting for about 40 percent of all nosocomial infections.

The organisms that commonly cause nosocomial infection have changed since the mid-1940s. Before antibiotics were developed, the largest proportion were streptococcal infections, but sulfonamides and penicillin effectively controlled these. In the 1950s and early 1960s, *Staphylococcus aureus* predominated, replaced by gram-negative organisms, notably *Escherichia coli, Proteus,* and *Pseudomonas* species in the late 1960s. Infections with yeasts and other spores have become commoner. These changes reflect the influence of increasingly powerful broad-spectrum antibiotics on the ecology of microflora in the gut and elsewhere in the human body. In the 1990s there has been a resurgence of virulent antibiotic-resistant streptococcal infection, including the so-called flesh-eating strep (a widespread necrotizing infection); although uncommon, this is dramatic and has drawn public attention to the problem of nosocomial (and other) routes of infection with these organisms.

The principal methods of spread of nosocomial infections are by direct contact and contaminated vehicles, including surgical instruments. Endoscopic procedures carry a high risk. Control is best achieved when the problem has been recognized and the hospital establishes an infection control committee with experts who investigate every recognized case of nosocomial infection. A combination of environmental measures and staff education helps to reduce the likelihood of similar occurrences in the future. Good hospital housekeeping, the use of disposable equipment, and centralized sterilizing services where disposable equipment is impracticable are all important measures contributing to control.

Food Poisoning

Contamination of food with bacteria or their toxins has always been common; most of us experience episodes of vomiting or diarrhea attributable to "food poisoning" from time to time. In the past this not infrequently caused death of infants, children, debilitated adults, and the frail elderly, and sometimes it still does. Outbreaks are occasionally due to chemical rather than bacterial poisoning; the epidemiologic features are similar whatever the cause. Episodes of food poisoning can be serious in modern urban societies, if food production or processing are highly centralized and contamination occurs at any stage between production and consumption. Chemical poisons that cause insidious onset of symptoms and signs are especially dangerous. A dramatic episode was traced to a batch of cooking oil in Spain in 1980.[24] The onset of symptoms was gradual and delayed, in some cases for weeks or even months after ingestion, and symptoms were unusual, affecting the respiratory and nervous systems, the liver, and the kidneys; there was a high mortality rate, but despite repeated, painstaking investigations the nature of the contaminant that caused the poisoning remains obscure.

Under everyday domestic circumstances, only small numbers are usually affected when there is a break in security against contamination during the preparation, processing, cooking, storage, or serving of foods. The resulting food poisoning may be due to bacteria (e.g., salmonella, shigella), bacterial toxins (e.g., staphylococcal enterotoxin—the commonest and best-known form of food poisoning), or viral, parasitic, or fungal organisms or their toxic products, or it may be chemical in origin (Table 3–5).

Some kinds of food poisoning have unmistakable symptoms and signs that make identification clinically easy. Staphylococcal food poisoning has an explosive onset within a few hours of ingesting staphylococcal enterotoxin; vomiting and prostration, sometimes with diarrhea, and without fever usually clinches the diagnosis. Many people can be affected at the same time, putting great strain on limited toilet facilities. One notorious outbreak affected almost all the passengers and most of the crew on a fully loaded widebody jet passenger airplane about halfway across the Pacific Ocean between

TABLE 3–5. Varieties of Food Poisoning

Disease	Etiologic Agent and Source	Incubation or Latency Period	Signs and Symptoms	Foods Involved
Staphylococcal in-toxication	Exoenterotoxins A, B, C, D, and E of *Staphylococcus aureus.* Staphylococci from noses, skin, and lesions of infected humans and animals	1–8 hr, mean 2–4 hr	Nausea, vomiting, retching, abdominal pain, diarrhea, prostration	Ham, meat, and poultry products, cream-filled pastry, food mixtures, leftover foods
Beta-hemolytic streptococcal infections	*Streptococcus pyogenes* from throat and lesions of infected humans	1–3 days	Sore throat, fever, nausea, vomiting, rhinorrhea, sometimes a rash	Raw milk, foods containing eggs
Bacillus cereus gastroenteritis	Exoenterotoxin of *B. cereus,* organism in soil	8–16 hr: rare reports of 2–4 hr	Nausea, abdominal pain, diarrhea; some reports of vomiting	Cereal products, rice, custards and sauces, meatloaf
Clostridium perfringens gastroenteritis	Endoenterotoxin formed during sporulation of *C. perfringens* in intestines. Organism in feces of infected humans, other animals, and in soil	8–22 hr, mean 10 hr	Abdominal pain, diarrhea	Cooked meat, poultry, gravy, sauces, and soups
Botulism	Exoneurotoxins A, B, E, and F of *Clostridium botulinum.* Spores found in soil and animal intestines	2 hr–8 days, mean 18–36 hr	Vertigo; double or blurred vision; dryness of mouth; difficulty in swallowing, speaking, and breathing; descending paresis; constipation; pupils dilated or fixed; respiratory paralysis. Gastrointestinal symptoms may precede neurologic symptoms. Frequently fatal	Home-canned low-acid foods, vacuum-packed fish, fermented fish eggs, fish, and marine mammals
Salmonellosis	Various serotypes of salmonella from feces of infected humans and animals	6–72 hr, mean 18–36 hr	Abdominal pain, diarrhea, chills, fever, nausea, vomiting, malaise	Poultry, meat and their products, egg products, other contaminated foods

(continued)

TABLE 3–5. *(continued)*

Disease	Etiologic Agent and Source	Incubation or Latency Period	Signs and Symptoms	Foods Involved
Vibrio parahaemolyticus gastroenteritis	*V. parahaemolyticus* from seawater or seafoods	2–48 hr, mean 12 hr	Abdominal pain, diarrhea, nausea, vomiting, fever, chills, headache	Raw seafoods, shellfish
Campylobacter gastroenteritis	*Campylobacter jejuni* from feces of domestic and wild animals and birds	2–10 days, mean 3–5 days	Diarrhea, abdominal pain, fever, nausea, vomiting	Unpasteurized milk, water, and various foods
Hepatitis A (infectious hepatitis)	Hepatitis A virus from feces, urine, blood of infected humans and other primates	10–50 days, mean 25 days	Fever, malaise, lassitude, anorexia, nausea, abdominal pain, jaundice	Shellfish, any food contaminated by hepatitis viruses, water
Trichinosis	*Trichinella spiralis* (roundworm) from flesh of infested swine, bear	2–28 days; mean 9 days	Gastroenteritis, fever, edema about eyes, muscular pain, chills, prostration, labored breathing	Pork, bear meat, walrus flesh
Scombroid poisoning	Histamine-like substance produced by *Proteus* spp. or other bacteria from histidine in fish flesh	Few minutes to 1 hr	Headache, dizziness, nausea, vomiting, peppery taste, burning throat, facial swelling and flushing, stomach pain, pruritus	Tuna, mackerel, Pacific dolphin
Chinese restaurant syndrome	Monosodium glutamate (MSG)	Few minutes to 1 hr	Burning sensation in neck, forearms, chest, tingling, flushing, dizziness, headache, nausea	Chinese food
Hemorrhagic[a] colitis	*Escherichia coli* O157:H7	2–9 days	Severe abdominal cramps, bloody diarrhea, nausea, vomiting, fever	Uncooked meats; most isolation from hamburger chain stores
Chemical food poisoning	Varies	Minutes to weeks, depending on agent	Varies: gastrointestinal, central nervous system, renal, etc.	Almost any food

[a] First reporting in 1982 in Canada and United States.
(Adapted from White FMM, Sweet L: Human Salmonellosis: Principles of Investigation and Control, Halifax, NS: Dalhousie University Press, 1985.)

Japan and the United States; fortunately one of the pilots remained well, having followed the rules and eaten different foods from everyone else.

Investigation of an outbreak of food poisoning is a common and important epidemiologic procedure. Table 3–6 shows the data from a typical outbreak, indicating how careful inquiry both among those who become ill and those who do not can help to identify the food that was the vehicle for the transmission of staphylococcal enterotoxin. In other forms of food poisoning, similar methods of investigation are used, but it can be difficult to trace the origin of the outbreak, especially when the incubation period is long and the affected individuals have scattered and have had time to forget details of what they had recently eaten. It is then difficult to obtain facts to calculate attack rates in relation to food items, a necessary prerequisite to identifying the origin of the outbreak.

Infectious Diseases of Children

Up to half the children ever born used to die before their fifth birthday, killed by measles, diphtheria, whooping cough, tracheobronchitis and croup, or infectious diarrhea, often when already weakened by malnutrition (see Chap. 5).

Since the late 19th century, mortality from these diseases has sharply de-

TABLE 3–6. Differences in Food-Specific Attack Rates in an Outbreak of Food-Borne Illness (Staphylococcal Enterotoxin in Barbecued Chicken)

Food	Persons Who Ate Specified Food				Persons Who Did Not Eat Specified Food				Difference in Attack Rates
	Ill	*Well*	*Total*	*Attack Rate (%)*	*Ill*	*Well*	*Total*	*Attack Rate (%)*	
Shrimp salad	8	4	12	67	15	21	36	42	+25
Olives	19	13	32	59	5	13	18	28	+31
Fried chicken	10	33	43	23	4	2	6	67	−44
Barbecued chicken	17	1	18	94	3	27	30	10	+84
Baked beans	12	13	25	48	12	10	22	55	−7
Potato salad	17	20	37	46	8	6	14	57	−11
Macaroni salad	9	15	24	38	15	10	25	60	−22
Root beer	23	23	46	50	0	2	2	0	+50
Bread	8	9	17	47	18	13	31	58	−11
Neapolitan cream pie	1	2	3	33	21	21	42	50	−17

(From Werner SB: Food poisoning. In Last JM (ed): Maxcy-Rosenthau Public Health and Preventive Medicine. 12th ed. E. Norwalk, CT: Appleton-Century-Crofts, 1986, p. 313.)

clined, to vanishing point in many rich industrial countries. An important reason has been ecologic changes associated with better living conditions, smaller family size (reducing infants' exposure to infections introduced into the household by older siblings), and improved nutritional status, which enhances resistance to infection. Childhood infectious diseases have been eliminated or further reduced by specific vaccines. Improved child health has enhanced national wealth. The economic drain of childhood sickness and premature death has disappeared, and the larger numbers living into healthy adult life have added to the labor force many millions who would in earlier generations not have been there.

Social, economic, and demographic changes since World War II have created new ecologic conditions favoring the spread of other infections among infants and young children. Rising proportions of single-parent families and families in which both parents are working have led to a considerable increase in the numbers of infants placed in day-care centers while their parents are working. By the mid-1970s, about 28 million children in the United States were taking part to some extent in day care, and 11 million spent more than 10 hours weekly in day-care centers.[25] The proportions are higher in many other countries. In China, day care is almost universal. Day-care centers are an excellent setting for the propagation of many kinds of infection: Respiratory infections; diseases transmitted by the fecal–oral route, including infectious diarrhea, hepatitis A, and giardiasis; skin infections such as impetigo, scabies, and head lice all occur. Transmission of many of these infections is likely because infants lack understanding of and training in elementary personal hygiene; the younger infants in day-care centers are not yet toilet-trained; most infants and young children are naturally affectionate and like to touch, hug, and kiss one another; and finally, staff in day-care centers often lack instruction in infection control. Rather similar problems of infection control occur in certain other institutional settings, notably mental hospitals and homes for the aged. Cytomegalovirus (CMV) and other previously uncommon infections have proliferated in day-care centers, reflecting changed work patterns (single-parent working mother, or both parents working). Breastfeeding plays a role, too, as CMV is excreted in milk.[26]

In developing countries about 12 million children still die every year from infectious diseases of childhood. Acute respiratory and gastrointestinal diseases kill about 4 million each. Measles is the most lethal vaccine-preventable disease, especially when combined with malnutrition (Chap. 5). Reduction and eventually elimination of measles is a target of the WHO Expanded Programme on Immunization. Because measles is common in developing countries, it is necessary to continue immunization programs in industrial nations where the disease has been reduced close to vanishing point. If we stop vaccinating infants and children in the United States and Canada when measles has been virtually eliminated from these nations, it could be reintroduced from the developing world, perhaps after herd immunity has declined and a generation of virgin susceptibles has grown up. This could be a scenario for disaster: History could repeat itself, even to the high mortality rates experienced by the aboriginal inhabitants of North America when measles was introduced by the European colonists several hundred years ago and had a mortality rate of up to 40 percent. Yet measles vaccination is not without adverse effects, so public health officials, family physicians, and pediatricians will face difficult choices when measles has been eliminated from nations like the United States, Canada, and the European Union (see Chap. 10).

Viral Hepatitis

Considerable progress has been made since the mid-1980s in identifying varieties of viral hepatitis. By late 1996, alphabetized varieties up to hepatitis g had been identified, but epidemiologic details not yet clarified. In the 1940s, hepatitis A ("infectious hepatitis") was differentiated from hepatitis B ("serum hepatitis"). Both are due to viruses, known as HAV and HBV, but hepatitis A has the epidemiologic features of fecal–oral transmission, whereas hepatitis B is blood-borne, transmitted by inadequately sterilized needles or in human blood or serum products, e.g., a batch of yellow fever vaccine. There is no cross-immunity. The incubation period of HAV is about 4 weeks, and that of HBV is 8 to 12 weeks.

Immunologic and molecular techniques have clarified the nature of hepatitis and made precise diagnosis possible. Development of immunoassay after the discovery of Australia antigen (HBsAg) allowed the detection of persons who were antibody-positive. Epidemiologic studies confirmed the pattern of spread of HBV by blood or other body fluids and as an STD among male homosexuals, a pattern later found also with HIV disease. HBV occurs in saliva, semen, and breast milk as well as blood. Maternal–fetal transmission also occurs. HBV is widely distributed in many developing countries, notably in Africa, East, Southeast, and South Asia, and has been associated with posthepatitis cirrhosis and with primary hepatocellular cancer. The high incidence of HBV in heavily populated areas of Asia and Africa explains the fact that primary hepatocellular cancer is the commonest cause of cancer death in these regions.

Genetic engineering techniques have reduced the cost of HBV vaccine; it is now advocated as a desirable if not essential routine immunization. It is desirable because the incidence of HBV, formerly low in industrial nations, is rising. Those at risk include all who receive transfusions of unscreened blood or blood products, and health care workers who come into contact with blood and blood products. In the United States, routine screening for HBsAg has been practiced by blood banks since the mid-1970s, and this has virtually eliminated HBV transmission via transfused blood. Transmission among illicit intravenous drug users by way of shared syringes and needles is still common.

Hepatitis C (HCV), formerly known as non-A non-B hepatitis, was differentiated as a parenterally transmitted hepatitis virus in 1989; it has an incubation period of 2 to 26 weeks, and infected persons may remain infective for life. It can be serious, even fatal. Like HBV, it is transmitted by contaminated blood and blood products and it has been a serious disease for hemophiliacs and others who received multiple transfusions of infected blood. The risk of transmission has declined since development of a test for HCV antibody and screening of blood and blood products.

Delta hepatitis is a parenterally transmitted virus, HDV, coated with HBsAg but with immunologically distinct internal antigen, thought to be transmitted similarly to, and sometimes with, HBV.

Hepatitis E virus is transmitted by the fecal–oral route, resembles HAV, and has a similar course and prognosis, except in pregnant women who have a case-fatality rate of up to 20 percent.

Tropical Infectious Diseases

Several important diseases of hot tropical countries have in common the feature of transmission dependent on vectors or passage through intermediate hosts, and their control may be easier to achieve by removing or reducing the vectors or intermediate hosts than by attacking the disease directly in the human population. Table 3–7 summarizes the host–parasite relationships of these diseases. I will not discuss parasitic worms; readers can refer to CCDM or sources cited at the end of this chapter.

Malaria

If a single disease could be said to have had the greatest impact on human well-being, this distinction belongs to malaria. It is out of control in much of Africa, where it causes more than a million deaths annually, barely controlled in parts of Asia and the tropical regions of the Americas, and is more difficult than ever to control because mosquitoes are increasingly resistant to pesticides and malaria parasites are increasingly resistant to antimalarials. Malaria has been the principal scourge of mankind in tropical regions and many damp, temperate zones since the beginning of recorded history. It contributed to the decline of the Roman Empire and may have been responsible for the collapse of civilizations in Southeast Asia and Central America. Until early in the 20th century, control measures did not exist because the nature of the disease was not understood. Cinchona bark, which contains quinine, has been known empirically since medieval times to relieve the symptoms of malaria and it can be lifesaving. Chloroquine, widely used in malaria prophylaxis, has chemical affinities with quinine; unfortunately, many varieties of malaria parasites have become resistant to chloroquine and to other antimalarials such as sulfadoxine and pyrimethamine (Fansidar).

Beginning in 1880 with Laveran's observation of malaria parasites in red blood corpuscles, the other essential features were worked out, culminating

TABLE 3-7. Features of Some Vectorborne Tropical Diseases

Disease	Vector	Control Measures
Malaria	Mosquito	Ecologic control often feasible Larvae, mosquito control Chemotherapy (chloroquine, etc.)
Schistosomiasis	Freshwater snails	Ecologic control difficult Molluscicides Chemotherapy not very effective
African trypanosomiasis (sleeping sickness)	Tsetse fly	Ecologic control very difficult— destroy fly habitat Education Chemotherapy[a]
Onchocerciasis (river blindness)	Blackfly (*Simulium*)	Ecologic control very difficult Protective clothing, repellants Larvicidal sprays Chemotherapy[a]
Chagas' disease	Cone-nose bugs	Residual insecticides; repair infested dwellings Chemotherapy[a]
Leishmaniasis	Sandflies (often mammalian host)	Ecologic measures vary Destroy sandfly habitat Control animal hosts Chemotherapy for human cases

[a]Chemotherapy is for treatment in selected cases, not for prophylaxis.

in the identification in 1897–98 by Ross and Grassi of the anopheline mosquito as the specific and only insect vector.

The causative organism, a protozoon, *Plasmodium,* passes the sexual phase of its life cycle in anopheline mosquitoes and an asexual phase in human liver and blood (Fig. 3–4).

Control requires reduction or preferably elimination of mosquitoes, or at least their removal from close contact with humans. This is best achieved where possible by ecologic approaches, i.e., elimination of mosquito breeding places, by draining swamps and careful management of other bodies of water in which mosquitoes can breed. Larvicides and oils to reduce surface tension of water so larvae cannot float and breathe are effective methods, but they cannot always be applied because the terrain or the ecology of local varieties of mosquitoes make these methods ineffective. Insecticidal sprays that kill adult mosquitoes are the next line of attack. Education aimed at reducing exposure to mosquito bites by the use of repellants, miminizing exposed skin surfaces, and mosquito nets are other important control measures.

Plasmodia can be directly attacked in the human host by antimalarial drugs. Chloroquine can be taken as a prophylactic measure in malarial areas. When there is evidence of chloroqine resistance, the preferred alternative is

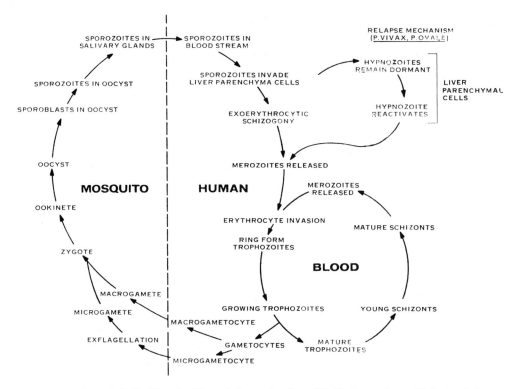

Figure 3–4. The life cycle of the malaria parasite. *(From Chin W. Diseases transmitted primarily by arthropod vectors—parasitic infections: Malaria. In Last JM (ed):* Maxcy-Rosenau Public Health and Preventive Medicine. *12th ed. E. Norwalk, CT: Appleton-Century-Crofts, 1986, p. 362.)*

sulfadoxine and pyrimethamine (Fansidar), but this can have severe side effects and the malaria parasite can develop resistance to this also. People who live permanently in malarial areas commonly get malaria and, if they recover, develop some immunity to reinfection. This observation raises the possibility that some form of artificial immunization might be developed, and research on this is an important aspect of the WHO/World Bank Tropical Disease Research Program. There is hope that early in the 21st century an efficaceous vaccine may be developed.

Other vectorborne diseases of great importance in tropical countries include schistosomiasis, in which freshwater snails are the intermediate hosts; onchocerciasis (river blindness) for which blackflies are the intermediate host; and trypanosomiasis (sleeping sickness), transmitted by the tsetste fly in much of the African savannah. This affects cattle, so it has considerable economic importance. The terrain, the economy, and the ecology of the intermediate hosts make control of these diseases generally more difficult than the control of malaria by ecologic means.

► **EMERGING AND REEMERGENT COMMUNICABLE DISEASES**

There are many millions of species of microorganisms. Most are unclassified, unnamed, and have never been studied. They could include myriads that have never encountered humans. As we have proliferated and spread to regions such as tropical rain forests that until recently were virtually uninhabited, it is hardly surprising that from time to time we encounter "new" species of microorganisms that can infect and kill us.

Several infectious diseases that have been recognized in the last two decades (whether really new or merely newly identified) illustrate vividly the unending challenges of communicable disease control. Some customs of modern society and some environmental changes have played a part in the emergence of several of these diseases as well as in the reemergence or appearance in new regions of old diseases. Table 3–8 is a list of some new ones, with the years in which they were identified. I will discuss a few that illustrate some of the challenges of communicable disease control.

TABLE 3–8. "New" and emerging infections

Year	Agent	Type	Disease, etc.
1973	Rotavirus	Virus	Infant diarrhea
1975	Parvovirus B19	Virus	Aplastic crisis in hemolytic anemia
1976	*Cryptosporidium*	Parasite	Acute or chronic diarrhea
1977	Ebola virus	Virus	Hemorrhagic fever
	Legionella	Bacterium	Legionnaires' disease
	Hantaan virus	Virus	Hemorrhagic fever and nephritis
	Campylobacter jejuni	Bacterium	Enteritis
1980	HTLV-1	Virus	T-cell leukemia and lymphoma
1981	Toxic staphylococcus	Bacterium	Toxic shock syndrome
1982	*Escherichia coli* O157:H7	Bacterium	Hemorrhagic colitis
	HTLV-2	Virus	Hairy-cell leukemia
	Borrelia burgdorferi	Bacterium	Lyme disease
1983	HIV	Virus	AIDS
	Helicobacter pylori	Bacterium	Peptic ulcer, gastrointestinal cancer
1986	*Cyclospora*	Parasite	Diarrhea
	BSE agent	Prion	Spongiform encephalopathy
1988	Herpesvirus 6	Virus	Exanthematous eruption
	Hepatitis E	Virus	Hepatitis
1989	Hepatitis C	Virus	Hepatitis
1991	Guanarito virus	Virus	Venezualan hemorrhagic fever
1992	*Bartonella henselae*	Bacterium	Cat-scratch disease
1993	Sin Nombre virus	Virus	Hantavirus pulmonary syndrome

AIDS = acquired immunodeficiency syndrome; BSE = bovine spongiform encephalopathy; HIV = human immunodeficiency virus; HTLV = human T-cell lymphotrophic virus.

Cholera is not a new disease of course; but new virulent strains of the cholera vibrio emerge from time to time, most recently in 1992 when a new strain of *Vibrio cholerae O139* was identified; it caused severe epidemics in Bangladesh and India. Severe epidemics have occurred in Central and South America in association with oscillations of the tropical Pacific current El Niño that led to blue-green algal blooms[27]: The cholera vibrio survives and breeds for lengthy periods in blue-green algae, which flourish in the warmer seas caused by El Niño oscillation. This epidemic in Peru, Ecuador, and Colombia caused nearly half a million cases and many thousands of deaths in 1990–92.

Toxic shock syndrome is not due to a recently discovered pathogen. This overwhelming staphylococcal septicemia–toxemia occurs most often among women who use absorbant vaginal tampons and keep them in for prolonged periods. In the early 1980s there was an "epidemic" of toxic shock syndrome associated with a new variety of absorbant vaginal tampon that the manufacturers advertised as suitable for working women to wear for 24 hours or more.[28] Prolonged stasis of menstrual fluid encouraged growth of toxin-producing staphylococci and sometimes streptococci.

Legionnaires' disease, a refractory, sometimes fatal variety of pneumonia, is a common vehicle infection in which the common vehicle is often moist air from air-conditioning systems.[29] The causative organism is the elusive gram-negative *Legionella pneumophila,*[30] discovered in 1977 after an epidemic among members of the American Legion who had attended a convention in a famous old hotel in Philadelphia. Another favored setting is the warm, moist environment of Turkish baths; some outbreaks have occurred in overheated hospitals.

Hemorrhagic dengue is occurring in worrying numbers in Mexico and the southern United States, following the arrival of a new and hardy species of urban culicine mosquito, *Aedes albopictus.* This migrated to the Americas from the Philippines in larval stage in pools of water in a shipment of used automobile tires imported for retreading—illustrating how international trade can lead to sudden change in the balance between humans and our microbial enemies.

Other communicable diseases have emerged or reemerged as a result of regional ecologic changes or because animal species that harbor dangerous pathogens have entered a new environment. Examples are Marburg disease and Ebola virus disease, which are caused by structurally unusual filamentous filoviruses.

Ebola virus disease, a highly lethal hemorrhagic fever of primates and humans, may be associated with changes in jungle ecosystems in equatorial Africa that have exposed significant numbers of people to an exotic pathogen species, although its epidemiology has not been worked out in detail. In 1989 there was an outbreak on the outskirts of Washington, D.C., in a colony of monkeys imported from the Philippines for medical research.[31] Fortunately, that strain of Ebola virus did not infect humans; if it had, there could have been a catastrophic epidemic in the nation's capital. There have been several sporadic cases and small outbreaks in Africa. In 1995 there was an epidemic in Zaire, with 316 cases and 245 deaths.[32] The reservoir for Ebola virus and its mode of transmission in nature remain unknown as of 1996.

Hantavirus pulmonary syndrome has emerged as a serious and highly lethal threat in the American West, where deer mice are carriers; with subtle shifts in climate and local ecosystems the likelihood of human infection has sharply increased in recent years. These and other emerging infectious diseases associated with climatic and ecologic changes have been reviewed in several recent articles[33] and other publications.[34]

► HIV/AIDS

The first cases of a disease characterized by opportunistic infections, such as *Pneumocystis carinii* pneumonia, immunodeficiency, and Kaposi's sarcoma, in young homosexual men were identified in Los Angeles in 1981[35]; in retrospect, cases dating back to the 1970s, perhaps earlier, were added. The features of the new disease were soon clarified. After the first case report, the number of cases increased sharply each year. At first, in industrial nations, male cases outnumbered female by about 16 to 1, reflecting the mode of transmission in the gay community; in Africa, the sex ratio has always been about equal, reflecting heterosexual transmission.

From the first report to clarification of AIDS epidemiology, identification of the causal organism, and development of serologic tests to detect HIV infection, progress was remarkably rapid, demonstrating the power of immunologic, molecular microbiologic, and epidemiologic methods. The HIV was identified by Luc Montagnier and others at the Pasteur Institute in Paris in 1983.[36] By 1985, there were reliable immunologic diagnostic tests and a screening test for HIV antibody.

In North American and European cases, the epidemiology at first resembled that of hepatitis B: The high-risk groups were male homosexuals who engaged in anal-receptive intercourse, illicit intravenous drug users, and persons such as hemophiliacs who received multiple blood transfusions. Health care workers known to have been accidentally exposed by needle stick have converted to HIV-positive, usually with a brief prodromal illness within weeks of infection. However, the risk of infection by accidental needle stick is relatively small, about 3 to 4 per 1000 episodes of needle stick.[37] As of December 1993, 128 definite and 113 probable cases of occupationally contracted HIV are known to have progressed to AIDS among health workers, mainly physicians and nurses.

Several cohorts of HIV-infected men have been followed long enough to suggest that the time from initial infection to frank AIDS can range from 3 to 20 years. Once AIDS develops, the course is usually rapid and inexorable; the mortality rate is virtually 100% and there is no effective treatment. The initial occurrence among promiscuous male homosexuals and illicit intravenous drug users led at first to considerable associated stigma. The grave prognosis caused AIDS to acquire an image of horror and dread not seen since the medieval epidemics of the Black Death, and as was the case then, initial societal and political reactions reflected fear and ignorance more than a rational response. HIV/AIDS is generally regarded as the gravest public health problem of the late 20th century. In the mid-1990s it generates tens of thousands of medical journal articles and popular press stories and hundreds of books every year, including frequent exhaustive accounts of the global HIV/AIDS situation. By January 1996, there were an estimated 30 million cases of HIV infection and over 9 million deaths worldwide.[38] By 2000, the world total of HIV infection is expected to exceed 40 million with 13 to 14 million deaths. In African urban centers the HIV seroprevalence rate among pregnant women in the early 1990s was 25 to 30 percent in Kigali, Rwanda; Kampala, Uganda; Lusaka, Zambia; and Blantyre, Malawi. In all cities the rate shot up very rapidly once infection was introduced; among sex workers, HIV seroprevalence rates of over 80 percent have been recorded in Ivory Coast and Kenya; elsewhere in Africa, the rates among pregnant women and sex workers are not quite so high but often exceed 50 percent. After a slow start, HIV disease soon became firmly established in India, Thailand, Burma, China, and other Asian and Pacific Rim countries. It has spread equally rapidly into Latin America and the Caribbean nations. It is associated everywhere with promiscuous sexual activity, sex tourism, and intravenous drug abuse. WHO's estimate of 40 million cases by 2000 could be low (Tables 3–9, 3–10, and 3–11).

TABLE 3–9.   Cumulative HIV Infections as of January 1, 1996, by Geographic Area of Affinity (GAA)[a]

GAA	Adults	Men	Women	Children[b]	Total
1 North America	1,269,000	1,087,000	181,000	18,000	1,286,000
2 Western Europe	829,000	691,000	138,000	9000	838,000
3 Oceania	31,000	28,000	3000	<1000	32,000
4 Latin America	1,477,000	1,182,000	295,000	79,000	1,556,000
5 Sub-Saharan Africa	16,550,000	7,881,000	8,670,000	2,672,000	19,222,000
6 Caribbean	467,000	280,000	187,000	36,000	503,000
7 Eastern Europe	37,000	34,000	3000	<1000	38,000
8 Southeast Mediterranean	76,000	63,000	13,000	<1000	77,000
9 Northeast Asia	179,000	149,000	30,000	2000	181,000
10 Southeast Asia	6,535,000	4,356,000	2,178,000	380,000	6,915,000
Total world	27,449,000	15,751,000	11,699,000	3,198,000	30,647,000

[a] Columns and rows may fail to sum because of rounding to the nearest 1000.
[b] HIV infection acquired before or at birth.
AIDS in the World II *survey.*

TABLE 3–10. Cumulative AIDS Cases as of January 1, 1996[a]

GAA	Adults	Men	Women	Children[b]	Total
1 North America[c]	443,000	380,000	63,000	7000	449,000
2 Western Europe	193,000	161,000	32,000	3000	195,000
3 Oceania	9000	8000	1000	<1000	9000
4 Latin America	518,000	414,000	104,000	62,000	579,000
5 Sub-Saharan Africa	6,367,000	3,032,000	3,335,000	2,046,000	8,413,000
6 Caribbean	133,000	80,000	53,000	27,000	160,000
7 Eastern Europe	7000	7000	<1000	<1000	7000
8 Southeast Mediterranean	12,000	10,000	2000	<1000	12,000
9 Northeast Asia	12,000	10,000	2000	<1000	12,000
10 Southeast Asia	332,000	221,000	111,000	206,000	537,000
Total world	8,024,000	4,321,000	3,703,000	2,351,000	10,375,000

[a] Columns and rows may fail to sum due to rounding to the nearest 1000.
[b] HIV infection acquired before or at birth.
[c] AIDS cases in North America have been estimated on the basis of the 1987 revised CDC AIDS surveillance case definition.
AIDS in the World II *survey.*

TABLE 3–11. Cumulative AIDS Deaths as of January 1, 1996, by Geographic Area of Affinity (GAA)[a]

GAA	Adults	Men	Women	Children[b]	Total
1 North America[c]	352,000	302,000	50,000	6000	358,000
2 Western Europe	141,000	118,000	24,000	2000	144,000
3 Oceania	7000	6000	<1000	<1000	7000
4 Latin America	458,000	366,000	92,000	60,000	518,000
5 Sub-Saharan Africa	5,611,000	2,672,000	2,939,000	1,999,000	7,610,000
6 Caribbean	115,000	69,000	46,000	27,000	141,000
7 Eastern Europe	5000	5000	<1000	<1000	5000
8 Southeast Mediterranean	7000	6000	1000	<1000	8000
9 Northeast Asia	6000	5000	1000	<1000	6000
10 Southeast Asia	231,000	154,000	77,000	194,000	425,000
Total world	6,933,000	3,702,000	3,231,000	2,289,000	9,223,000

[a] Columns and rows may fail to sum due to rounding to the nearest 1000.
[b] HIV infection acquired before or at birth.
[c] AIDS cases in North America have been estimated on the basis of the 1987 revised CDC AIDS surveillance case definition.
AIDS in the World II *survey.*

Social and cultural factors and work patterns influence the way HIV disease has spread. In Thailand it has been customary for young girls from rural areas to work for a few years in brothels in Bangkok to earn their dowry before returning to their villages to marry. In Bangkok they use intravenous drugs, which was the initial mode of transmission; HIV/AIDS is now solidly established in rural Thailand. In many parts of Africa, the men go to the cities to work and are infected with HIV by prostitutes (it can cost less to hire a prostitute for a few minutes than it costs to buy a condom!). The men infect their wives when they go back to their villages. As the men and women get AIDS and die, they leave a generation of orphans to be reared by grandparents and no one to till the fields and grow and harvest the crops. High proportions of urban, educated office workers and professional men in many African countries have long been promiscuous, and HIV/AIDS has devastated the civil service, banking, and other administrative structures—and produced a generation of orphans, many of whom are also HIV-positive.

The diagnostic screening test identifies persons who are HIV-positive, and cohort studies have clarified the natural history; the annual rate of progression from HIV-positive to overt AIDS is about 1 to 3 percent in the first few years after conversion to HIV-positive, perhaps higher subsequently.

Isolation and identification of HIV raised hopes that a vaccine would soon be developed, but a unique feature of AIDS is the disruption of immune defences, so immunization could prove difficult. The search for effective prevention, an HIV vaccine, and for curative treatment has been unrelenting, but so far the chemotherapeutic weapons can offer only reduced rate of progress from HIV infection to frank AIDS and probably reduced risk of mother-to-infant transmission. By far the best preventive strategy remains safe-sex practices, preferably monogamous sexual partnership, and strict avoidance of contact with blood or other body fluids from HIV-positive or suspected positive persons.

Public health authorities in many countries have developed guidelines for AIDS prevention. WHO guidelines are as follows:

HIV is spread from person to person in three ways: (1) through sexual contact with an infected person; (2) direct contact (inoculation) with infected blood or blood products; or (3) from infected mother to child before, during, or after birth.

1. To prevent sexual spread, limit the number of sexual partners; avoid sexual relations with persons at high risk and who have many sexual partners; avoid anal intercourse; use a condom, which may help reduce the risks of spread during both homosexual and heterosexual intercourse.

2. To prevent spread by contact with blood or blood products, test donations of blood for transfusion; do not use HIV-positive blood for patients; use transfusions only when medically necessary; treat special blood products (such as clotting factor) to destroy HIV; ensure that

needles and other instruments that pierce the skin, whether medically or for other reasons (e.g., tattooing), are clean and sterile; take
particular care to sterilize when needles must be reused.

3. To reduce mother-to-infant transmission, advise infected women
   about the risks for themselves and for their infants if they become
   pregnant.

▶ CONCLUSION

I have alluded to historic trends and to ecologic changes. I have emphasized
the complex and ever-changing relationship of humans and pathogenic microorganisms. This cannot be ignored if we want to maintain and improve
control of communicable diseases. We have made great progress in control
measures during the 20th century, but we have not eliminated threats to
health and long life from infectious pathogens. I doubt if we ever will, because there are so many more varieties of microorganisms than there are humans. Our best hope is to regard microorganisms in their ecologic perspective and to work with, rather than against, the ecosystems that include
humans and pathogenic organisms.

▶ REFERENCES

1. Robertson SE, Hull BP, Tomori O, et al.: Yellow fever: A decade of reemergence.
   JAMA 276:1157–1162, 1996.
2. *MMWR* 45:693–697, 1996.
3. Benenson AS (ed): *Control of Communicable Diseases Manual,* 16th ed. Washington,
   DC: American Public Health Association, 1995.
4. Hamer W: *Epidemic Disease in England: the Evidence of Variability and of Persistency of
   Type.* (Milroy Lectures, 1906). London: Bedford, 1906.
5. Greenwood M: *Epidemics and Crowd Diseases.* London: Williams & Norgate, 1935.
6. Bailey NTJ: *The Mathematical Theory of Epidemics.* London: Griffin, 1957.
7. Hamer W: Epidemic disease in England. *Lancet* 1:733–739, 1906.
8. Anderson RM, May RM: *Infectious Diseases of Humans: Dynamics and Control.* Oxford: Oxford Science Publications, 1992.
9. Ewald PW: *Evolution of Infectious Disease.* New York: Oxford University Press, 1994.
10. Fine PEM: Herd immunity: history, theory, practice. *Epidemiol Rev* 15:2:265–302,
    1993.
11. Schulte PA, Perera FP: *Molecular Epidemiology: Principles and Practices.* Orlando, FL:
    Academic Press, 1993.
12. Frank A, Frank OH, Pressler M (ed/trans): *The Diary of a Young Girl.* New York:
    Doubleday, 1991.
13. *MMWR* 45:SS1, 1995.
14. Soper FL: *Proposal of the Director of the Pan American Sanitary Bureau Regarding a Pro-
    gram for Cooperation of the Bureau in the Eradication of Smallpox in the Americas.* Sev-

enth meeting of the Executive Committee, Pan American Health Organization, OSP, CE7, W-15. Washington, DC: PAHO, 1949.

15. Beveridge WIB: *Influenza: The Last Great Plague.* New York: Prodist, 1977.

16. Neustadt R, Fineberg H: *The Epidemic that Never Was: Policy-making and the Swine Flu Affair.* New York: Vintage, 1983.

17. Langmuir AD, Bregman DJ, Kurland LT, et al.: An epidemiologic and clinical evaluation of Guillain-Barré syndrome reported in association with administration of swine influenza vaccines. *Am J Epidemiol* 119:841–879, 1984.

18. John Bunyan (1628–1688): *The Life and Death of Mr. Badman.* Bristol: Smith and Son, 1680.

19. Dubos R, Dubos J: *The White Plague: Tuberculosis, Man and Society.* Boston: Little, Brown, 1952.

20. Frost WH: The age selection of mortality from tuberculosis in successive decades. *Am J Hyg* 30:91–96, 1939.

21. Porter JDH, McAdam KPWJ: The re-emergence of tuberculosis. *Annu Rev Public Health* 15:303–323, 1994.

22. Zelnik M, Kim Y: Sex education and its association with teenage sexual activity, pregnancy, and contraceptive use. *Fam Plann Perspec* 14:117–126, 1982; and many subsequent replications of this study, all showing exactly the same.

23. Haley RW, Culver DH, White JW, et al.: The nationwide nosocomial infection rate: A new need for vital statistics. *Am J Epidemiol* 121:159–167, 1985.

24. Kilbourne EM, Rigau-Perez JG, Heath CW, et al.: Clinical epidemiology of toxic-oil syndrome. *N Engl J Med* 309:1408–1414, 1983.

25. Goodman RA, Osterholm MT, Granoff DM, et al.: Infectious diseases in child day care. *Pediatrics* 74:134–139, 1984.

26. Stagno S, Cloud GA: Working parents: The impact of day care and breast feeding on cytomegalovirus infections in offspring. In Roizman B (ed): *Infectious Diseases in an Age of Change.* Washington, DC: National Academy Press 1995; pp. 15–30.

27. Huq A, Colwell RR, Rahman R, et al.: Detection of *Vibrio cholerae* 01 in the aquatic environment by fluorescent monoclonal antibody and culture methods. *Appl Environ Microbiol* 56:2370–2373, 1990.

28. Davis JP, Chesney PJ, Wand PJ, et al.: Toxic shock syndrome: Epidemiologic features, recurrence, risk factors and prevention. *N Engl J Med* 303:1429–1435, 1980.

29. Fraser DW, Tsai TF, Orenstein W, et al.: Legionnaires' disease: Description of an epidemic of pneumonia. *N Engl J Med* 297:1189–1197, 1977.

30. McDade JE, Shepard CC, Fraser DW, et al.: Legionnaires' disease: Isolation of a bacterium and demonstration of its role in other respiratory disease. *N Engl J Med* 297:1197–1203, 1977.

31. Update: Filovirus infection in animal handlers. *MMWR* 39:221, 1990; see also the best-seller, *The Hot Zone,* by Richard Preston, New York: Bantam.

32. World Health Organization: *World Health Report 1996.* Geneva: WHO, 1996.

33. Patz JA, Epstein PR, Burke TA, et al.: Global climate change and emerging infectious disease. *JAMA* 275:217–223, 1996.

34. Levine MM, Thacker SB (eds): Emerging and reemerging infections. *Epidemiol Rev* 18:1:1–97, 1996.

35. Centers for Disease Control: *Pneumocystis* pneumonia—Los Angeles. MMWR 30:250–252, 1981.

36. Barre-Sinoussi F, Cherman JC, Rey F, et al.: Isolation of a T-lymphotropic retro-

virus from a patient at risk for acquired immune deficiency syndrome (AIDS). *Science* 220:868–871, 1983.

37. Heptonstall J, Gill ON: Occupational exposures and medical responsibilities. *Lancet* 346:578–579, 1995; Fitch KM, Alvarez LP, Medina RDA, et al.: Occupational transmission of HIV in health care workers: A review. *Eur J Public Health* 5:175–186, 1995.

38. Mann J, Tarantola D (eds): *AIDS in the World, II.* New York: Oxford University Press 1996, pp. 5–40.

4

Environmental
Health

Environmental health is concerned with all the factors, circumstances, and conditions in the environment or surroundings of humans that can influence health and well being. A clearly defined aspect of the environment is the workplace, where many kinds of exposures to hazards have been identified. Another is best described as the built environment, a term that encompasses domestic housing conditions and the environment in public spaces such as office buildings, hotels and other institutions, and enclosed sports arenas.

Occupational medicine is a branch of medical specialization; physicians have well-defined roles and responsibilities in many industrial settings. Other health-related professions such as occupational safety, industrial hygiene, occupational therapy, aspects of engineering, architecture, and other skills are also involved. I will emphasize occupational aspects of environmental health but refer to broader environmental issues and make no distinction between occupational and environmental health problems and issues in some of the following sections. Many conditions that are due to environmental factors affect people both within and outside the workplace. There is growing concern about the ill effects of environmental pollution, not only on human health, but on all living things. To a considerable extent my remarks apply to health problems associated with the built environment, especially in cities.

Environmental medicine impinges on every clinical specialty and on all the basic biomedical sciences. A popular convention is to group together the conditions associated respectively with metals, dusts, chemicals, and physical agents, but it would be as sensible to classify environmental diseases according to their mode of clinical presentation. I will briefly describe some common hazardous exposures and general principles of prevention and control, but this is not a comprehensive survey; readers should consult the reference texts listed at the end of the chapter for further information.[1-5]

► HISTORY

Our knowledge of some industrial diseases is ancient. Pliny the Younger (A.D. 23–79) described lead poisoning and recognized its connection with lead-based paints. The medieval guilds understood that some trades were hazardous and accordingly advised their members. In 1700 Bernardino Ramazzini published *De Morbis Artificum*[6] (Diseases of Workers), a systematic treatise that is as fascinating to read today as when it was first written. Today many of us are curious enough about how other people live and work to provide a secure market for books on the subject. Several 19th-century writers, notably Charles Dickens and Henry Mayhew, aroused the social conscience of their times with their vivid and moving accounts of the appalling conditions under which many people worked and so paved the way for much-needed reform. The growing political power of trade unions contributed to further improvement of working conditions in mines and factories, beginning early in the 20th century. Scientific discoveries have rapidly expanded our understanding, first in toxicology and pulmonary pathophysiology, more recently in epidemiology and molecular biology.

Laws and regulations protect workers against many workplace hazards, making previously dangerous trades safer than in the past. Protection against environmental hazards outside the workplace is often still inadequate, rudimentary, or nonexistent. Investigative journalism, nowadays on television, can be a useful form of leverage on lawmakers and regulatory agencies.

► ENVIRONMENTAL EPIDEMIOLOGY

An important use for epidemiology is surveillance of persons exposed to known or suspected toxic substances, both within and outside the workplace. Epidemiologic methods can clarify cause–effect relationships as a prelude to preventive programs and can be used to evaluate control measures.

There are many important questions. Does exposure to herbicides increase the risk of birth defects?[7] Is there a level of exposure to ionizing radiation below which cancer risks are virtually nonexistent?[8] Does ureaformaldehyde foam insulation emit formaldehyde gas in sufficient quantities to consitute a health hazard?[9] Do people living close to high-voltage electric power lines suffer adverse health effects?[10] Many questions and the methodologic problems that arise when we try to answer them demonstrate that environmental epidemiology has difficult features, some arising also in toxicology (Box 4–1).

The ambient levels and body burdens of many toxic substances can be measured only with difficulty and often at great expense. At times a substance itself is not toxic, but its metabolic breakdown products are. Measurements rarely begin at the time of first exposure to a presumed toxic substance. The dose–response relationships may be uncertain, variable, and

---

BOX 4–1. **Epidemiologic and Toxicologic Problems in Environmental Health**

Ambient levels of toxic substances may be difficult to determine
Body burdens may be difficult to determine
Measurements seldom begin soon enough
Long latency or incubation time
Ill-defined clinical effects
Variable dose–response relationship
Low incidence of serious adverse effects
 Confounding effects resulting from exposure to several toxic
 substances
Occupations and exposures change
Workers may be migratory
Which denominator, which numerator should be used?

---

poorly understood. Sometimes, although there may be intuitive grounds for believing that long-term low-level exposure is hazardous, it is impossible to demonstrate clinical, physiologic, or pharmacologic effects. There may be a long incubation time between first exposure and the onset of clinically apparent effects. For example, the latency period for both tobacco-related and asbestos-related lung cancer is 20 to 30 years. There may be a low incidence of adverse effects among those exposed, perhaps one in a thousand or even less. If only small numbers are exposed, it may be many years before the health hazard is even suspected, let alone identified. Sometimes people are exposed to multiple environmental toxins, making it difficult to incriminate a particular agent. A case of lung cancer may be due to workplace exposure or to smoking; the gastrointestinal or hepatotoxic effects of a pesticide may be aggravated by alcohol consumption or by exposure to volatile solvents used in a basement home–hobby workshop. Meticulously detailed histories of all exposures, whether work-related or not, are needed to identify such confounding effects, and even then it may not be possible to state with confidence that a condition is due to a particular exposure.[11,12]

The affected populations may be transient workers. Many people work for a time in an industry with certain exposures, then move to another with different risks. Migratory agricultural workers exposed to a multiplicity of pesticides are very difficult to study for this reason. High dropout rates from some industries and from cohort or follow-up studies undermine the stability of numerators and raise questions about which number to use for the denominator. Some of these difficulties are overcome if there is a large population available for study, and if a record linkage system[13] and a mortality database such as the National Death Index (Chap. 2) can be used.

A challenging problem is that the population being studied may be members of a labor union, but the necessary information about exposures can come only from management, which might resist disclosure in order to protect trade secrets. Mutual suspicions between these traditional adversaries, especially if complicated by intervention of the media or government regulatory agencies, can introduce political and emotional issues that add further to the difficulty of objective epidemiologic study (see Chap. 10).

Finally in this catalogue of difficulties, we must include the possibility that the power of suggestion is the cause of at least some symptoms and signs. "Behavioral epidemics" are well documented: They can include obvious physical signs like skin rashes, as well as headaches, nausea, and similar symptoms that are often labeled "emotional" in origin. There have been several epidemics of vague symptoms among office workers in modern sealed buildings, in which air is recirculated through the heating and cooling system to conserve energy.[14,15] It can be difficult to determine whether these epidemics are behavioral or environmental in origin (more discussion of this follows).

Despite these difficulties, there have been many notable epidemiologic discoveries about environmental disease. Some have depended on observation of an increase in the incidence of what was previously a very rare condition. Mesothelioma of the pleura following exposure to asbestos[16] and hemangiosarcoma of the liver among those working with vinyl chloride are well-known examples. The first four cases of hemangiosarcoma of the liver in vinyl chloride workers were observed over an 8-year period in a workforce of 500, representiong a relative risk about 5000 times higher than in the general population.[17] Case-control or cohort studies have identified many other occupational or environmental hazards. The Canadian Mortality Data Base and record linkage[18] (Chap. 2) have been powerful tools in important studies of occupational and environmental exposures, e.g., to ionizing radiation, agricultural pesticides, and formaldehyde.[19] In some studies of environmental exposure, e.g., to ionizing radiation downwind from the atomic weapons testing sites in Nevada[20] and near a nuclear power station at Sellarfield in England, reports of increased childhood cancer incidence and mortality rates have been topics of controversy.[21] Methods must be carefully chosen and research protocols must be adhered to very strictly. Impaired neuropsychologic development was observed among children exposed in utero and in infancy to polybrominated biphenyls (PBBs) in one investigation but not in another.[22–24] Flawed epidemiologic methods, inadequate measurements, and inappropriate statistical methods can invalidate results and conclusions and lead to either needless anxiety or a false sense of security. Good epidemiologic studies can allay fear and abate rumors, as well as measure accurately the incidence rates of outcomes in exposed and unexposed populations.[25]

Because of all these difficulties, analysis of mortality data by occupational categories has often been relied on for surveillance, but this is a blunt instrument: Occupational details on death certificates are scanty and do not provide any information about exposures, which have to be inferred. Death may not occur until many years and several occupational changes after the exposure to risk. Moreover, the information is too late to be of value to the deceased and often is too late to help others exposed to the same risks.

Another tool used in environmental epidemiology is analysis of mortality by cause and area. This can provide much interesting information. Regional variations in cancer mortality have been mapped in the United States, Canada, China, Japan, and many other nations.[26] This has drawn attention to the existence of high-risk regions, where either environmental or occupational factors can be further investigated. An interesting example of regional variation is that of cardiovascular mortality in relation to drinking water quality; this has been observed in several countries. It remains uncertain whether the presence in hard water of certain salts has a protective effect, the absence of some factor from soft water should be incriminated, or whether the evidence has been spuriously inflated in importance by the use of inappropriate statistical methods.[27]

► CARCINOGENIC CHEMICALS

Much of the evidence on chemicals as causes of cancer in the workplace and in the general environment comes from epidemiology or toxicology. The National Research Council reviewed the value of these topics in 1991.[12] Molecular epidemiology has opened the way to precise identification of carcinogens and how they work.[28] Genetic studies can identify high-risk groups and individuals, though the use of genetic tests for this purpose is controversial: It could justify or encourage discriminatory hiring practices.[29]

Percivall Pott, a London surgeon (Pott's disease and Pott's fracture are named for him), reported in 1775 that chimney sweeps were prone to cancer of the scrotum; he correctly attributed this to lodgement of soot in the rugae of the scrotal skin. The responsible chemical carcinogen was identified nearly 200 years later by Kennaway: It is a polycyclic hydrocarbon of the dibenzanthracene family. Many other chemicals in this group are carcinogenic and occur in other important substances besides coal tar. The tar of tobacco smoke is the best known. Industrial chemicals of many varieties contain (or are themselves) chemical carcinogens. They include aniline dyes, bis(chloromethyl) ethers, benzidine, 2-naphthylamine, vinyl chloride, and many others. There are carcinogens in certain foodstuffs or produced in the body by digestion of organic substances in foods (aflatoxins, nitrosamines).[30]

Aniline dye workers have long been known to have a high incidence of bladder cancer. Derivatives of 2-naphthylamines, which are widely used industrially, e.g., as antioxidants in the rubber industry, can undergo metabolic transformation in vivo to form actively carcinogenic 2-naphthylamine. This is the mechanism for bladder cancer, which is an occupational risk in rubber tire, insulating cable, and other industries using rubber. Much of our knowledge of carcinogenic chemicals has come from epidemiologic studies (Table 4–1).

TABLE 4–1. Industrial Processes, Occupations, and Chemicals Classified by an IARC ad hoc Working Group as Definitely or Probably Carcinogenic (Evidence Strong) for Humans

	Neoplasm
Definitely Carcinogenic for Humans	
Industrial Processes and Occupational Exposures	
Auramine manufacture	Bladder
Boot and shoe manufacture and repair	Bladder, nasal
Furniture manufacture	Nasal
Isopropyl alcohol manufacture (strong acid process)	Paranasal sinuses
Nickel refining	Nasal, lung
Ionizing radiation	Leukemia, others
Rubber industry	Bladder, others
Underground hematite mining (with exposure to radon)	Lung
Chemicals and Groups of Chemicals	
4-Aminobiphenyl	Bladder
Arsenic and arsenic compounds	Lung, skin
Asbestos	Lung, mesothelioma
Benezene	Leukemia
Benzidine	Bladder
Bis(chloromethyl) ether and technical-grade chloromethyl methyl ether	Lung
Chlorophenoxy herbicides	Soft tissue sarcoma
Chromium and certain chromium compounds	Lung
Mustard gas	Lung
2-Naphthylamine	Bladder
PCBs	Various sites
Soots, tars, and oils	Skin, lung, bladder
Vinyl chloride	Liver (angiosarcoma)
Probably Carcinogenic for Humans, Evidence Strong	
Occupational Exposures	
Manufacture of magenta	Bladder
Chemicals and Groups of Chemicals	
Acrylonitrile	Lung, others
Benzo[a]pyrene	Skin, lung, bladder
Beryllium and beryllium compounds	Lung
Diethyl sulfate	Larynx
Dimethyl sulfate	Lung
Nickel and certain nickel compounds	Lung, sinonasal
Ortho-toluidine	Bladder

(Adapted from International Agency for Research on Cancer: IARC Monographs on the Evaluation of the Carcinogenic Risk of Chemicals to Humans [suppl. 4]. Lyon, France: IARC, 1982 and updated.)

► METALS

Many metals, even when essential to life, like iron, copper, zinc, and magnesium, are toxic at high doses or in some compound formulations.[31] I will discuss only a few important varieties; details can be found in books listed in the references. Some exposure standards appear in tables. It is fitting to consider first the two oldest known poisonous metals: lead and mercury. The discussion illustrates some important general principles.

Lead

Lead has been an environmental contaminant and a cause of disease since ancient times. By the Middle Ages, lead was already being deposited in Greenland ice, carried there by the wind over previous centuries from mining and smelting operations in Europe dating back to Roman times.[32] The Roman domestic economy made extensive use of lead; mild mental impairment resulting from chronic low-level lead poisoning has even been suggested as a factor in the decline and fall of the Roman Empire.

Metallic lead has many uses, ranging from malleable piping to storage batteries; lead salts are ingredients in paint, lead is a contaminant in many other metal ores and concentrates, and tetraethyl and tetramethyl lead have been widely used as antiknock additives in gasoline. Inhaling or ingesting lead or its compounds causes lead poisoning. The pathogenesis is not fully understood; there is interference with essential enzyme systems, causing damage to central and peripheral nervous systems, bone marrow, kidneys, and other organs and tissues. Lead poisoning can present clinically in many ways, including lead encephalopathy, peripheral neuritis, lead colic, nephritis, anemia, and spontaneous miscarriage. Organic lead poisoning and acute lead poisoning in children are very dangerous, with predominantly neurologic effects, including Korsakoff's psychosis and lead encephalopathy.[32]

Occupational groups at risk include lead miners and smelters, paint manufacturers, battery makers and breakers, gasoline suppliers, and many others. Small children can be at special risk of environmental lead poisoning because their high metabolic activity enhances susceptibility of vulnerable enzyme systems.[33] Environmental contamination with lead occurs in some urban areas as a result of emission from factory smelters or leaded gasoline. This can cause chronic low-level lead intoxication, which is a cause of intellectual impairment ranging from slight reduction of I.Q. to mild mental retardation. The effects are long lasting, persisting through at least middle childhood even after removal from exposure.[34]

Prevention of environmental lead poisoning of children requires elimination of lead emissions from smelter stacks and elimination of lead additives in gasoline. Prevention of occupational lead poisoning is a textbook illustration of the principles of industrial hygiene. Education of workers on the importance of cleanliness (washing hands to get rid of lead dust before eating);

"good housekeeping" in the workplace to avoid build-up of toxic concentrations of dust; the use of exhaust ventilation and work processes to exclude workers from contact with lead fumes, all play a part. Surveillance of potentially exposed workers is also important. Women in the reproductive years are at risk of miscarriage as a result of lead intoxication; lead compounds have long been used to induce abortions. No one should be exposed to such high concentrations of lead in the workplace as to reach lead levels that could cause miscarriage; but the protection of women who are or could become pregnant is especially important. Some industries have instituted a "fetal protection policy" that excludes women of reproductive age from work in places where lead levels may be high, but this policy begs the question of adequately protecting other workers against the risk of lead poisoning and against the reproductive effects of lead on male workers.

Mercury

Metallic mercury is a heavy liquid at room temperature and gives off small amounts of mercury vapor, which is toxic. The inorganic and organic compounds in common use are also toxic. Metallic mercury is used in many scientific instruments; inorganic mercury compounds include vermillion, a pigment; fulminate, used in detonators; and mercuric oxide, an antifouling additive in marine paints. Organic mercurials are used in fungicides, medicinals, and surgical dressings. Mercury batteries are widely used in electronic equipment. Mercury compounds are found in some industrial effluents, e.g., from pulp paper manufacture. Some of these compounds are metabolized in marine ecosystems, making edible crustacea, shellfish, and fish toxic to humans. A dramatic example was the crippling condition that occurred in the 1950s among people living along the shore of Minamata Bay in Japan,[35] which was polluted by organic mercury salts in industrial effluent. This condition affected persons of all ages, including developing fetuses, leading to the birth of severely retarded and deformed offspring. Organic mercury poisoning has occurred in other dramatic episodes, e.g., in Iraq in 1956 when several hundred farmers and their families ate seed corn that had been treated with ethyl mercury, a fungicide. Like Minamata disease, this damaged the fetus. However, no clinically recognizable cases of Minamata disease have occurred outside Japan, even among Canadian Indians in communities where extremely high levels of mercury in fish and in human blood and hair samples have been recorded. Mercury was formerly an ingredient in popular remedies for irritability associated with teething in infancy, and this caused "pink disease" until the cause was recognized in 1959. Until then, children's hospitals, such as one where I was an intern briefly in 1950, had enough cases to justify special wards for the care of infants with pink disease.

The clinical manifestations of mercury poisoning differ among metallic, inorganic, and organic compounds. Metallic mercury and inorganic salts cause neurologic symptoms, dermatitis, gingivitis, and ocular damage. Organic mercurials cause predominantly neurologic damage.

Occupational groups at risk include miners and refiners, scientific instrument makers, felt hat makers (hence the saying "mad as a hatter"), and workers with dyestuffs, pharmaceuticals, and certain pesticides.

Prevention of mercury poisoning requires the complete enclosure of industrial processes to avoid all contact between the mercury and the worker, with use of respirators also as indicated. Rigorous environmental control, e.g., prohibition of mercurial fungicides and of the mercury compounds known as slimicides, used to treat softwood in the pulp paper industry, is also required.

Aluminum

Aluminum, the most plentiful metal in the earth's crust, was until recently regarded as innocuous. But aluminum dust causes aluminosis, a form of pneumoconiosis. Patients on renal dialysis develop neurotoxic symptoms and dementia resulting from accumulation of aluminum.[36] It has been observed that patients with Alzheimer's disease have high concentrations of aluminum in brain tissue, but despite much research,[37] no connection has been found to aluminum ingestion (e.g., as a trace contaminant that might escape from aluminum pots or related to alum used as an antiflocculant in reservoir water supplies). Occupational exposure occurs in industries using aluminum or its compounds, including petroleum refining, where aluminum chloride is used.

Arsenic

Compounds of arsenic are used as pigments, fungicides, and insecticides. Arsenic salts also contaminate gold, copper, and silver ores and are an important toxic ingredient of smelter stack emissions, causing environmental contamination. Acute arsenic poisoning is often fatal. Chronic effects include dermatitis, peripheral neuritis, and malignant changes in skin, lung, and liver. Organic arsenicals include Ehrlich's "magic bullet," the first effective antisyphilitic, and its derivatives used to treat syphilis for half a century before penicillin. Antisyphilitic organic arsenicals can cause dermatitis, but if they are carcinogens, many more cases of cancer ought to have been observed among the innumerable patients treated for syphilis in the prepenicillin era. Other arsenicals, notably arsenic trioxide, are known carcinogens. Those who work with sheep dip are at risk and arsenic fumes in smelter stack emissions aggravate lung and skin cancer risks. Angiosarcoma is another end result. More frequent effects of chronic arsenical poisoning are dermatitis and polyneuritis. Acute arsenic poisoning is fatal, as several famous murders have demonstrated.

Beryllium

Alloys of beryllium with copper, nickel, aluminum, etc. have many uses. Beryllium was used in fluorescent tubes until its severe toxic effects led to replacement by other substances that fluoresce when an electric current is passed through a vacuum tube. Chronic beryllium disease is a granulomatous condition resembling sarcoid with effects on many body systems and organs. Workers' families are affected by dust brought home on work clothing (family contact disease) and people living near factories may also get beryllium disease unless strict control measures are enforced.

Cadmium

Nickel–cadmium storage batteries are an important industrial use of this metal. Resistance to corrosion makes cadmium a suitable coating for many other metallic surfaces. Cadmium also occurs in factory-cured cigarette tobacco. Both acute and chronic cadmium poisoning can occur. Chronic cadmium poisoning causes pulmonary emphysema and renal tubular damage, sometimes with secondary hypertension. Heavy cigarette smokers may absorb enough cadmium to cause chronic poisoning, because the rate of excretion is very low. Cadmium occurs as a contaminant in oil refining and can get into aquifers from the effluent in petrochemical plants. Some evidence suggests that in regions with high cadmium concentration in groundwater, there are elevated incidence and mortality rates from carcinoma of the prostate.[38] Occupational risk groups include workers with various alloys, refiners, and battery and paint makers. Exposure limits are given in Table 4–2.

Chromium

This is mainly used as chromium plating and in alloys with steel, which are particularly strong. Chromium plating is an electrolytic process that emits chromium fumes; these and the salts are irritants, producing deep cutaneous ulcers and intense tracheobronchial and conjunctival irritation. Lung cancer, resulting from exposure to the trivalent form, is common among chromium workers (Table 4–2). Occupational groups at risk include various metal workers, electroplaters, and welders.

Nickel

The principal uses are in alloys with copper, stainless steel, cobalt, etc. The Mond nickel production process involves treatment of impure nickel powder with carbon monoxide to produce nickel carbonyl, from which very high-grade pure metallic nickel is precipitated. Nickel carbonyl is highly toxic, producing acute hemorrhagic pneumonitis and tracheobronchitis. Chronic

TABLE 4-2. **Safety Standards: Some Carcinogenic Metals and Organic Chemicals**

Substance	Number Exposed in U.S.	Safety Standards
Trichlorethylene (liver carcinogen in animals)	290,000	PEL 100 ppm 8-hr TWA (OSHA)
Ethylene dibromide (animal carcinogen)	108,000	0.13 ppm/15 min (NIOSH) PEL 20 ppm (OSHA)
Chrome pigment (lead chromate is a human carcinogen)	?	0.2 mg/m^3 lead 0.5 mg/m^3 chromium
Asbestos (brake and clutch assembly and service)	?	100,000 fibers/m^3 for 8-hr TWA
PCBs	12,000	PEL 1 µg/m^3
Chloroform	40,000	PEL 2 ppm 60-min ceiling
Radon daughters	?	4 working-level mo/yr
Inorganic arsenic	?	2 µg As/m^3
2-Naphthylamine (known human carcinogen)	15,000	Minimize or prohibit exposure (NIOSH)
Tetrachlorethylene (potential human carcinogen)	Dry-cleaning ? many thousands	50 ppm for 10-hr workday
Vinyl halides (vinyl chloride is a human carcinogen)	2.5 million	Lowest possible exposure
Formaldehyde	1.6 million	PEL 3 ppm 8-hr TWA (OSHA)
Ethylene dibromide (potential carcinogen)	108,000	20 ppm 8-hr TWA (OSHA)
2,3,7,8-TCDD (known carcinogen)	?	Decontamination procedures
Cadmium		PEL 40 µg/m^3 10-hr TWA
Methyl halides (potential carcinogens)	146,000	No exposure desirable

NIOSH = National Institute for Occupational Safety and Health; OSHA = Occupational Safety and Health Administration; PCB = polychlorinated biphenyl; PEL = permissible exposure limit; TCDD = tetrachlorodibenzo-*p*-dioxin; TWA = time-weighted average. *(From MMWR vol 35 (suppl), September 26, 1986.)*

nickel exposure, e.g., to nickel dust or fumes, produces dermatitis and also causes cancer of the nasal sinuses and lungs. Nickel in rice paper used to make cigarettes may contribute to the risk of lung cancer among cigarette smokers, although the tobacco contains more than enough carcinogens. Improved, enclosed processing methods have reduced the occupational hazards of nickel and nickel carbonyl. Exposed groups include battery, sparkplug, and paint makers.

Other metals that can cause disease include antimony, cobalt, copper, iron, manganese, platinum, selenium, thallium, tin, vanadium, and zinc. Details can be found in the reference books listed at the end of this chapter.

▶ OCCUPATIONAL RESPIRATORY DISEASES

Environmental conditions in the workplace and outside of it often lead to inhalation of dusts that can cause chronic obstructive pulmonary disease (COPD). The combination of moist, humid climatic conditions and atmospheric pollution with oxides of sulfur and nitrogen and with solid particles of carbon can produce chronic bronchitis and emphysema—although pollution of inspired air with tobacco smoke is a more common and serious cause of COPD (Box 4–2).

The respiratory tract is equipped with ciliated epithelium and mucus secretions that successfully trap and sweep out many small particles. However, particles smaller than 5 to 7 μ can penetrate to the alveoli, where they remain or are absorbed by phagocytes and are transported to interalveolar

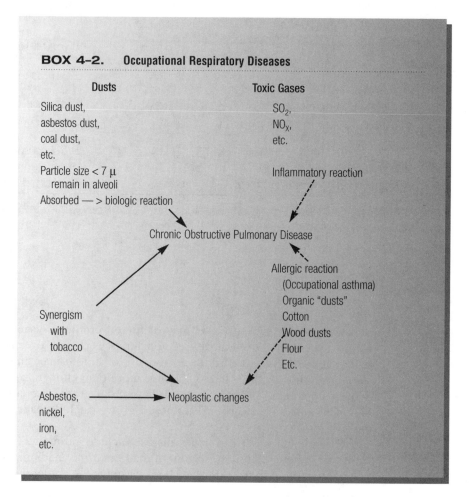

BOX 4–2. **Occupational Respiratory Diseases**

Dusts	Toxic Gases
Silica dust,	SO_2,
asbestos dust,	NO_x,
coal dust,	etc.
etc.	
Particle size < 7 μ remain in alveoli	Inflammatory reaction
Absorbed —> biologic reaction	

Chronic Obstructive Pulmonary Disease

Synergism with tobacco

Allergic reaction
(Occupational asthma)
Organic "dusts"
Cotton
Wood dusts
Flour
Etc.

Asbestos, ⟶ Neoplastic changes
nickel,
iron,
etc.

spaces.[39] Asbestos, silica, coal dust, and various organic substances and microorganisms are the right size to reach the alveoli. Once these small particles reach the alveoli, the bodily response produces specific diseases.

Asbestos Disease

Asbestos is a fibrous material, formerly widely used as insulation and for many other purposes because of its fire-resistant and seemingly inert nature. Unfortunately, it is anything but inert inside the human body.[40] The fibers consist of microscopic fibrils, which under the electron microscope are seen to consist of very small fibers in the Angstrom unit size range. These very small fibers do the damage, probably at the intracellular level. The exact pathogenesis is not known. Asbestos produces three distinct pathologic conditions: asbestosis; cancer, especially of the lung but also the larynx and gastrointestinal tract; and mesothelioma.

Asbestosis is a chronic progressive pulmonary fibrosis that causes impaired respiratory function, cor pulmonale, and death from respiratory or right-sided heart failure or from secondary bronchopneumonia. It is caused by heavy exposure to asbestos dust and has a short latent period, often less than 10 years.

Lung cancer occurs often among asbestos workers since working conditions have improved enough to lead to reduced incidence of asbestosis—more workers live long enough to get cancer. Histologically it resembles tobacco-related lung cancer but is more often seen in the periphery of the lung than close to the hilum, and in the lower lobes. These are the same areas affected by asbestosis, making early detection by x-ray examination more difficult.

In one large cohort study of asbestos workers in the United States and Canada, the mortality rate from lung cancer among men with more than 20 years exposure to asbestos was five times higher than would be expected in the general population (Table 4–3).

There is a powerful synergistic effect of cigarette smoking: an asbestos worker who also smokes has approximately 50 times the risk of dying of lung cancer, compared to a nonsmoker not exposed to asbestos. This fact led some employers to establish a policy of hiring nonsmokers only. The latency period for asbestos-related lung cancer is usually in the range of 20 to 35 years but can be as short as 10 years.

Mesothelioma is malignant change of pleural or peritoneal membrane. It is uniquely associated with exposure to asbestos, as Table 4–3 shows. Almost no cases are known in which there is no confirmed history of exposure to asbestos. In one series, exposure was definite in 69 out of 70, and probable in the 70th case.[41]

Exposure to asbestos sufficient to cause mesothelioma may not be occupational: Cases have occurred among family members of asbestos workers, wives and children who have handled clothing heavily contaminated with as-

TABLE 4–3. Deaths Among 17,800 Asbestos Insulation Workers in the United States and Canada, Jan. 1, 1967–Dec. 31, 1976

	Within 20 Years of First Exposure		20 or More Years After First Exposure	
Number of men	12,683		12,051	
Man-years observation	89,462		77,391	
	Expected	Observed	Expected	Observed
Total deaths	282.9	325	1376.0	1946
Lung cancer	11.9	36	93.7	450
Mesothelioma	0	5	0	170
Stomach and bowel	5.6	5	46.7	76
All cancer	42.6	83	277.1	912
Asbestosis	0	8	0	160

(From Selikoff, IJ.[41])

bestos dust, and among persons living in neighborhoods where asbestos dust occurs in the air. Very small quantities of asbestos fibrils may suffice to initiate malignant change. Asbestos is used in brake shoes of automobiles, so asbestos occurs in the air wherever automobiles are used, especially in big cities. Mesothelioma is increasingly common; it could become a serious public health problem.

Control measures for asbestos exposure are seldom adequate. The U.S. and Canadian standard is a permitted exposure of 2 fibers per mL per 8-hour shift. This translates to 2 million fibers per cubic meter, and a worker inhales about 8 to 10 cubic meters of air in a working day. Moreover, it is not microscopically visible fibers that do the damage but fibrils visible only under the electron microscope. Stricter exposure limits have been set in other countries. Exhaust ventilation, cleaner work habits, and enclosed work areas permitting no exposure have led to some improvement in risk.

Since the beginning of the 1980s there has been a dramatic reduction in production and use of asbestos. Several lawsuits in the industry in which workers sought compensation for occupationally related cancers led one large corporation to file for bankruptcy. There is heightened awareness of the risks of asbestos as a building material; it has been removed from many public buildings at great trouble and expense and replaced with other insulating materials. Unfortunately, some other insulating materials, e.g., glass fiber, are proving also to be hazardous.

Silicosis

Silica, or silicon dioxide, constitutes much of the Earth's crust. Natural forces and man-made processes such as mining and grinding convert silica particles to a fine dust that, when inhaled, produces progressive pulmonary fibrosis and respiratory failure, or clinical silicosis.[42] It has been a common industrial disease since explosives have been used in underground mining. It is a serious risk for others occupationally exposed to silica dust, e.g., sandblasters, knife grinders. Exposure also occurs in the manufacture of abrasive soaps and in many other occupations.

Silicosis is a common industrial disease in nations where control measures in underground mining and in foundries were not applied when the hazard was first recognized. These nations include Germany, India, the United States, and Canada. Once silicotic nodules form, they progress even after exposure ceases and eventually disable the victim and often cause death. Tuberculosis is a frequent complication, even when this is rare in the general population. Early radiologic signs are diagnostic, and removal from further exposure then should be mandatory. The best method of prevention is exclusion from exposure. There are many variations of classic silicosis, e.g., resulting from exposure to diatomaceous earth, volcanic clay, or bentonite, which also contains asbestos.

Coal Worker's Pneumoconiosis

Underground mining is a hazardous occupation, coal mining especially so, because the risk of being crushed in a collapsing mine shaft is at least equaled by the risk of asphyxiation or death in explosion of gas (e.g., methane) or an atmospheric suspension of coal dust. Coal miners who avoid serious injury or death in such disasters may die more slowly of coal worker's pneumoconiosis (CWP). This can be due to inhalation only of coal dust, but often the coal dust is mixed with silica, to produce an even more disabling silicoanthracosis. Either is commonly called "black lung" and is characterized by fibrosis, destruction of alveoli, cavitation, and progressive impairment of respiratory function, often complicated by secondary infection and terminating in cor pulmonale and death in heart failure or pneumonia[43] (Fig. 4–1).

Occupational Chronic Bronchitis

Exposure to many varieties of dusts, fumes, and vapors can irritate and inflame the lungs. These substances may be inorganic or organic. The latter include many varieties of allergens that cause occupational asthma and a few organic fibers such as those of cotton and sugarcane, which cause byssinosis and bagassosis, respectively. Some inhaled organic matter is actually alive, e.g., molds from hay, which produce farmer's lung, and amebae from water coolers and air conditioners, which can cause a form of asthma. Often, exposure to organic dusts produces allergenic responses that make permanent removal from exposure necessary. For example, bakers can develop allergy to flour that is severe enough to force a change of occupation.

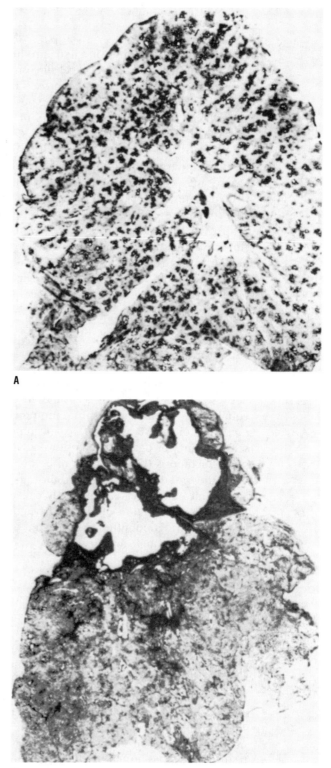

Figure 4–1. A. Whole lung section
showing simple coal worker's
pneumoconiosis (CWP) with associated
focal emphysema but otherwise
preserved lung architecture. **B.** Whole
lung section showing progressive
massive fibrosis with cavitation involving
the superior segments of the lung on a
background of simple CWP and extensive
emphysema. *(From Merchant JA:*
Occupational Respiratory Diseases. *In
Last JM (ed): Maxcy-Rosenau Public
Health and Preventive Medicine. 12th ed.
E. Norwalk, CT: Appleton-Century-Crofts,
1986, p 549.)*

Control of Occupational Respiratory Diseases

Prevention of occupational respiratory disease is difficult. In general, control measures are best based on exclusion from exposure: exhaust ventilation, work processes that segregate workers from dust, and use of respirators. Miners often will not wear respirators in stuffy underground mines. Wet processes damp down the dust but may make extraction of ore more difficult. Clearing mine shafts after blasting to allow dust to settle is desirable, but it reduces productivity. Better ventilation of mine shafts and better engineering controls are helpful measures in many mines. Medical surveillance of miners with respiratory function tests, regular x-rays, and exclusion of miners with damaged lungs is most used. Similar measures apply to other dusty industries.

▶ CHEMICALS

The technologic advances of the 20th century have included development of innumerable new chemical substances. Most are organic chemicals, many produced during petroleum refining or as by-products of the petrochemical industry. They include substances of enormous economic importance: dyestuffs, organic solvents, pesticides, and plastics. Some of these substances are toxic and others have toxic contaminants, waste products, or by-products.

Toxicologists have not managed to keep pace with these developments. Approximately 55,000 chemicals are in use in the United States; of these, 1000 to 1500 are hazardous, but only about 450 have established threshold limit values (TLVs) and adequate toxicity testing. Several hundred new chemicals come into use each year, basically untested. Only drugs, food additives, and pesticides are required by law to have premarket toxicity tests; the rest are merely reported to the Environmental Protection Agency (EPA); if EPA does not ask for toxicity tests within 90 days, the chemical enters the marketplace. This conforms to the requirements of the Toxic Substances Control Act (TOSCA). The Agency for Toxic Substances and Disease Registry (ATSDR) fights a difficult battle in the teeth of these adversities (Box 4–3).

When testing is required, it is usually for acute and chronic health effects. Manufacturers voluntarily carry out in vitro tests for short-term toxic effects and also do Ames tests for mutagenicity before premarket notification to EPA. Tests for carcinogenicity and teratogenicity are, however, rarely done.

Regarding existing chemicals, under law, EPA cannot have more than 50 chemicals on its priority list for testing at any given time, so many chemicals in common use have never been tested for health effects. Methods and procedures of toxicity testing often do not detect important effects, especially those that are long-delayed or slowly cumulative. There is disagreement about purported toxic effects among industrialists, union members, community residents, environmental activists, politicians, economists, biologists, and physicians. Conflicting opinions from self-appointed or dubiously reliable "experts"

> **BOX 4-3.**   **Toxicity Testing and Control of Chemical Substances**
>
> 55,000 chemicals in use in United States
> Major hazards from 1000 to 1500
> TLVs for about 450
> Premarket toxicity tests required only for drugs, food additives, and
>   pesticides
> Manufacturers do routine (voluntary) toxicity tests
>   For short-term effects
>   For mutagenicity (Ames test)
> No routine tests for carcinogenicity or teratogenicity
> At any one time, EPA cannot have more than 50 chemicals on priority list for
>   toxicity testing
> NO ADEQUATE SAFEGUARD AGAINST LATENT OR CUMULATIVE EFFECTS

can make objective appraisal of the evidence difficult. There is a long and dismal record in the United States and many European nations of inaction, indifference, prevarication, deceit, and even corruption before, in some instances, public opinion has been aroused enough to produce pressure for control of long-known environmental hazards. Every month brings new disclosures by investigative journalists, nowadays as often on television as in print; but although sensational and apparently accurate accounts (for instance of the possible effects toxic chemicals that mimic sex hormones might have on fertility and spermatozoa counts)[44] arouse much public concern, governments are often slow to react with adequate safeguards against environmental contamination.

Organic Solvents

Economically important petroleum or coal-tar derivatives include alcohols, ketones, ethers, aldehydes, glycols, aromatic hydrocarbons, carbon disulfide, etc. Some are carcinogenic, and several have unique toxic properties. Strictly speaking, not all are solvents but it is convenient to consider them with solvents because they are chemically related. Several chemicals in this group illustrate the range of chemical and pathophysiologic effects (Box 4-4).

Volatile solvents such as some alcohols, ethers, chloroform, trichlorethylene, etc. are central nervous system (CNS) depressants that penetrate myelin sheaths and interrupt neural transmission. Some have a narcotic or anesthetic effect.

Benzene, an aromatic hydrocarbon, is an acute CNS depressant and narcotic. Chronic low-level toxicity causes severe bone marrow depression and can cause leukemia or aplastic anemia.

BOX 4-4.   Volatile Solvents—A Few Examples

	Exposure	
	Acute	**Chronic**
Chloroform	Narcosis	Bone marrow depression, cancer
Benzene	Toxic psychosis	Leukopenia
Carbon tetrachloride	Respiratory and/or cardiac arrest	Leukemia
Carbon disulfide		Liver damage
Vinyl chloride		Liver damage
		Acroosteolysis
		Scleroderma
		Eosinophilic bronchitis
		Hemangiosarcoma
Formaldehyde	Respiratory irritation	?Carcinoma

Halogenated hydrocarbons include chloroform, carbon tetrachloride, and vinyl chloride. In addition to its former use as an anesthetic agent, chloroform is a useful solvent, but it is also a confirmed carcinogen. In chlorinated water supplies with a high content of organic matter, chloroform can be produced in trace amounts. This and other halogenated compounds that occur as pollutants produce trihalomethanes, which as trace contaminants of drinking water supplies are implicated as a potential and perhaps an actual cause of certain cancers.[45]

Carbon tetrachloride is a liver poison. It is used in the manufacture of other chemicals, e.g., fluorocarbons. It escapes to the environment in industrial effluent that enters rivers and lakes, where it kills wildlife as well as harming human health.

Vinyl chloride is used to make the useful plastic polyvinyl chloride. In the early 1970s it was found to be responsible for a peculiar syndrome of acroosteolysis (atrophy of terminal phalanges), skin changes resembling scleroderma, and eosinophilic bronchitis. Soon afterwards, as described earlier, some cases of hemangiosarcoma of the liver were observed and found to be attributable to vinyl chloride; cirrhosis of the liver also occurs among vinyl chloride workers.

Carbon disulfide is a volatile liquid used to make viscose rayon and cellulose. Acute inhalation may be rapidly fatal because of CNS depression; encephalopathy and toxic psychosis occur with subacute exposure; chronic exposure disrupts peripheral nerve transmission, may produce hypertension, and also depresses or inhibits spermatogenesis.

Formaldehyde is a highly irritant colorless gas that has many uses, both as a component in numerous industrial processes and as an ingredient in inks, resins, and adhesives. It is also used as a preservative, e.g., by embalmers and pathologists, and as a fungicide and disinfectant. it was used for some years to make urea-formaldehyde foam insulation (UFFI); this was suspected of emitting toxic concentrations of formaldehyde inside sealed buildings insulated with UFFI. The suspicion was charged with emotions because of the evidence from animal studies that high concentrations of formaldehyde cause nasal and paranasal cancer; however, several epidemiologic studies of occupational groups who are exposed to high concentrations of formaldehyde failed to demonstrate an increased cancer risk.[46] Formaldehyde is emitted in trace amounts inside modern sealed buildings, not only from UFFI but also from carpet adhesives and particleboard. It is a component of wood smoke and tobacco smoke—it is responsible for much of the irritant effect of secondhand smoke. But no carcinogenic effect has been demonstrated.[47]

Nitrosamines are formed by reaction of organic amines and nitrous acid (or nitrites and acid), which occurs most commonly in production, preparation, and digestion of various foodstuffs. Nitrosamines were shown to be hepatotoxic, then carcinogenic. They are incriminated in several varieties of cancer, e.g., cancer of the esophagus, which is endemic in parts of China, where animals and poultry as well as humans are affected. The epidemiologic detective work that clarified the cause of cancer of the esophagus in Lin Xian province, China, is a fascinating story. Several factors are involved: A soil deficiency leads to high nitrite content of green leaf vegetables, a staple diet in the area; this is the environmental factor; the behavioral factor is the local custom of preferring to eat moldy bread, the source of the amines.[48]

Halogenated Polyaromatic Hydrocarbons

This group includes polychlorinated biphyenyls (PCBs), polybrominated biphenyls (PBBs), chlorinated dibenzo-*p*-dioxins (dioxins), and chlorinated dibenzofurans. These substances have great public health importance. They cause both acute and chronic diseases, the latter including cancer and birth defects. Some chemicals in this group have also had great economic importance or are toxic by-products of subtances that are economically important. Some have been widely distributed in food chains and, because they are very persistent (not biodegradable), their effects could be felt for generations even though production and distribution have ceased. Their pathophysiologic effects are mostly similar, although their toxicity varies. Acute effects include chloracne, neurologic and psychiatric disorders, liver damage, and reproductive dyscrasia—dysmenorrhea, oligospermia, small-for-dates offspring, mental retardation of offspring,[49] and miscarriage. In experimental animals and perhaps in humans, they are carcinogenic, teratogenic, and mutagenic (Box 4–5).

BOX 4-5.   PCBs, PBBs, and Dioxins

Environmentally persistent
Biologically active
Found in tissue samples worldwide
Concentrated in some food chains
Excreted in breast milk
Fetotoxic
Chronic effects:
  Chloracne
  Liver damage
  Cancer
  Birth defects
  Neuropsychologic damage

PCBs have been used as insulation in electrical equipment, wood sealants, plasticizers, in carbonless copy paper, and for many other industrial purposes. Concern about environmental contamination with PCBs led to suspension of manufacture in the United States in 1975, but hundreds of thousands of tons of PCBs are contained in products still in use, and these can be released into the environment in various ways. Disposal is a problem; PCBs can be destroyed, i.e., degraded to harmless components, by high-temperature incineration, but no one wants a disposal plant or a PCB dump site in their neighborhood, so local political pressures tend to keep PCBs moving about. There have been several episodes of mass poisoning. In Yusho, Japan, in 1968, a batch of cooking oil was contaminated with PCBs.[50] Thousands of people developed chloracne, a persistent, disfiguring skin eruption with pigmentation, neurologic symptoms; girls and women developed dysmenorrhea; babies of affected women were small-for-dates, heavily pigmented, and many suffered intellectual impairment.

PBBs were widely used as fire-retardants, to impregnate fabrics so that they would not burn or ignite easily, until their carcinogenic effect on animals was demonstrated. In 1973, a batch of cattle feed in Michigan was accidentally contaminated with PBBs. Dairy cattle fed on this developed gross abnormalities including muscle weakness, abortion, loss of milk, and lesions of the hide and hoofs; the farm families who used the milk from these cows, and in some instances ate meat of slaughtered cattle, suffered vague symptoms unlike any known illness: lassitude, defective memory, loss of ability to do the simple arithmetic required for farm bookkeeping, inability to recognize infrequently seen close relatives, loss of libido.[15]

Was this a "behavioral epidemic," caused not by a chemical but by the power of suggestion? It is very unlikely. Some of those affected were quite isolated, belonging to no social network in common with other affected families. The question is, of course, important and must always be asked in the event of such an outbreak. Clearly some physicians initially thought it was a "behavioral epidemic," an example of mass hysteria. Neurologic tests and tests of intellectual ability gave equivocal results; the school performance of children from the affected regions was consistently below the state average. These effects seem to be persistent. A shameful aspect of this episode was the failure of the state agricultural or public health authorities to react appropriately to repeated calls for help; there almost seemed to be an epidemic of official indifference to the occurrence of an obviously serious environmentally induced epidemic in farm animals and people. This led, among other things, to wide dissemination of dairy products contaminated with PBB. It is estimated that these products may have been consumed by 40 million people.[52]

Dioxins, chlorinated dibenzo-*p*-dioxins, include in particular 2,3,7,8-tetrachlorodibenzo-*p*-dioxin (TCDD), which is the most toxic of all man-made chemicals. Dioxins are not manufactured but occur as by-products or trace contaminants in such economically important substances as the herbicides 2,4,5-T and 2,4-D. One industrial process in particular, that used to make Agent Orange (a form of 2,4,5-T), produced high concentrations of contaminating 2,3,7,8-TCDD, and there is suggestive anecdotal evidence that servicemen exposed to Agent Orange in Vietnam, and the Vietnamese, suffered severely. Many developed chloracne, and a history of cancer and of birth defects among offspring is frequently found. Initial case-control studies of Vietnam veterans in the United States[53] and Australia[54] failed to find definite evidence of elevated cancer incidence or elevated birth defect incidence among offspring; however, later cohort studies of other groups, for instance U.S. agricultural workers[55] and Canadian farmers,[56] have found elevated incidence and mortality rates from non-Hodgkin's lymphoma and other soft-tissue malignancies. Other epidemiologic studies in Sweden and in New Zealand have shown a weak association between soft tissue sarcoma and lymphoma and past history of exposure to 2,4,5-T; these studies are based on small numbers but the consistent results must be respected.

There have been several acute environmental disasters with dioxin; the best-known was an explosion in a chemical factory in Seveso, Italy, in 1976.[57] There is, however, little evidence of permanent damage to human health in Seveso. The women in the town who were pregnant at the time almost all had therapeutic abortions, and examination of the abortuses did not reveal severe malformations.[58] In Love Canal, a dump site at Niagara Falls, N.Y., and at Times Beach, Mo., soil contamination with dioxins was a cause célèbre, generating great local and national anxiety;[59] but analysis of the data has not revealed evidence of lasting adverse effects on human health in either instance; adverse effects with long latency remain possible.

Dioxins and PCBs are nearly all very stable chemicals that persist in the environment. Because they are structurally similar to chemicals in essential enzyme systems of plants and animals and are fat-soluble, they enter food chains and, with progressive concentration, they can cause specific environmental catastrophes. For instance, in the early and mid-1970s, herring gull colonies in Lake Ontario suffered an epidemic of embryonic death (hatching failure) and high mortality of chicks associated with gross congenital malformations. The evidence implicates dioxins and PCBs. These were concentrated in the food chain that terminates with herring gulls, which had as much as 140 parts per million of PCBs in the liver and egg yolk.[60] This episode illustrates the way in which observation of wildlife populations can be used to monitor environmental concentrations of toxic chemicals.

Were human health and reproductive performance affected? Stillbirth statistics and available information on spontaneous miscarriage among families around the Great Lakes, particularly Lake Ontario, did not show miscarriages or stillbirths in excess of normal expectations. But the numbers were too small to generate stable rates, and reporting of miscarriages was incomplete and after the fact. Epidemiologic studies in situations such as this are very difficult; before we can conduct effective environmental monitoring, we need more complete information than was available to investigate this episode. Human tissue samples from many parts of the United States and Canada have been examined, and trace amounts ranging up to about 12 parts per billion have been found in fat; no demonstrable adverse effects on human health have been reported in association with occurrence of these toxic substances, but the period of observation is so far quite brief.

Pesticides

These are toxic substances that are deliberately added to the environment to do away with pests—insects, rodents, weeds, fungi, etc. They are a diverse group of chemicals, ranging from simple inorganic salts to complex compounds. Some have had far-reaching ecologic impact; for instance, dichlorodiphenyltrichloroethane (DDT), which is very persistent in the environment. Their economic benefits and often their beneficial effect on human health, as in the control of malaria and other mosquito-borne diseases, justify the claim that discovery and use of pesticides are among the most important contributions to improvement of the human situation in the 20th century. But many pesticides also have acute or chronic toxic effects on humans, or species we value. Their adverse effects, as well as their benefits, have been felt most acutely in the developing nations.[61] The toxicology and public health aspects have to be considered separately for each variety of pesticide (Box 4–6).

Organophosphorus compounds include parathion and malathion, which act by inhibiting acetyl cholinesterase. They are therefore neurotoxins. Both arthropods and humans can absorb these percutaneously. They cause

---

BOX 4–6. **Toxicology of Important Pesticides**

Organophosphorus compounds	Acute neurotoxic effects
Parathion, malathion	Anticholinesterase inhibition
Chlorinated hydrocarbons	Stored in fat
DDT	Concentrated in food chains
Hexachlorobenzene	Excreted in breast milk
Chlordecone (Kepone)	Severe toxicity
2,4-D and 2,4,5-T	2,4,5-T often contains dioxins
Paraquat	Lung and liver damage
DBCP	Spermatocidal

---

death by respiratory failure, preceded by restlessness, anxiety, convulsions, and coma. Parathion is so toxic that its use has been discontinued. Malathion, used to eradicate DDT-resistant mosquitoes in Pakistan, caused an episode of poisoning in nearly 3000 out of 7500 sprayers in 1975. Prevention of such episodes requires education of exposed workers and the use of protective clothing. Delayed neurotoxity, with symptoms and signs resembling multiple sclerosis, occurs with some organophosphorus compounds. The best known of this family of chemicals is not an insecticide but a plasticizer and cylinder lubricant, triorthocresylphosphate (TOCP), which has caused several epidemics of paralysis and death when it has contaminated food or cooking oil. There were 5000 cases and several hundred deaths in one episode in Morocco in 1959.

Chlorinated hydrocarbons include DDT, one of the first and best-known effective insecticides. The precise mode of action is unknown. Absorption may be percutaneous or by ingestion, and the lethal effect on insects is primarily neurotoxic. DDT is a CNS stimulant in fish, mammals, and birds. It is permanently stored in fat as dichlordiphenylethylene (DDE) and concentrated in food chains, including several terminating with humans. Fat metabolism in birds' and reptiles' eggs is impaired, endangering some species. The long-term effect of DDT on mammals is unknown, but it is unlikely to be good. Despite these reservations, DDT has had spectacular beneficial effects on human health, as the first successful means of controlling arthropod vectors of disease. During the Allied advance through Italy in World War II, a potentially deadly epidemic of louse-borne typhus was stopped in its tracks in Naples in 1943, and all over the tropical world, beginning soon after the end of World War II, malaria eradication campaigns depended heavily on residual spraying with DDT. It has been estimated that 20 million lives a year were saved and 100 million cases prevented by DDT in the early years of the campaign, which brought malaria under control for the first time ever in much of the world; with proliferation of DDT-resistant strains of mosquitoes, this approach no longer works, but it provided precious time and energy for affected countries to develop other control methods.

Hexachlorobenzene, another chlorinated hydrocarbon, is a fungicide, used to treat grain to prevent it rotting. In Turkey in 1956 it caused an epidemic of acquired porphyria cutanea tarda, with heavy fetal loss and infant mortality and morbidity. Hexachlorobenzene is produced as a by-product in other chlorinated hydrocarbon processes and is widespread as an environmental contaminant. It is also one of several important toxic substances that have been detected in human breast milk.[62] Chlordecone (Kepone) is a highly toxic chlorinated hydrocarbon insecticide developed in the late 1960s. It was being manufactured at a plant in Virginia in the early 1970s until about half the workforce developed bizarre and serious neurologic and psychiatric symptoms; many also had oligospermia or became sterile. Kepone is an animal carcinogen and may be a mutagen. Its production has ceased.

Herbicides include phenol derivatives, phenoxyaliphatic acids, and bipyridine. Phenol derivatives act by uncoupling oxidative phosphorylation, thus interfering with cellular respiration. The best known is 4,6 dinitro-*o*-cresol (DNOC); these are effective herbicides but can cause acute poisoning.

The **phenoxyaliphatic acids** include two well-known and widely used broadleaf herbicides, 2,4,5-T and 2,4-D. These are economically very important herbicides, which have been used worldwide since the mid-1940s. Concern about their possible adverse effect on human health arises because of the presence of dioxins, especially 2,3,7,8-TCDD, as contaminants of the manufacturing process. After carefully reviewing the evidence, a British scientific advisory committee in 1980 concluded that with the probable exception of the toxic effects of Agent Orange, there was little or no convincing evidence to justify banning or restricting herbicides of this variety, provided that adequate safeguards were employed to eliminate dioxin contaminants before distribution.[63] In view of the economic benefits from use of phenoxyaliphatic herbicides, this recommendation seems sensible. Even so, 2,4,5-T has been prohibited in many jurisdictions since the purported harmful effects of Agent Orange were publicized.

Bipyridyl herbicides include paraquat, which is medically important because its accidental or suicidal ingestion causes slow, agonizing death from progressive necrotizing pulmonary fibrosis. It has been used to spray illegal plantations of marijuana, and this may have led to a few cases of paraquat poisoning among persons who smoked the leaves retrieved before they had been destroyed by the spray.

Dibromochloropropane (DBCP) is a soil fumigant and nematocide. But it also kills human spermatozoa. The result is aspermia and sterility, which may be irreversible.

There is a perceptible body burden of many pesticides because of their ubiquitous use, their environmental persistence, and the tendency for some to be concentrated in food chains that include humans. The long-term effects are often difficult to study for the reasons already discussed and also, in the case of some that may be mutagenic, because of the length of human generations. No one is happy about the dissemination of so many toxic chemicals, but our civilization seems to have decided, at least by default, that the economic benefits outweigh the risks.

Toxic and Irritant Gases and Fumes

Some very important chemicals that make air unsafe to breathe are included in this group. Most occur in industrial and related settings and some as environmental pollutants.

Carbon dioxide is a simple asphyxiant when its concentration rises above 20 to 30 percent in respired air. It is colorless and odorless and can cause unconsciousness and death from asphyxia even though it is not really a toxic gas.

Carbon monoxide, on the other hand, is extremely toxic, combining with hemoglobin to form stable carboxyhemoglobin. It is a very common constituent of industrial emissions as well as exhaust fumes from internal combustion engines. It, too, is colorless and odorless but often occurs with other exhaust gases that provide warning of its presence.

Ozone is an irritant and toxic gas that causes inflammation of mucous membranes and conjunctiva. Chronic exposure may cause pulmonary fibrosis, and in animals it causes chromosomal damage. It is used as an oxidizing agent, a disinfectant, and deodorizer and has a number of other industrial uses.

Sulfur dioxide is an irritant gas, forming sulfurous acid on contact with moisture such as mucous membranes. It is the active ingredient in many smogs and is the principal component of industrial emissions responsible for acid rain. It is used in the manufacture of several economically important sulfur compounds, as a fumigant, and as a preservative.

Ammonia is irritant for the opposite reason: It forms a strong caustic alkali, ammonium hydroxide, on contact with mucus surfaces. Its industrial uses are numerous and so are many possible occupational exposures; it is the source for nitrogen in many compounds such as fertilizers, synthetic dyes, and plastics.

Phosgene decomposes to form hydrochloric acid, and this delayed effect leads to inhalation of potentially lethal amounts before the acute respiratory symptoms warn the victim. Phosgene is used to make dyes, to synthesize isocyanates, polycarbonates, and other economically important chemicals. It may have been one of the ingredients released to the atmosphere in the Bhopal disaster in 1984, in addition to methyl isocyanate.

Oxides of nitrogen include nitrous oxide, nitric oxide, and nitrogen dioxide, as well as various other combinations. Nitrous oxide is the anesthetic gas, but nitrogen dioxide and nitric oxide are irritant gases that form nitric and nitrous acid on contact with moisture. These are ingredients of

TABLE 4–4. ACGIH Standards for Irritant Gases

Gas	Time-Weighted Average (ppm)
Ammonia	25
Sulfur dioxide	5
Chlorine	1
Phosgene	0.1
Bromine	0.1
Ozone	0.1
Nitrogen dioxide	5

ACGIH = American Conference of Government Industrial Hygienists
(From Frank AL: Diseases associated with exposure to chemical substances—toxic and irritant gases. In Last JM (ed): Maxcy-Rosenau Public Health and Preventive Medicine. 12th ed. E. Norwalk, CT: Appleton-Century-Crofts, 1986, p. 684.)

some industrial smogs, notably in Los Angeles. Oxides of nitrogen are emitted in many industrial processes besides combustion of various fuels.

Table 4–4 gives the safety standards for toxic gases.

► AIR POLLUTION

A relationship between atmospheric pollution and respiratory disease has been consistently observed worldwide. Increasingly the main source of urban air pollution is not solid particulates and sulfur emissions from combusted coal, but oxides of carbon and nitrogen, aldehydes, and ozone from combusted petroleum fuels.[64,65] When coal is the principal industrial and domestic fuel, sulfur dioxide and solid particles are the pollutants, with smaller amounts of carbon and nitrogen oxides. Weather conditions can produce episodes of severe smog (smoke and fog) when warm, moist air loaded with pollutants is trapped below a layer of cold air. This combination produces acute, subacute, and chronic lower respiratory tract disease. The best known episode was the London smog of 1952, which lasted almost a week. I was in London then. It was an eerie sensation navigating the streets in fog that sometimes was so dense I could barely see my own feet (which were not far away; I am quite short). The acrid sulfurous fumes made my eyes sting, my throat burn, and induced a tickling cough that lasted until long after the fog dispersed. That episode of London smog caused a sharp increase in the number of deaths from respiratory disease (Fig. 4–2)[66]; the association with sulfur dioxide concentration was especially close, as the figure shows. Similar episodes, all with high sulfur dioxide concentrations, have occurred in many places, e.g., Donora, Pennsylvania; the Ruhr and Meuse valleys; and Tokyo. Clinical, experimental, and epidemiologic studies show that the most consistent relationship to chronic bronchitis and to acute inflammatory changes is with sulfur dioxide.

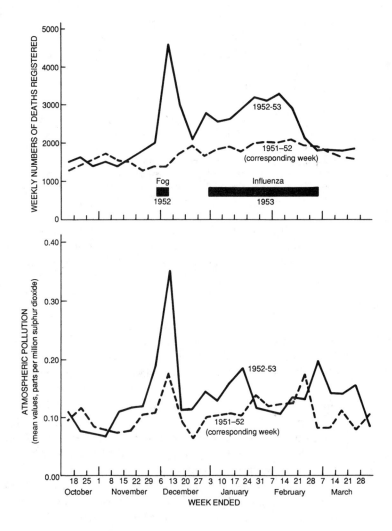

Figure 4–2. The great fog, or "smog," of December 1952. Weekly numbers of deaths registered in Greater London (*top*) in relation to levels of air pollution indicated by SO_2 (*bottom*), including all causes of death for all ages, both sexes. The 1953 influenza epidemic is also shown. *(From Morris JN:* Uses of Epidemiology. *2nd ed. Edinburgh: Livingstone, 1964, p 200.)*

The infamous Los Angeles smog, now appearing in many other congested urban environments with heavy automobile traffic, has a different origin and chemistry. Atmospheric inversions trap oxides of nitrogen (mainly from automobile exhausts), which undergo degradation by ultraviolet light from the sun to produce nitrogen dioxide, a brownish gas that is very irritant to the upper respiratory tract and conjunctiva. Ozone is also produced in toxic amounts.

Smoke abatement policies in Britain, largely in response to the 1952 smog episode, dramatically improved air quality. It is too soon to say whether there has been an associated decline in the incidence and mortality from chronic bronchitis; the confounding effect of cigarette smoking and the reduced prevalence of smoking also make it difficult to be sure.

The relationship between air pollution and respiratory cancer is difficult to determine for the same reason. Lung cancer incidence and mortality rates are higher in communities whose air is heavily polluted; but these are mainly working-class communities, where cigarette smoking has high prevalence, so the relationship of air pollution to lung cancer is almost impossible to unravel because of the confounding effect of smoking.

Air pollution is largely due to incomplete combustion of fossil fuels; if efficient furnaces and fuel-efficient cars and buses are used, there is much less release of solid particles and oxides of carbon, sulfur, and nitrogen. Other toxins, e.g., cadmium oxides, are also present in emissions from inefficient furnaces. Other components are benz(*a*)pyrene and anthracene carcinogens; these reach especially high concentrations in emissions from wood and other biomass fuels. A better solution for the problem of atmospheric pollution with combusted carbon-based fuels would be to develop alternative energy sources such as solar power and hydrogen-based fuels; even perfect combustion of carbon-based fuels does not reduce the greenhouse burden of carbon dioxide.

Indoor Air Pollution

Indoor air pollutants are biologic, physical, or chemical.[67] The important varieties, their sources, and some reported concentrations are shown in Table 4–5. Hazards to health come from several toxic gases, respirable suspended particulates, ionizing radiation, notably radon and its "daughters," and, of course, tobacco smoke, which may be the most important; in homes where parents or others smoke, children have significantly higher prevalence of respiratory disease than in homes where parents are nonsmokers, and the non-smoking spouses of smokers have higher rates of bronchitis and respiratory cancer than those whose spouses do not smoke.[68]

Radon and its radioactive daughter emissions can be a cause of respiratory and other cancers; an estimated 14,000 deaths each year in the United States might be attributable to radon.[69] The U.S. Environmental Protection Agency regards removal of radon from homes as a public health priority.[70]

Tragedies sometimes occur when carbon monoxide accumulates, for instance if insufficient exhaust ventilation is provided for indoor heating stoves. In developing countries, where cooking is often done over open wood

TABLE 4–5. Sources and Possible Concentrations of Some Indoor Pollutants in the United States

Pollutant	Sources of Indoor Pollution	Possible Indoor Concentrations	Location
Carbon monoxide	Combustion equipment, engines, faulty heating system	115 mg/m^3	Skating rinks, offices, cars, shops, homes
Respirable particles	Stoves, fireplaces, cigarettes, condensation of volatile substances, aerosol sprays, resuspension, cooking	100–500 μg/m^3	Homes, offices, cars, public facilities, bars, restaurants
Organic vapors	Combustion, solvents, resin products, pesticides, aerosol sprays	NA	Homes, restaurants, public facilities, offices, hospitals
Nitrogen dioxide	Combustion, gas, cookers, water heaters, dryers, cigarettes, gasoline engines	200–1000 μg/m^3	Homes, skating rinks
Sulfur dioxide		20 μg/m^3	Removal inside by absorption on surfaces
Suspended particulate matter (without smoking)	Combustion, resuspension, heating system	100 μg/m^3	Homes, offices, transportation, restaurants, native huts
Formaldehyde	Insulation, product binders, particle board	0.06–1.3 mg/m^3	Homes, offices
Radon and "daughter" products	Building materials	0.1–30 nCi/m^3	Homes, buildings
Asbestos	Fireproofing	< 1 fiber/cm^3	Homes, schools, offices
Mineral and synthetic fibers	Various products, cloth, rugs, wallboard	NA	Homes, schools, offices
Carbon dioxide	Combustion, humans, pets	5400 mg/m^3	Homes, schools, offices
Viable organisms	Humans, pets, rodents, insects, plants, fungi, humidifiers, air conditioners	NA	Homes, hospitals, schools, offices, public facilities
Ozone	Electric arcing, UV light sources	40–400 μg/m^3	Offices, airplanes

(From Global Environmental Monitoring System [GEMS]: Estimating Human Exposure to Air Pollutants. Geneva: WHO Offset Publication No. 69, 1982.[64])

fires inside village huts, toxic emissions from biomass fuels are an important cause of chronic respiratory damage and sometimes of respiratory cancer. About 400 million women in developing countries may be affected by this environmental health problem—the commonest occupational health problem of women in the world[71] (Table 4–6).

The biologic hazards in the indoor environment include many molds and other organic matter that is often allergenic; legionella, which may live

TABLE 4–6. Indoor Air Pollution from Biomass Fuel Combustion in Developing Countries

Location	Suspended Particulate Matter (mg/m³)	BaP (ng/m³)	CO (ppm)	Other
Nigeria, Lagos	—	—	940	NO₂: 8.6 ppm SO₂: 28 ppm Benzene: 86 ppm
Papua New Guinea, eastern highlands	0.84	—	31	HCHO: 1.2 ppm
Kenya, highlands	4.0	145	—	BaP: 224 ng/m³ Phenols: 1.0 µg/m³ Acetic acid: 4.6 µg/m³
Guatemala, two villages				
Poorly ventilated	—	—	26–50	
Well ventilated	—	—	15–31	
India, Ahmedabad				
Cattle dung fuel	16.0	8250	—	NO₂: 144 µg/m³ SO₂: 242 µg/m³
Dung plus wood fuel	21.2	9320	—	NO₂: 326 µg/m³ SO₂: 269 µg/m³
India, Gujarat	2.7–10.0	2220–6070	—	
Monsoon conditions	56.6	19,300	—	

BaP = Benz(a)pyrene; HCHO = Carbonic acid; NO₂ = Nitrogen dioxide; SO₂ = Sulfur dioxide.
(From Last JM: Housing and Health. In Last JM (ed): Maxcy-Rosenau Public Health and Preventive Medicine. 12th ed. E. Norwalk, CT: Appleton-Century-Crofts, 1986, p. 893, as modified from de Koning HW, et al: Biomass Fuel Combustion and Health. Bulletin WHO 63:11–26, 1985.)

in water-cooled air conditioning systems; and many varities of pathogenic microorganisms. *Mycobacterium tuberculosis* can survive for long periods in dark, dusty places. Infections of all kinds are spread more readily when homes are dirty, dusty, verminous, and rat-infested.

Ecologic Effects of Air Pollution

Human health in regions close to heavy industrial sites is allegedly "protected" by using tall smokestacks to dispel and supposedly dilute harmful emissions high in the atmosphere. This merely moves the pollutants to places farther away. The effects on the environment remain serious. Sulfur and nitrogen oxides combine with water vapor to produce sulfuric and nitric acid, which fall as acid rain. In upstate New York, Ontario, and Quebec downwind from the industrial coal-burning areas in the Ohio Valley, the rain has a pH as low as 4.0. This has a very damaging effect on freshwater ecology, killing many small forms of aquatic life. It also causes dieback at the tips of growing tree branches, and in time it kills the trees. Acid rain also damages the fabric of many public buildings as well as private dwellings. There are, perhaps unfortunately, no obvious ill effects on human health—if there were, we might take action against acid rain before all the lakes and forests in the affected areas are dead. Acid precipitation does, however, cause some respiratory damage: Especially in the form of acid fog, it increases the incidence of asthma and acute bronchitis.[72]

Increased combustion of fossil fuels since the beginning of the 20th century has led to an increase in the atmospheric concentration of carbon dioxide from about 200 to well over 300 parts per million. Reduction of forested areas (where carbon dioxide is metabolized to cellulose) has contributed to the buildup. By the mid-1990s, a scientific consensus has emerged that the increased concentration of atmospheric carbon dioxide is altering the climate[73] (see Chap. 11).

► WATER AND SOIL POLLUTION

"Environmental pollution" includes contamination of water and soil (and, of course, food). In the past, the most frequent harmful contaminant was human excreta, and this is still the case in many parts of the developing world. In the industrial nations we are more concerned about the dangers of local or widespread pollution resulting from a seemingly limitless variety of toxic chemicals described earlier. Since the 1986 Chernobyl disaster, contamination of the environment with radioactive material has been uppermost in many people's minds. The subject is too large to be dealt with in detail here; only highlights can be mentioned.[74]

Human excreta fouled the habitat of primitive peoples, fostering the spread of fecal–oral infections in the early days of human settlements. Excreta can be safely disposed of in a water-carried sewage disposal system, a septic tank, a chemical closet as used in commercial aircraft, or a pit privy. Details can be found in the references listed at the end of this chapter.

Water purification, meaning elimination of pathogenic organisms, is achieved in large water storage systems by filtration, both a mechanical and a biologic process, and chlorination; other procedures are sometimes also used; the chemical and engineering aspects are complex and interesting; see the references at the end of this chapter for details.

Industrial toxic wastes are the main cause of concern. Some have been alluded to already. Disposal is one of the emerging technologies, barely keeping pace with the proliferation of toxic substances, only some of which are covered by the provisions of the Toxic Substances Control Act in the United States and similar legislation in other countries. There are at least 10,000 hazardous waste dump sites in the United States that pose a threat to the public health and perhaps almost half a million altogether in which some potentially or actually toxic substances may be penetrating to aquifers. There is a casual attitude to disposal of chemicals, which are sometimes surreptitiously tipped into a sewer or allowed "accidentally" to leak from a tanker truck. The Superfund in the United States is aptly named: Super amounts of funds are needed to clean up contaminated environments. In some of the worst-affected parts of the world, e.g., many places in the former Soviet Union, the money simply is not available. The details are discussed in several of the references listed at the end of this chapter.

▶ PHYSICAL HAZARDS IN THE ENVIRONMENT

Under this heading we include ionizing and nonionizing radiation, heat and cold, and sound and pressure.

Ionizing radiation is part of the normal environment—cosmic and background radiation affects us all. The principal manmade source of radiation is x-rays; nuclear radiation is an increasingly important source and could become a major environmental hazard in the future, owing to problems of disposing of nuclear waste products and industrial accidents at nuclear power plants.

Ionizing radiation is mutagenic, carcinogenic, and teratogenic. It also causes cataracts, sterility or impaired fertility, alopecea, and other biologic effects such as premature aging.[75] Radiation-induced cancer follows exposure after a latent period of as little as 2 to 5 years for leukemia and 5 to 25 years in the case of other malignancies. Current evidence suggests that there is no threshold dose below which there is no risk of malignancy. Far smaller doses than those considered carcinogenic, when given to developing human embryos in the form of diagnostic x-rays that may be medically indicated for their mothers, have consequences that collectively can be described as premature aging.[76] Allowable exposure limits for those occupationally exposed to ionizing radiation are arbitrary. It is calculated that the current allowable limit of 0.02 to 0.026 rem per year may be responsible for 20 to 60 additional cancers per year among the 7.7 million persons occupationally exposed to radiation in the United States, whose annual cancer incidence is about 22,000 cases. This is considered an acceptable price in human lives for the benefits conferred by radiation, although the affected radiation workers doubtless take a different view of it.

The Chernobyl nuclear reactor disaster in 1986 led to a small number of immediate deaths among workers and those who attempted to contain the radiation leakage. By early 1996 the death toll from thyroid cancer and leukemia was mounting, especially among people who had been living at the time in the regions of heaviest radiation contamination[77] (Fig. 4–3, Table 4–7).

Since the collapse of the former Soviet Union, more information has come to light about serious radiation contamination in the period 1949 to 1956 near the Mayak complex, a plutonium production plant in the Ural Mountains; several other regions of the former Soviet Union were severely

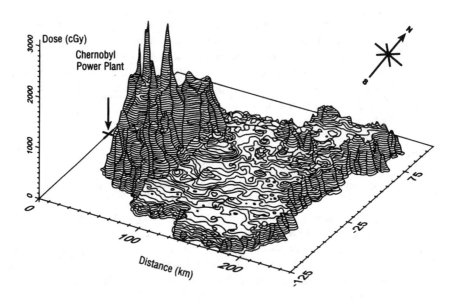

Figure 4–3. Average distribution of thyroid doses in children born in 1986, Chernlgovskaya region, Ukraine. *(Used with permission from Wld Hlth Statist Quar, 49, 1996.)*

contaminated by nuclear radiation and toxic chemical spills. Ultimately, many thousands of premature deaths will be attributable to these environmental disasters. Disposal of radioactive waste in all countries with nuclear power industries, not only in the former Soviet Union, is rapidly emerging as a serious, indeed intractable problem that will challenge environmental engineers in the early 21st century.

Ultraviolet (UV) radiation has several important biologic effects. It causes tanning by its effect on melanocytes and causes skin cancer, especially among fair-skinned people. Two varieties, nonmelanoma skin cancer and malignant melanoma, are both caused by UV radiation. The mechanism is activated through Langerhans cells in the dermis.[78] Langerhans cells play a crucial role in cell-mediated immunity as receptors for immunoglobulin (Ig) G molecules and interaction with CD4 and CD1 lymphocytes. Probably skin cancer of both types results from disruption of this process. Increased UV radiation could impair other immune responses such as reactions to immunizing agents, in this way adding to the risk of epidemic disease as a consequence of global change (see Chap. 11). The attenuation of stratospheric ozone is allowing increased surface-level UV radiation flux that is likely to lead in future years to increased incidence of skin cancer, both melanotic and nonmelanoma cancers. UV radiation also increases the risk of cataracts.

TABLE 4–7. The Structure of Cancer Mortality (Russian Population and Tartar–Bashkir Population)

	Russian Population				Tartar–Bashkir Population			
	Number of Cases		Standardized Mortality Rate per 100,000 PY		Number of Cases		Standardized Mortality Rate per 100,000 PY	
Site	Control	Exposed	Control	Exposed	Control	Exposed	Control	Exposed
All neoplasms	2980	611	113 (109–117)	143 (132–155)	425	163	86 (78–95)	133 (113–155)
Oral and pharynx	50	12	1.7 (1.3–2.2)	2.7 (1.4–4.7)	2	3	0.4 (0.05–1.41)	2.5 (0.52–7.3)
Esophagus	103	13	3.7 (3.0–4.5)	3.0 (1.6–5.1)	74	30	15.1 (11.9–18.9)	24.4 (16.5–34.9)
Stomach	1010	104	37.4 (35.1–39.8)	42.0 (34.2–51.1)	122	44	25.2 (20.9–30.1)	35.4 (25.7–39.2)
Other organs of GI tract	371	76	13.7 (12.3–15.2)	17.2 (13.5–21.6)	54	19	11.1 (8.4–14.5)	15.3 (9.2–23.9)
Lung and bronchus	499	98	18.6 (17.0–20.3)	22.4 (18.2–27.2)	72	21	14.9 (11.6–18.8)	17.2 (10.6–26.3)
Bone	47	7	1.9 (1.4–2.5)	2.0 (0.8–4.1)	7	0	1.4 (0.6–2.9)	0
Skin	24	8	0.8 (0.5–1.2)	1.8 (0.8–3.5)	0	4	0	3.6 (0.9–8.4)
Female breast	47	10	1.9 (1.4–2.5)	2.3 (1.1–4.2)	8	3	1.9 (0.8–3.7)	2.4 (0.5–7.0)
Uterine corpus and cervix	367	98	14.3 (12.8–15.9)	23.0 (18.7–27.9)	31	17	6.6 (4.5–9.4)	13.4 (7.8–21.4)
Other urogenital organs	173	38	6.4 (5.5–7.1)	8.7 (6.2–11.9)	25	7	5.3 (3.4–7.8)	5.7 (2.3–11.7)
Leukemia	64	19	3.2 (2.5–4.9)	5.6 (3.4–8.7)	6	8	1.3 (0.5–2.8)	6.8 (2.9–13.4)
Other gemo-blastoses	34	10	1.5 (1.0–2.1)	2.3 (1.1–4.2)	3	2	0.7 (0.14–2.0)	1.5 (0.2–5.4)
Other	191	38	7.8 (6.8–8.9)	10.5 (7.4–14.4)	21	5	2.2 (1.4–3.4)	5.3 (1.7–12.3)

Note: 90 percent confidence given in parentheses.
(From World Health Statistics Quarterly, 49, 1996.)

Infrared radiation produces thermal burns and can also cause cataracts. It is an occupational risk of workers in foundries and other hot environments.

Microwave radiation is the wavelength used for radar and in microwave ovens and shoplifting detection devices. This wavelength can cause deep tissue burns and can also disrupt the activity of cardiac pacemakers.[79] Prolonged exposure to microwave radiation, as among radar operators, may be associated with impaired fertility. Eastern European investigators have described vague intellectual and emotional disturbances associated with prolonged exposure to microwave radiation.

Lasers are pulsed electromagnetic waves, i.e., light waves in which all waves are in phase. They have several important scientific and industrial uses. Lasers can cause irreparable retinal damage and severe burns.

Video display terminals (VDTs) have become almost universal in offices throughout the industrial world. Do they emit radiation or have other harmful effects on health? Rigorous tests have failed to demonstrate evidence of emitted radiation. The harmful effects are ergonomic, a result of improper positioning of the screen in relation to the worker's head and hands; and visual, eyestrain caused by prolonged use of the video screen in situations where there is much reflected light. There are also psychologic effects, the result of heavy, monotonous workloads; a feeling of captivity by the keyboard; and perhaps insufficient work breaks. Box 4–7 summarizes what is known about the biologic effects of various forms of electromagnetic radiation.

Heat and cold effects are important in many occupational settings. Heat is generated by metabolic action and muscular effort and lost by radiation, convection, and conduction, and evaporant cooling associated with sweating.

BOX 4–7.   Effects of Electromagnetic Radiation

Frequency (Hertz)	Wavelength (Meters)	Type of Radiation	Effects
10^{22}–10^{18}	10^{-13}–10^{-10}	Gamma	Intracellular damage to chromosomes or mitochondria (high doses lethal) Neoplasia
10^{20}–10^{16}	10^{-12}–10^{-8}	X-rays	Premature aging
10^{17}–10^{16}	10^{-8}–10^{-7}	Ultraviolet	Tanning Melanoma Skin cancer Cataract Immune deficiency
10^{15}	10^{-6}	Visible light	Required to maintain life
10^{14}–10^{12}	10^{-6}–10^{-2}	Infrared	Cataract Tissue warming
10^{11}–10^{9}	10^{-2}–10^{-1}	Microwaves	Deep tissue damage ?Neuropsychic effects ??Carcinogenic
10^{12}–10^{2}	10^{-4}–10^{6}	Radio waves	No confirmed effects

In a hot environment these natural processes may be inadequate, and body temperature then rises. Electrolyte loss in sweat is another result of working in a hot environment. Heat exhaustion and heatstroke are serious medical emergencies, preventable by appropriate measures to maintain the working environment within the limits of physiologic adaptation. Similarly, exposure to a very cold environment can exceed the limits of physiologic adaptation, and hypothermia results.

Sound consisting of very loud noise, above 115 to 120 decibels, can damage the cochlea and permanently impair hearing. (See Fig. 4–4.) The damage to the cochlea depends on the duration and intensity of noise: It may lead to generalized hearing loss or impaired hearing over specific sound frequencies. Noise-induced hearing loss typically begins with loss at the 4000 Hz frequency. In an occupational setting, loud noise is also a hazard because it limits ability to hear warning signals. In many industries, a standard of 85 to 90 decibels is accepted as the upper limit of occupational exposure, above

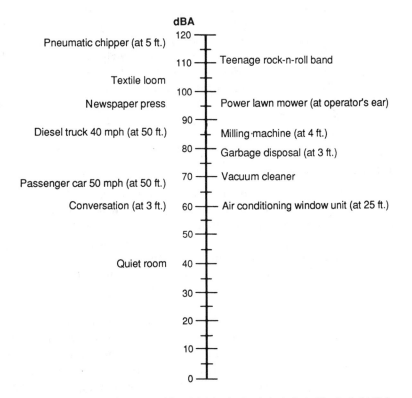

Figure 4–4. Occupational hazards—typical A-weighted noise levels in decibels: The decibel (dB) is a logarithmic measure of sound intensity. The "A-weighted scale" is used to weigh the various frequency components of the noise to approximate the response of the human ear. *(From MMWR Annual Summary 1984. Atlanta: Centers for Disease Control, 1986.)*

which ear protectors are required. The Occupational Safety and Health Administration (OSHA) standard is 90 decibels over an 8-hour time-weighted average. Ground crews at airports, exposed to 110 to 120 decibels, normally wear ear protectors. Patrons and employees in discotheques exposed to similar levels do not, and some have hearing loss in consequence. The prolonged, often irregular and unpredictable noise to which people who live under flight paths of busy airports or adjacent to busy highways or roadworks are exposed can cause sleeplessness, irritability, general malaise, perhaps impaired sexual function[80]—yet more discontents of modern civilization imposed upon us by the way of life we have chosen.

Pressure is also a physical environmental hazard. Extreme variations of atmospheric pressure are tolerable if the oxygen supply is maintained. Under high pressure, more oxygen and nitrogen are dissolved in blood and body tissue. Under extremely high pressure, e.g., scuba diving below 100 meters, so much nitrogen is dissolved that nitrogen narcosis results, with disorientation and loss of consciousness. This is preventable by replacing nitrogen with helium. Sudden reduction of pressure leads to release of dissolved gases from blood and tissues, with formation of bubbles—"the bends," so-called because of the acutely painful effect on joints. Under low pressure, vital processes are oxygen-starved. Prolonged life at high altitude (above 3000 meters) leads to physiologic adaptation—polycythemia, raised hemoglobin concentration, etc. Brief exposure to high altitudes of people acclimatized to sea-level atmospheric presure causes mountain sickness, a condition attributable to oxygen starvation, with cardiovascular, respiratory, and other systemic effects.

Occupational Injury

Some trades are dangerous and carry a high risk of death or disability from injury. Examples include mining, construction, forestry, deep-sea fishing, and road transport. Workers in these trades and in various other heavy industries have mortality rates three or more times higher than the national average because of injury. Epidemiologic study confirms that most occupational injuries occur under predictable circumstances and could be prevented by appropriate action. One obvious example is eye injury, especially corneal foreign bodies, one of the commonest of all occupational injuries. Most of these injuries would not have occurred if workers had been wearing protective goggles. Provision of safety equipment and making workplace environments safer are an important but regrettably often ignored responsibility of employers.

Many injuries in factories and on construction sites occur because of untidy working conditions. "Good housekeeping" can prevent many of these. Education of workers about safe and desirable work practices can prevent other injuries. For example, simple instruction about how to lift heavy weights can significantly reduce the incidence of incapacity resulting from injured backs, another high-incidence industrial injury. This is a very common occupational injury among nurses, who often have to lift heavy patients under ergonomically awful conditions.

Even office work can be hazardous, sometimes literally so because of indoor air pollution from tobacco smoke, photocopier solvents, and other pollutants, sometimes because of ergonomic problems, sometimes because of sexual harassment and intimidation.[81]

Industrial Dermatitis

This is the commonest of all occupational diseases. In surveys of workforce populations it accounts for up to 40 percent of the total occupational conditions.

The skin is a sensitive organ, easily and often damaged by solvents that remove protective natural secretions, by grease that clogs sebaceous glands, by chemicals that cause contact dermatitis, by abrasion, and in a variety of other ways. Some toxic chemicals, e.g., dioxins and PCBs, cause severe cutaneous reactions (chloracne) and many industrial chemicals cause various forms of dermatitis, which is a cutaneous manifestation of a systemic response. "Industrial" dermatitis is a common condition among women exposed to domestic detergents and other solvents, paints, etc. used in the home. Domestic work is, of course, among the most demanding, is unpaid, and often amounts to thankless lifelong drudgery.

Psychologic Factors

Only a minority of people in an industrial society enjoy their work. For many, work is just a necessity, providing an income to pay for food, shelter, and clothing. Lack of pleasure in achieving or having something to show for one's efforts can be depressing, demoralizing, and if sustained, can cause emotional, even perhaps physical illness. This is responsible at least in part for much industrial unrest. It is difficult to demonstrate the relationship by epidemiologic study, but suggestive evidence includes significant reduction in absenteeism and minor illness on the job when boring, repetitive assembly line work is changed to introduce variety, challenge, and an opportunity to use more initiative.

▶ PREVENTION AND CONTROL OF OCCUPATIONAL HEALTH PROBLEMS

This subject is best considered under the headings of environmental modification, personal protection, environmental monitoring, worker education, medical intervention, and government regulation.

Environmental Modification

This is the best option, because it directly addresses the hazards in and related to the workplace. Although opposed by some industrial and commercial interests on the grounds of expense, it may in the long run prove a good way to save money. For instance, efficient fuel consumption saves fuel as well as reducing environmental pollution. Enclosure of hazardous processes—where possible, their complete exclusion from human contact—is a worthwhile safety measure even when not essential to safeguard life and health. Guarding dangerous moving parts of machines falls into the same category. Some processes, e.g., work with explosive materials, can be isolated from other activities, so that the minimum number of workers will be at risk should mishaps occur. Extremely high-risk processes, such as work with radioactive substances, should be remote controlled. Wherever possible, hazardous substances and processes should be replaced with others that are safe, while achieving the same ends.

Ventilation—but not of toxic waste gases to the neighborhood of the factory—and removal of dusts, etc., from the air in the workplace is another form of environmental control.

Personal Protection

This is less satisfactory than the first option, because it does not eliminate the hazard and also depends on the compliance of those exposed to make use of protective equipment. There are many varieties of protective eqipment—respirators, safety glasses, ear protectors, safety gloves, hard-capped shoes, repellent clothing, worker-operated shielding devices between the worker and the hazardous process, etc.

Environmental Monitoring

An important component of industrial hygiene is measuring (monitoring) the levels of toxic substances, noise, etc., in the workplace. Workplace surveillance involves such practices as air quality monitoring to ensure the maintenance of levels of toxic contaminants, such as noxious gases, below the maximum allowable concentration or threshold limit value. Surveillance of workers may be a variation of this theme, as when workers exposed to ionizing radiation wear dosimeters that are periodically checked. Maintenance of safety standards in the workplace includes routine testing and maintenance of safety equipment. "Good housekeeping" ensures that the work environment is uncluttered, clean, well lit, that electric power outlets, gas taps, piping, etc., are secure and safe.

Worker Education

Most occupational risks can be reduced by knowledge and awareness. Instruction as to correct methods of lifting heavy weights helps to prevent back

injuries. Knowing that a substance is toxic may be sufficient incentive to follow the prescribed safety procedures. The educational message must be
transmitted intelligibly, and it is important to evaluate its effectiveness by ob-
serving the behavior of workers and the reduction of adverse outcomes. Management and labor can achieve most by working together, for instance on
preparing and conducting formal or informal educational programs. As well
as dealing with safe work practices and the need for personal hygiene, worker
education should include instruction in emergency measures such as first aid
(including resuscitation of the unconscious), discussion of the legal rights of
workers, and the facts about "right to know" legislation.

Many state and local laws have been enacted in the United States since
the first community right-to-know law was passed in Philadelphia in 1981.
These laws ensure that information about toxic and hazardous substances is
passed on from manufacturers to employers and, most importantly, to potentially or actually exposed workers and others who live in communities where
these substances are produced or used. The importance of such laws is that
they affirm the duty of employers and manufacturers to provide information
about risks, without a specific request from those who are or may be exposed
to risk. Under the Medical Access Rule of OSHA, employers must release
both medical and exposure data, but only on request. This is powerful protection if workers know about it.

Medical Intervention

Under this heading we can consider screening and periodic monitoring of
workers for exposure-specific health effects and routine surveillance of workers' health. A common form of surveillance is regular routine medical examinations, conducted with the aim of detecting early departures from normal
values, e.g., of hemoglobin or respiratory function. This is a poor substitute
for improving safety standards in the workplace but if for some reason that is
impracticable, routine examination of workers is a second-best option. This
approach has been used often in the past, e.g., to detect early evidence of
lead poisoning and occupational respiratory disease such as asbestosis and
silicosis.

► THE PHYSICIAN'S ROLE IN OCCUPATIONAL HEALTH

Physicians can become involved in occupational health in several ways. They
may be asked to examine workers or prospective workers and evaluate their
medical fitness for the job; they may be asked to determine whether an injury
or illness is work related. More formally, they may be asked to advise management or labor as to the medical safety of working conditions. Physicians who
perform such tasks may be paid a sessional fee by the employer; paid on a
fee-for-service basis by the employer, a union, or individual workers; work on

salary or contract for an industrial organization; or they may be paid by the insurer for a Worker's Compensation Board.

In many of these situations, a "third party" pays for the services that physicians render in their personal encounters with patients or clients. How does this modify the confidentiality of the doctor–patient relationship? The answer is that, strictly speaking, there is no alteration in the confidentiality of the doctor–patient relationship, no matter who pays for the service. If physicians are full-time salaried staff members working for an industry, their medical records must be kept in locked files, accessible only to authorized medical staff, not accessible to industrial management, labor union representatives, officials from the Worker's Compensation Board, or anyone else. At times, the physician may have to reassure patients or clients that the confidentiality of their relationship remains inviolable. Among other considerations, the adversary relationship that sometimes exists between management and labor may make it necessary for the doctor to demonstrate conspicuous impartiality. (See also Chap. 10.)

Of course doctors are required to state their medical opinion when asked (and paid) to do so. Before revealing to a third party any clinical details, such as precise results of physical examination or the diagnosis, the doctor must obtain the consent of the patient, i.e., the worker. This consent may be implied and is often explicit, in a consent form signed by the patient. The previously mentioned ethical issues are dealt with in a Code of Ethical Conduct for Physicians Providing Occupational Medical Services that was adopted by the American Occupational Medical Association in 1976 (Box 4–8). A similar code of conduct was approved by the International Commission on Occupational Health in 1992 (see Chap. 10).

In cases involving claims for worker's compensation it is even more important than at other times to maintain accurate and complete medical records. If a claim is contested, physicians can harm patients if their records are inadequate and lawyers find fault with them—and the physician can be humiliated by a cross-examining lawyer.

An increasingly wide range of diseases, as well as injuries sustained on the job, are subject to worker's compensation. Some of these diseases, such as poisoning by lead and certain chemicals, several kinds of occupational respiratory diseases, certain cancers, and many skin eruptions, are well recognized as occupational in origin, although the "legal" definition of compensable occupational disease varies from one jurisdiction to another, from time to time, and as determined by legal precedent or legislation.

An important responsibility of the physician is always to take a complete medical history. It may happen that a person is incapacitated by chronic respiratory disease that progresses relentlessly for years after employment in the dusty occupation that caused the disease has ceased. This would not be discovered by the physician whose curiosity ended with the question "What's your job?" It is necessary to ask about previous occupations, progressing methodically back to the beginning of the person's working life. If this is not

BOX 4–8. Code of Ethical Conduct for Physicians Providing Occupational Medical Services (Adopted by the Board of Directors of the American Occupational Medical Association, July 23, 1976)

These principles are intended to aid physicians in maintaining ethical conduct in providing occupational medical service. They are standards to guide physicians in their relationships with the individuals they serve, with employers and workers' representatives, with colleagues in the health professions, and with the public.

Physicians should:

1. accord highest priority to the health and safety of the individual in the workplace
2. practice on a scientific basis with objectivity and integrity
3. make or endorse only statements that reflect their observations or honest opinion
4. actively oppose and strive to correct unethical conduct in relation to occupational health service
5. avoid allowing their medical judgment to be influenced by any conflict of interest
6. strive conscientiously to become familiar with the medical fitness requirements, the environment, and the hazards of the work done by those they serve and with the health and safety aspects of the products and operations involved
7. treat as confidential whatever is learned about individuals served, releasing information only when required by law or by overriding public health considerations or to other physicians at the request of the individual according to traditional medical ethical practice; and recognize that employers are entitled to counsel about the medical fitness of individuals in relation to work but are not entitled to diagnoses or details of a specific nature
8. strive continually to improve medical knowledge, communicate information about health hazards in a timely and effective fashion to individuals or groups potentially affected, and make appropriate reports to the scientific community
9. communicate understandably to those they serve any significant observations about their health, recommending further study, counsel, or treatment when indicated
10. seek consultation concerning the individual or the workplace whenever indicated
11. cooperate with governmental health personnel and agencies and foster and maintain sound ethical relationships with other members of the health professions
12. avoid solicitation of the use of their services by making claims, offering testimonials, or implying results that may not be achieved; but they may appropriately advise colleagues and others of services available.

done, patients (sometimes their next of kin) can be deprived of compensation to which they are entitled.

Government Regulation

In the United States, several government agencies are concerned in surveillance and control of environmental and occupational health problems. These include the Environmental Protection Agency (EPA), OSHA, and the National Institute for Occupational Safety and Health (NIOSH). NIOSH recommends standards and exposure levels and OSHA sets them through a public policy-making process. The result can be standards that differ from the NIOSH recommendation. Many laws have been passed that relate to safety and hazard control in the workplace and the environment, e.g., the Toxic Substances Control Act.

Exposure Standards

Experience and laboratory tests have been the main bases for empirically determined exposure standards, i.e., amounts or concentrations of toxic substances that can be safely tolerated. The most commonly used scales of measurement are maximum allowable concentration (MAC), TLV, and permissible exposure limits (PEL). The choice of the scale is determined by the combination of toxic properties, e.g., whether the effects of the substance are or are not cumulative, and by other aspects of the work situation. The values for MAC, TLV, or PEL change from time to time as criteria are revised. These criteria are published in criteria documents for each of the substances concerned.[82]

► ENVIRONMENTAL DISASTERS

With disturbing frequency, mechanical or technical failure or human error cause serious dangers to health not only in industrial settings, but often also in the vicinity of industrial plants or related activities. The disaster may be acute, as at Seveso, Italy (1976), when a chemical explosion released highly toxic dioxins, or in Bhopal, India, in 1984, when a chemical factory accident released deadly methyl isocyanate, which killed several thousand persons and blinded or otherwise permanently maimed several thousand more (the largest industrial accident recorded anywhere so far). The already-mentioned explosion and meltdown at the Chernobyl nuclear power generating station in the former Soviet Union in 1986 caused about 30 immediate deaths, many cases of severe exposure to ionizing radiation, and made necessary the evacuation from their homes of scores of thousands of people. Each year since, the toll from radiation-induced cancers of the thyroid and from leukemia has mounted inexorably. These and other such disasters capture world attention and make headlines. They are one variety of disaster for which well-organized community-wide planning is required and should be in place permanently (see Chap. 8).

A different type of disaster that may proceed unnoticed by the public or the news media until its consequences become obvious, perhaps years after it begins, is insidious poisoning of environments by toxic chemicals. One such episode already alluded to was pollution of the Niagara River and subsequently of Lake Ontario with toxic chemicals from a dump site in Niagara Falls, N.Y., that led to a reproductive catastrophe among herring gull colonies on Lake Ontario in the early 1970s. Another toxic waste dump site in the same area, Love Canal, got much more publicity when toxic chemicals leaked into aquifers, were believed to have caused much ill-health and perhaps some cancer deaths, and led eventually to the evacuation of homes in the area. There have been several other episodes of this nature, e.g., Times Beach, Mo., where the soil was contaminated with dioxins; and Suffolk County, N.Y., and Woburn, Mass., where aquifers and wells were contaminated with a variety of chemicals, including leaded gasoline, ethylene dioxide, and carbon tetrachloride. In Woburn, pollution of wells is suspected as a causal factor in a local cluster of malignancies. Sometimes, as in Pelham, Minn., toxic chemicals have been dumped and forgotten for many years and cause harm when inadvertantly uncovered—in that instance, causing arsenic poisoning among those exposed. In all industrial nations there are now innumerable, often undocumented dump sites containing huge quantities of toxic materials of all kinds, from radioactive waste material with a half-life of thousands of years to chemicals that may combine with other seemingly innocuous substances with deadly consequences. Our descendents, perhaps many generations in the future, may have much cause to indict us for our criminal negligence in disposing so recklessly of these toxic wastes.

▶ HEALTH AND THE BUILT ENVIRONMENT

Throughout this chapter I have referred to ways in which the environment in the industrial and postindustrial age has exposed us to innumerable new health hazards: smog and other varieties of air pollution; toxic chemicals that foul the air, sea, and land; ionizing radiation, etc. Many of these hazards are an even greater danger to millions living in periurban slums and shanty towns in the developing world than they are in rich nations, a fact vividly illustrated in *World Resources, a Guide to the Global Environment 1996–97*.[83] This report is packed with valuable facts and figures as well as with graphic photos that tell far more eloquently than words ever can how bad living conditions are for half or more of the human race, and how health is affected thereby. I urge my readers to peruse this report. I use the term "built environment" to cover urban planning, domestic housing, public buildings, and enclosed sports facilities such as indoor skating arenas and enclosed sports stadiums. The health hazards associated with these diverse varieties of living and working spaces are many and various, and here there is space only to mention a few highlights. Some aspects have already been dealt with in earlier sections of this chapter. My focus is on health and ways to protect it rather than on diseases that arise because of unhealthy living and working environments.

The Health Promotion initiative of the World Health Organization had as one of its useful by-products, the "Healthy Cities" projects.[84] The aim of these projects is to improve the urban environment, quality of life, provide amenities for healthy living, and ensure that infrastructures necessary for health are in place and well maintained. The first "Healthy Cities" included

Toronto, Düsseldorf, Liverpool, and others—cities that were at one extreme already well managed and pleasant to live in and, at the other, urban "disasters" with blighted industrial areas, high unemployment, poor facilities, and inadequate, obsolete, or decayed infrastructure for health, education, social support, etc.

The American Public Health Association has published several editions of *Model Standards*[85] that spell out desirable, practical, and affordable standards for regional and local public health services, and these have included public health standards for housing and public use buildings, with details about needed facilities for provision of pure water, storing and preparing food, space required for office workers, domestic living conditions, and much more. These are intended as a guide to public health administrators and practitioners, but they do not have the force of law—although local political pressure can help to ensure that communities achieve the specified standards.

Public occupancy spaces such as enclosed sports stadiums are usually adequately lit, ventilated, and maintained so as not to present a danger to health. But occasional disasters still occur, for instance from collapse of tiered grandstands that crush spectators. Sometimes emergency exists are inadequate or are blocked and many people can die when a fire or other emergency leads to the need for rapid evacuation of a cinema, theater, or nightclub. Inspection and maintenance of such facilities is a joint responsibility of public health and fire department officials in some jurisdictions—a useful coalition that benefits all.

► OCCUPATIONAL HAZARDS IN THE HEALTH PROFESSIONS

The poet John Keats, a medical student, died of tuberculosis; so did innumerable other medical and nursing students, up to my own student days 50 years ago. Four students in a class several years ahead of mine were infected with tuberculosis, just before streptomycin and other antibiotics removed this threat. Other infections have always been common, often in the past ending in fatal septicemia after streptococci or other pathogens got into the body through punctures made by needle or scalpel. Nowadays the most feared infection is HIV; but hepatitis B and C are other risks, some preventable by vaccines that, it can be argued, should be given to all exposed medical and nursing students. All health professionals at all times are exposed to risks of infections with any of innumerable pathogenic microorganisms.

In the early days of x-rays, many doctors were exposed to excessive radiation, and many paid the price for this in cancer or leukemia; until recently, the mortality rates from these conditions were significantly higher among specialists in radiology than among specialists not exposed to radiation, such as psychiatrists. Knowledge of the hazards of ionizing radiation has led to use of radiopaque shields to protect radiologists and radiographers, and dosimeters show that their exposure to ionizing radiation is now no greater than that of anyone else in the health professions.

Exposure to anesthetic gases is associated with increased incidence of spontaneous miscarriage and birth defects among the offspring of operating room personnel and dentists. Occupationally exposed male workers have the same high incidence among offspring as female workers, suggesting that whatever is responsible must act by damaging chromosomes.

Physicians work under stressful conditions; sometimes they may have personality traits (perhaps related to their choice of a medical career) that render them susceptible to emotional disturbances. These factors could help to account for the high rates of suicide, alcoholism, and substance abuse that exist. Members of the medical profession have easy access to supplies of addictive drugs. Doctors also have a high rate of marital breakdown and of separations and divorces. To a lesser extent these problems are observed also among members of other health professions—dentists, pharmacists, and nurses. All of us lead such stressful professional lives that it's hardly surprising our personal and family lives sometimes get caught in the crossfire of conflicting claims on our emotions.

► **REFERENCES**

1. Guidotti TL, Cowell JWF, Jamieson GG, et al. (eds): *Occupational Health Services; A Practical Approach.* Chicago: American Medical Association, 1989.
2. Key MM, Henschel AF, Butler J, et al. (eds): *Occupational Diseases: A Guide to Their Recognition.* Washington, DC: U.S. DHEW, U.S. PHS, CDC, NIOSH, 1977.
3. Rom WN (ed): *Environmental and Occupational Medicine.* 2nd ed. Boston: Little, Brown, 1990.
4. World Health Organization: *Early Detection of Occupational Disease.* Geneva: WHO, 1986.
5. Raffle PAB, Adams PH, Baxter PJ, et al. (eds): *Hunter's Diseases of Occupations.* 7th ed. London: Arnold, 1994 [You should also consult earlier editions of this classic work, written solely by Donald Hunter, who wrote beautifully and gave many fascinating historical and anecdotal details based on cases he had seen and treated.]
6. Ramazzini B, Wright WC (trans): *De Morbis Artificum* (Diseases of Workers). Chicago: University of Chicago Press, 1940.
7. Townsend JC, Bodner KM, van Peene PFD, et al.: Survey of reproductive events of wives of employees exposed to chlorinated dioxins. *Am J Epidemiol* 115:695–713, 1982.
8. United Nations Scientific Committee on the Effects of Atomic Radiation: *Sources of Effects of Ionizing Radiation.* New York: United Nations, 1994, E.94.IX.11.
9. Harris JC, Rumack BH, Aldrich FD: Toxicology of ureaformaldehyde and polyurethane foam insulation. *JAMA* 245:243–246, 1981.
10. Easterly CE: Cancer link to magnetic field exposure. A hypothesis. *Am J Epidemiol* 114:169–174, 1981.

11. Armstrong BK, White E, Saracci R (eds): *Principles of Exposure Measurement in Epidemiology.* Oxford: Oxford Medical Publications, 1992.
12. National Research Council, Committee on Environmental Epidemiology (Miller AB, chairman): *Environmental Epidemiology; Public Health and Hazardous Wastes.* Washington, DC: National Academy Press, 1991.
13. Briggs D, Corvalán C, Nurminen M (eds): *Linkage Methods for Environment and Health Analysis.* Geneva: WHO, UNEP, USEPA, 1996.
14. Robertson AS, Burge PS, Hedge A, et al.: Comparison of health problems related to work and environmental measurements in two office buildings with different ventilation systems. *Br Med J* 291:373–376, 1985.
15. Hicks JB: Tight building syndrome. *Occup Health Saf* 51:1–7, 1984.
16. Wagner JC, Sleggs CA, Marchand P: Diffuse pleural mesothelioma and asbestos exposure in the Northwest Cape Province. *Br J Ind Med* 17:260–271, 1960.
17. Creech JL Jr, Johnson MN: Angiosarcoma of the liver in the manufacture of polyvinyl chloride. *J Occup Med* 16:150, 1974.
18. Smith ME, Newcombe HB: Use of the Canadian Mortality Data Base for epidemiologic follow-up. *Can J Public Health* 73:39–46, 1982.
19. Levine RJ, Andjelkovich DA, Shaw LK: The mortality of Ontario undertakers and a review of formaldehyde-related mortality sutdies. *J Occup Med* 26:740–746, 1984.
20. Lyon JL, Klauber MR, Gardner JW, et al.: Childhood leukemias associated with fallout from nuclear testing. *N Engl J Med* 300:397–402, 1979.
21. Black D, Adelstein AM, Berry RJ, et al.: Investigation of the possible increased incidence of cancer in West Cumbria; A report of an independent advisory group. London: HMSO, 1984. See also Gardner MJ, Snee MP, Hall AJ, et al.: Results of a case-control study of leukemia and lymphoma among young people near Sellarfield nuclear plant in West Cumbria. *Br Med J* 300:423–429, 1990.
22. Seagull EAW: Developmental abilities of children exposed to polybrominated biphenyls (PBB). *Am J Public Health* 73:281–285, 1983.
23. Schwartz EM, Rae WA: Efect of polybrominated biphenyls (PBB) on developmental abilities of young children. *Am J Public Health* 73:277–281, 1983.
24. Nebert DW, Elashoff JD, Wilkox KR, et al.: Possible effects of polybrominated biphenyl exposure on the developmental abilities of children. *Am J Public Health* 73:286–289, 1983.
25. Neutra R: Roles of epidemiology. The impact of environmental chemicals. *Environ Health Perspect* 48:99–104, 1983.
26. Kurihara M, Aoki K, Hisamichi S: *Cancer Mortality Statistics in the World 1950–1985.* Nagoya, Japan: UICC and University of Nagoya Press, 1989. See also Aoki K, Kurihara M, Hayakawa N, et al. (eds): *Death Rates for Malignant Neoplasms for Selected Sites by Sex and Five-Year Age Group in 33 Countries.* Nagoya, Japan: UICC and University of Nagoya Press, 1992.
27. Comstock GW: Water hardness and cardiovascular disease. *Am J Epidemiol* 110:375–400, 1979.
28. Schulte PA, Perera FP: *Molecular Epidemiology: Principles and Practices.* Orlando, FL: Academic Press, 1993.
29. Seller MJ: Genetic Counselling. In Gillon R (ed): *Principles of Health Care Ethics.* Chichester: John Wiley & Sons Ltd, 1994; pp. 961–992.
30. Monson RR: Occupation; Willett WC: Diet and Nutrition. In Schottenfeld D, Fraumeni JF (eds): *Cancer Epidemiology and Prevention.* 2nd ed. New York: Oxford University Press, 1997, pp. 373–405; 438–461.

31. Grandjean P: Health significance of metals. In Last JM, Wallace RB (eds): *Maxcy-Rosenau-Last Public Health and Preventive Medicine*. 13th ed. E. Norwalk, CT: Appleton & Lange, 1992, pp. 381–401.
32. Nriagu JO: A History of Global Metal Pollution. *Science* 272:223–224, 1996.
33. Needleman HL: Lead at low doses and the behavior of children. *Acta Psychiatr Scand* 67 (suppl):26–37, 1983.
34. Tong S, Baghurst P, McMichael A, Sawyer M, Mudge J: Lifetime exposure to environmental lead and children's intelligence at 11–13 years: The Port Pirie cohort study. *Br Med J* 312:1569–1575, 1996.
35. Tsubaki T, Trukayama K: *Minamata Disease*. Tokyo: Kodansha; Amsterdam: Elsevier, 1977.
36. Wills MR, Savory J: Aluminum poisoning. Dialysis encephalopathy, osteomalacia and anemia. *Lancet* 2:29–34, 1983.
37. Breteler MMB, Claus JJ, Van Dvijn CM, Lavner LJ, Hofman A: Epidemiology of Alzheimer's Disease. *Epidemiol Rev* 14:59–82, 1992.
38. Bako G, Smith ESO, Hanson J, et al.: The geographical distribution of high cadmium concentrations in the environment and prostate cancer in Alberta. *Can J Public Health* 73:92–94, 1982.
39. Kilburn KH: Pulmonary responses to organic chemicals. In Last JM (ed): *Maxcy-Rosenau Public Health and Preventive Medicine*. 12th ed. E. Norwalk, CT: Appleton & Lange, 1986, pp. 562–569.
40. Kilburn KH: Asbestos and other fibers. In Last JM, Wallace RB (eds): *Maxcy-Rosenau-Last Public Health and Preventive Medicine*. 13th ed. E. Norwalk: Appleton & Lange, 1992, pp. 343–361.
41. Selikoff IJ, Hammond EC, Seidman H: Mortality experience of insulation workers in the United States and Canada 1943–1976. *Ann NY Acad Sci* 3301:91–116, 1979.
42. Lilis R: Silicosis. In Last JM, Wallace RB (eds): *Maxcy-Rosenau-Last Public Health and Preventive Medicine*. 13th ed. E. Norwalk: Appleton & Lange, 1992, pp. 371–379.
43. Merchant JA: Coal worker's pneumoconiosis. In Last JM, Wallace RB (eds): *Maxcy-Rosenau-Last Public Health and Preventive Medicine*. 13th ed. E. Norwalk, CT: Appleton & Lange, 1992, pp. 365–370.
44. Colborn T, Myers JP, Dumanoski D: *Our Stolen Future*. New York: Dutton, 1996.
45. Marrett LD, King WD: *Great Lakes Basin cancer risk assessment: A case-central study of cancers of the bladder, colon, and rectum*. Ottawa: Bureau of Epidemiology, LCDC, Health Canada, 1995.
46. Acheson ED, Barnes HR, Gardner MJ, et al.: Formaldehyde in the British chemical industry. An occupational cohort study. *Lancet* 1:611–616, 1984.
47. Flamm WG, Frankos V, Acheson ED, et al: Formaldehyde. In Wald NJ, Doll R (eds): *Interpretation of Negative Evidence for Carcinogenicity*. Lyon, France: IARC and WHO, 1985, pp. 85–100. IARC Monograph No. 65.
48. Li MX, Cheng SJ: Carcinogenesis of esophageal cancer in Lin Xian, China. *Chi Med J (Engl)* 97:311–316, 1984.
49. Jacobson JL, Jacobson SW: Intellectual impairment in children exposed to polychlorinated biphenyls in utero. *N Engl J Med* 335:783–789, 1996.
50. Kuratsune M: Yusho. In Kimbrough ED (ed): *Halogenated Biphenyls, Terphenyls, Naphthalenes, Dibenzodioxins and Related Products*. Amsterdam: Elsevier, 1980, New York: Oxford University Press, 1980.

51. Anderson HA, Lilis R, Selikoff IJ, et al.: Unanticipated prevalence of symptoms among diary farmers in Michigan and Wisconsin. *Environ Health Perspect* 23:217–226, 1978.

52. Fischbein A, Bekesi JG, Tsang P: Polybrominated biphenyls (PBBs). In Last JM, Wallace RB (eds): *Maxcy-Rosenau-Last Public Health and Preventive Medicine.* 13th ed. E. Norwalk: Appleton & Lange, 1992, pp. 444–445.

53. Erichson JD, Mulinare J, McClain PW, et al.: Vietnam veterans' risk of fathering babies with birth defects. *JAMA* 252:903–912, 1984.

54. Donovan JW, MacLennan R, Adena M: Vietnam service and risk of congenital anomalies; A case-control study. *Med J Aust* 140:394–397, 1984.

55. Hoar SK, Blair A, Holmes FF, et al.: Agricultural herbicide use and the risk of lymphoma and soft-tissue sarcoma. *JAMA* 256:1141–1187, 1986.

56. Wigle DT, Semeciew RM, Wilkins K, et al.: Mortality study of Canadian male farm operators. Non-Hodgkin's lymphoma mortality and agricultural practices in Saskatchewan. *J Natl Cancer Inst* 82:575–582, 1990.

57. Fuller JG: *The Poison that Fell from the Sky.* New York: Random House, 1977.

58. Caramaschi F, del Corrno G, Favaretti C, et al.: Chloracne following environmental contamination by TCDD in Seveso, Italy. *Int J Epidemiol* 10:135–143, 1981.

59. Highland JH, Fine ME, Harris RH, et al., Environmental Defense Fund: *Malignant Neglect: Cancer and Environmental Pollution in the U.S.A.* New York: Knopf, 1979.

60. Peakall DB, Fox GA, Gilman AP, et al.: Reproductive success of herring gulls as an indicator of Great Lakes water quality. In Afghan BK, Mackay D (eds): *Hydrocarbons in the Aquatic Environment.* New York: Plenum, 1980.

61. *Impact of Pesticide Use on Health in Developing Countries;* Proceedings of a symposium held in Ottawa, Canada, 17–20 September, 1990. Ottawa: International Development Research Center, 1991.

62. Rogan WJ, Bagniewska MA, Damstra T: Pollutants in breast milk. *N Engl J Med* 302:1450–1453, 1980.

63. Advisory Committee on Pesticides: *Further Review of the Safety for Use in the UK of the Herbicide 2,4,5-T.* London: Ministry of Agriculture, Fisheries and Food, 1980.

64. Global Environmental Monitoring System (GEMS): *Estimating Human Exposure to Air Pollutants.* Geneva: WHO Offset Publication No. 69, 1982.

65. Seatton A: Particles in the air; The enigma of urban air pollution. *J Roy Soc Med* 89:604–607, 1996.

66. Morris JN: *Uses of Epidemiology.* 2nd ed. Edinburgh: Livingstone, 1964.

67. World Health Organization: *Indoor Air Pollutants: Exposure and Health Effects.* Copenhagen: WHO Reg *Publ Eur Series,* 1982. No. 78.

68. Office on Smoking and Health: *The Health Consequences of Involuntary Smoking: A Report of the Surgeon General.* Rockville, MD: U.S. Public Health Service, 1986.

69. Samet JM, Hornung R: Workshop on indoor air quality: Review of radon and lung cancer risk. *Risk Anal* 10:65–75, 1990.

70. *Radon: A Physician's Guide.* Washington, DC: U.S. EPA, 1993.

71. de Koning HW, Smith KR, Last JM: Biomass fuel combustion and health. *Bull World Health Organ* 63:11–26, 1985.

72. Bates DV, Sizto R: Air pollution and hospital admissions in Southern Ontario; The acid summer haze effect. *Environ Res* 43:317–331, 1987.

73. Intergovernmental Panel on Climate Change: *Climate Change 1995;* Vol. 1: *The Science of Climate Change;* Vol. 2: *Impacts, Adaptation and Mitigation of Climate Change.* Cambridge: Cambridge University Press, 1996.

74. Okun DA: Water quality management; Tanaka M, Takatsuki H, Itokawa Y: Solid waste disposal; pp 649–658; Dvorak V: Radioactive waste disposal. In Last JM, Wallace RB (eds): *Maxcy-Rosenau-Last Public Health and Preventive Medicine.* 13th ed. E. Norwalk, CT: 1992, pp. 619–648; 649–658; 659–660.

75. National Academy of Sciences: *Health Effects of Exposure to Low Levels of Ionizing Radiation.* Washington, DC: National Academy Press, 1990.

76. Meyer MB, Tonascia J: Long-term effects of prenatal X-ray of human females. *Am J Epidemiol* 114:304–336, 1981.

77. Health Consequences of the Chernobyl accident and other radiological events. *World Health Stat Q* 49:1:2–71, 1996. [Papers presented at an international conference held in Geneva, Switzerland, November 20–23, 1995.]

78. McKenzie RC, Sauder DN: Ultraviolet radiation: Effects on the immune system. *Ann Roy Coll Phys Surg Can* 27:20–26, 1994.

79. Environmental Protection Agency: *Biological Effects of Radiofrequency Radiation.* Research Triangle Park, NC: EPA, 1984.

80. Fay TH (ed): *Noise and Health.* New York: NY Academy of Medicine, 1991.

81. Stellman J, Henifin MS: *Office Work Can Be Dangerous to Your Health.* New York: Pantheon, 1983.

82. Revisions are published from time to time in *Morbidity and Mortality Weekly Reports.*

83. World Resources Institute, UN Environment Programme, UN Development Programme, World Bank: *World Resources: A Guide to the Global Environment, 1996–97.* New York: Oxford University Press, 1996.

84. Ashton J (ed): *Healthy Cities.* Milton Keynes, England: Open University Press, 1992.

85. *Healthy Communities 2000; Model Standards. Guidelines for Community Attainment of the Year 2000 National Health Objectives.* 3rd ed. Washington, DC: APHA 1991.

5

Food and Nutrition

The quality and quantity of food are important determinants of individual and community health. Disease can occur if food is contaminated by pathogenic microorganisms, toxic chemicals, or any of innumerable adulterating substances. Health is also endangered if we do not get enough to eat or if food lacks essential ingredients such as vitamins or minerals. The nutritional needs of pregnant and lactating women, of infants, and of growing children are of special concern. Other groups whose nutrition often needs careful management include postoperative patients, people who suffer from disorders of absorption or metabolism of food, and elderly people, particularly if they live alone and do not have help from family, friends, or neighbors.

At the cusp of the millenium, there is rising concern about global food security. With the population increasing by about 85 million a year, declining fish stocks in many formerly bountiful coastal and ocean fishing zones of the world, a stationary or falling yield of many grain crops,[1] and intimations of further decline that might accompany global warming, there are renewed doubts about the Earth's carrying capacity (see Chap. 11). Food security is rightly regarded as a matter of national importance in virtually all countries in the world. Disruption of food supplies by destruction of crops, blockade, attacks on supply lines, etc., has been a weapon of war at least since the time of Thucydides in the golden age of Athenian civilization. Pests and natural disasters like floods and droughts, too, can devastate food supplies and cause famine, have done so repeatedly from biblical times to the present day, and doubtless will again in the future.

▶ FOOD QUALITY

Increasing urbanization and mechanization of agriculture have led to the separation of producing regions from consuming populations. After food has been grown and harvested or slaughtered, it must be processed, packed, transported, stored, and sold through wholesale and retail outlets. The processing often takes place in a factory, but it is sometimes done in small-scale farm-based settings where control over possible contamination is difficult to ensure. This is especially true when these settings are in another country. Food production is an international activity, partly controlled by transnational corporations, but mainly conducted by innumerable independent growers, processors, shippers, etc. Depending on seasonal fluctuations, people in North America or Western Europe eat fruit and vegetables, meat and fish grown and prepared for the market in Africa, Latin America, the Middle and Far East. We are dependent on food hygienists and inspectors in all parts of the world and sometimes rely on attenuated lines of transport and communication. There are seemingly endless possibilities for harm from impure food, notably gastrointestinal infection caused by exotic pathogens[2]; yet serious episodes of food-borne disease occur rarely, mild and moderate episodes infrequently. How so?

The potential hazards to health at all stages between production and consumption are nearly all well controlled by a combination of legislated surveillance and self-regulation by the food industry. National legislation dealing with safety, purity, and wholesomeness of foods is reinforced by local ordinances in many states and municipalities. Inspection, particularly of meat and dairy products and certain processed foods, is conducted at national and local levels. When food is transported interstate, there is often another stage of state inspection between federal and local levels. The surveillance of local food outlets, dairies, slaughterhouses, bakeries, restaurants, hospital and other institutional kitchens, etc., is conducted by health inspectors who are usually employed by the local health department (see Chap. 8). Unsanitary premises can be closed and the proprietors can be fined or even charged with a criminal offence for violating health laws and regulations.

The food industry—producers, processors, shippers, wholesale and retail dealers—share a powerful economic incentive to reduce loss from spoilage, contamination, and deterioration. Moreover, there is a strong incentive to promote attractiveness, wholesomeness, and long shelf life. All these factors lead to an efficient series of self-regulatory measures by the food industry, and most of these measures—but not all of them—are in the public interest.

▶ FERTILIZERS, GROWTH REGULATORS, AND PESTICIDES

Production of food by mechanized agriculture is heavily dependent on the use of fertilizers, growth-enhancing substances, and many kinds of pesticides. Some of these can have adverse effects on human health (see Chap. 4).

Fertilizers are not harmful to human health. Whether naturally occurring or artificially produced, nitrogenous chemicals are metabolized the same way by vegetable and grain crops. There is no intrinsic difference in the quality of bread, for instance, attributable to its production from grain that was fertilized "naturally" with manure or "artificially" with chemicals produced in a factory. Of course human or animal excreta used as fertilizer can contain pathogens, and these can contaminate the surface of plants, fruits, and vegetables; but the pathogens do not become an intrinsic part of the plant itself.

Growth-enhancing substances include antibiotics and hormones. Antibiotics are added to animal feed to reduce or eliminate animal pathogens that might otherwise cause cattle, pigs, poultry, etc., to be sickly and undersized. The growth of the animals is thereby made more rapid and vigorous. However, antibiotic residue can persist in the carcass, and this can cause symptoms in persons who are sensitive to the antibiotic; it also contributes to the development of resistant strains of human pathogens. For these reasons, the use of antibiotics to enhance growth of animals used as human food is illegal in many jurisdictions. Meat from animals treated with antibiotics in places where this is legal may not be imported into places, such as the United States, where it is not.

Many pesticides are used at several stages between the production and consumption of food. Some of these can have adverse effects on human health. Herbicides include 2,4,5-T, which may contain trace amounts of toxic dioxins (see Chap. 4). This hazard has led to the prohibition of 2,4,5-T in many parts of the world; only the less toxic herbicide 2,4-D is now permitted. Fungicides include mercurials used to treat seed corn; a lethal epidemic of mercury poisoning occured in Iraq in 1956 when seed corn treated in this way was eaten during a famine. Captan has been used as a fungicidal spray on crops such as strawberries grown close to the ground; it is a suspected animal mutagen and carcinogen; its use is restricted or prohibited in many states. Some insecticides, including dichlorodiphenyltrichloroethane (DDT), are very persistent and may be concentrated as they move through the food chain that ends with humans. This and other pesticides, especially in the chlorinated hydrocarbon family, are stored in fat and excreted in human milk. The economic and health-related benefits of many pesticides are undeniable. Their potentially or actually harmful effects on human health are usually slight, although some effects, and especially the delayed ones, are poorly understood. There is enough uncertainty to justify caution in using pesticides in situations where they may contaminate or otherwise enter foods that humans eat. Those that have a chemical structure resembling naturally occurring components of metabolic or enzyme transformations in the human body are likely to remain permanently in the human body or to have a very long half-life. Those that are excreted in breast milk can expose newborn infants to high concentrations, because infants are at the end of the food chain in which these chemical contaminants are concentrated.[3] Fat-soluble polychlorinated biphenyls (PCBs) can be ingested in large quantities from certain foods, notably lake fish; PCBs pass through the placental barrier to the developing fetus and are excreted in breast milk, too, so breast-fed infants can absorb excessive quantities that remain permanently in their fatty tissues—and brain. Children exposed to PCBs in this way can suffer intellectual impairment.[4] PCBs and certain pesticides that structurally resemble and therefore mimic natural hormones ("environmental estrogens") may be responsible for empirically observed declining sperm counts and other potentially harmful effects on human reproduction[5] (see Chap. 4).

▶ TRANSMISSION OF DISEASE BY FOOD

Contamination of food with raw sewage or with human excreta containing pathogens often occurs when vegetables are grown in unsewered or poorly sanitated communities. If these vegetables are eaten raw, fecal–oral transmission of disease is almost certain to occur. The only effective protection is cooking. Thorough washing with a disinfecting solution may be an acceptable alternative for vegetables normally eaten raw, such as lettuce; but where there is any possibility of contamination with pathogens such as *Salmonella typhi* or the cysts of amebic dysentery, washing with a disinfectant, however thoroughly, gives quite inadequate protection.

Disease can be transmitted by food in many other ways. Pathogenic microorganisms can gain access to food that is not screened from flies, e.g., uncovered food displayed in open markets. Food handlers can pass on infection, such as shigella and salmonella, via their hands or clothing and can transmit tuberculosis, diphtheria, streptococcal infection, etc.

Meat Hygiene

Meat may come from diseased animals and be capable of causing human disease. The most important disease in this category is tuberculosis. Certain parasitic helminths in which the stages of the parasite's life cycle are passed in different animals also fall into this class. Trichinosis, beef and pork tapeworm, and the fish tapeworm are examples. Table 5–1 summarizes the important helminth parasites that can be transmitted by food, their distribution, and control measures. Meat inspectors in abbatoirs condemn animals that are identified as diseased before slaughter, and carcasses found to be diseased after slaughter. The health of abbatoir workers is also monitored both in the public interest and for the sake of the workers themselves; they are at risk of several diseases, notably Q fever and brucellosis.

Sanitary Control of Milk

Milk and milk products are peculiarly susceptible to contamination with pathogenic microorganisms. Some pathogens can be excreted in the milk of the diseased cow, e.g., bovine tuberculosis and streptococcal infections; others are introduced into the milk by dairy workers, e.g., diphtheria, typhoid,

TABLE 5–1.   **Helminth Parasites Transmitted by Food**

Parasite	Infection Source	Condition Caused	Distribution	Control
Nematodes				
Hookworms	Larvae penetrate skin	Enteritis Anemia	Tropics, subtropics	Sanitation Wearing shoes
Pinworms	Fecal–oral	Pruritus ani	Worldwide	Hygiene Sanitation Education

Ascaris
  (roundworms)
	Fecal–oral,
	  e.g., vegetables
		Enteritis
		Pneumonitis
			Worldwide	Sanitation

Trichinella	Undercooked meat,
	  especially pork
		Trichinosis	Worldwide	Abbatoir
				  inspection
				Cooking

Dracunculosis	Intermediate host in drinking water	Skin sores	Tropics	Sanitation Safe water Education
Trematodes (Flukes)				

Fasciola
  hepatica
	Vegetables, grass,
	  watercress
		Hepatitis	Worldwide	Sanitation
				Education
				Eradicate
				  from pigs

Clonorchis *sinensis*	Undercooked fish	Hepatitis	China, SE Asia	Sanitation Education Thorough cooking
Heterophyes *heterophyes*	Undercooked fish	Enteritis	N. Africa, SE Asia	Sanitation Thorough cooking
Paragonimus *westermani*	Undercooked crab	Pulmonary cysts	SE Asia	Education Thorough cooking

Schistosoma	Larvae penetrate
	  skin
		Enteric or
		  vesical
		  inflammation
			Far East, Africa	Sanitation
				Eradicate snails
				Education

Cestodes **(Tapeworms)**				
Taenia solium	Undercooked pork	Enteritis	Worldwide	Sanitation Education Thorough cooking
Taenia saginata	Undercooked beef	Enteritis	Worldwide	Sanitation Education Thorough cooking

Echinococcus
  granulosus
	Eggs in dog feces	Cysts in lung,
		  liver, etc.
			Worldwide	Education
				Dispose of offal
				  away from dogs

Diphyllobothrium	Undercooked fish	Enteritis, anemia	N. Europe N. America	Education Cooking

and streptococcal and staphylococcal infections. Milk is an excellent culture medium for many microorganisms, and this accounts for the frequency with which it is the vehicle for transmission of infection (Table 5–2).

The best and most widely used method of making milk safe is pasteurization; boiling is a method of sterilization. Several pasteurization techniques are used, with different combinations of time and temperature to kill pathogens without altering the flavor or consistency of the milk. Pasteurization is often combined with other processes such as homogenization to improve the appearance and ostensibly the flavor of milk. Other ways to safeguard milk products include freeze-drying and condensing. Sweetened condensed milk, like other sweet preparations, relies on the high sugar concentration to kill pathogens.

▶ **FOOD POISONING**

There are several varieties of food poisoning (Box 5–1).

1. **Infection with pathogenic organisms.** These include viruses, bacteria, and parasites. Examples include viral gastroenteritis, e.g., resulting from rotavirus infection, salmonellosis, shigellosis, and trichinosis. Epidemics or sporadic cases can occur with most of these; their investigation is an important and frequent task of epidemiologists (see Chap. 3).

2. **Bacterial food poisoning.** The disease here is due to a toxic product or metabolite of the microorganism that has contaminated food. Examples are staphylococcal enterotoxic gastroenteritis and botulism. Staphylococcal food poisoning is common, usually attributable to

TABLE 5–2. Important Milk-Borne Diseases

Contained in cow's milk
  Tuberculosis
  Streptococcal infections
  Staphylococcal infections
  Brucella abortus
  Milk can also contain pesticides, antibiotic residue, PCBs, dioxins, radioactive trace elements

Contained in goat's milk
  Brucella

Transmitted by milk handlers
  Typhoid
  Diphtheria
  Staphylococcal, streptococcal infections
  Numerous *Salmonella*

PCBs = polychlorinated biphenyls.

BOX 5–1.   **Features of Varieties of Food Poisoning**

Type	Features
Infection (bacterial, viral, etc.)	Vomiting, nausea, diarrhea Systemic symptoms (fever, etc.) Variable incubation and duration Transmissible to others
Bacterial toxins	
Staphylococcal enterotoxin	Explosive onset after short incubation Vomiting predominates Few or no systemic symptoms Not transmissible
Botulism	Slow onset Neurotoxic symptoms Not transmissible
Plant, animal poisons	Short incubation Dramatic symptoms, usually gastrointestinal
Chemical contamination	Variable incubation—minutes to days Widespread systemic effects

storage of food for a few hours or longer after preparation but before consumption under conditions that enable the staphylococcus to proliferate and produce its enterotoxin. This toxin is heat stable and has no detectable flavor or odor. Botulism, produced by the toxin of *Clostridium botulinum,* is far more serious. *Clostridium botulinum* is anaerobic, and its growth produces a foul odor as well as the extremely powerful toxin that causes botulism.

3. **Chemical food poisoning.** Most often this follows accidental contamination of food with chemicals, but sometimes food is deliberately adulterated. There have been many famous episodes, some with large numbers affected and tragic consequences. Any kind of chemical may be involved; if it is one with few initial symptoms or signs and a slow onset or prolonged latent period before adverse effects are apparent, large numbers of people can be affected and it can be difficult to trace the origins of the episode. Table 5–3 lists some well-known episodes of chemical food poisoning. The Spanish cooking oil disaster was particularly difficult and unpleasant.[6] It had several unique features: a long, variable incubation time up to several weeks and symptoms affecting variously the renal, respiratory, and central

TABLE 5–3. Some Episodes of Chemical Food Poisoning

Year	Place	Source	Numbers Affected
1951	Provence, France	Ergot in flour	c. 600
1955	Minamata, Japan	Seafood, methylmercury	c. 1000 Brain damage
1959	Morocco	TOCP	c. 10,000 Many permanently disabled
	Iraq	Ethylmercury (in corn)	c. 1000
1968	Yusho, Japan	PCBs	c. 1700 Some permanent disability
1971	Iraq	Methylmercury (in corn)	50,000 Many permanent
1981	Spain	Toxic oil	12,000 Many deaths

PCBs = polychlorinated biphenyls; TOCP = Triorthocresylphosphate.

and peripheral nervous systems. It is still not known what toxin caused this, although there is no doubt that it occurred in a batch of rapeseed oil, either as a contaminant or as a result of biologic interaction. As well as adulteration of food with toxic chemicals, chemical food poisoning can arise because utensils or containers are contaminated, if the chemical is very toxic and only small quantities are required to cause harm; sometimes the utensils themselves may be toxic or interact with the food being stored or prepared. George Baker investigated Devonshire colic in an early epidemiologic study,[7] in 1767. He showed it to be due to poisoning with lead salts produced in acidic cider by chemical interaction with the lead-lined cider vats. Episodes of lead or antimony poisoning are still caused this way occasionally.

4. **Poisons of plant or animal origin.** Poisonous shellfish and fungi are sometimes eaten in the mistaken belief that they are edible. This is most likely to happen when people are unfamiliar with local hazards, so travelers and immigrants are at high risk. In 1951, in a rural general practice in South Australia, I had to deal with an unforgettable and dramatic medical emergency when an entire large family of immigrants new to the community cooked and ate a basket of the local toadstools, which resembled edible fungi familiar to them in Europe. They were all very ill with symptoms of muscarine toxicity. Fortunately all recovered; and, wiser after the event, the family warned other immigrants about their unhappy experience.

► METHODS OF MAKING FOOD SAFE

Cooking

The discovery that some foods, especially meat, taste better and are more easily digested when they have been cooked is so ancient that the genius responsible cannot be commemorated. It is pleasant to reflect on the likelihood that this discovery, like the other great ancient discovery of agriculture, was among the contributions to improvement of the human condition made by women, while their menfolk were off hunting and gathering. Almost incidentally it is worth adding that cooking exposes most pathogens in food to enough heat to kill them.

Freezing, Drying, Preserving

Pickling food in brine or vinegar makes an inhospitable environment for most pathogens. Similarly, a dry environment is inhospitable, inhibiting reproduction of many pathogens. Freezing suspends bacterial multiplication and kills many but not all pathogens. Frozen food, once thawed out, can again become a vehicle for bacterial multiplication and food poisoning. Typhoid bacilli are among the pathogens that survive freezing, so ice cream is occasionally incriminated as the source of an outbreak. Frozen foods in general must be considered potentially contaminated in places where food safety cannot be guaranteed.

Irradiation of Food

Ionizing radiation is another way to kill microorganisms, both pathogens and nonpathogens. This process is a by-product of the nuclear power industry. It is an effective way to preserve the natural color and flavor of foods such as strawberries and other delicate fruits. There is no residual ionizing radiation in irradiated food, but this method of preservation is distrusted by some people because of irrational fears about radiation.

Chemical Preserving

Several chemicals create an environment hostile to pathogens. Pickling in brine or vinegar or suspension in a supersaturated sugar solution (syrup) are traditional forms of chemical preservation that have been used for over 2000 years. Sulfur dioxide, benzoic acid, and carbon dioxide are among widely used modern chemical preservatives. There is no hazard to consumers of food preserved in these ways. Sulfites were banned by the Food and Drug Administration (FDA) in 1986: They can cause severe reactions in some people who consume food that contains or is contaminated by sulfites.

Canning

Commercial canning of foods is accompanied by heating to a temperature sufficient to kill pathogens, and the canned food is then sealed to exclude air. The process renders almost all foodstuffs safe for prolonged periods; cans as old as 50 years may be opened and their contents eaten safely, provided the can has remained intact. Occasional hazards arise from additives intended to preserve or enhance the color or flavor of the food. In the past some canning processes that involved the use of lead or antimony seals exposed people to the risk of lead or antimony poisoning. A more serious risk, especially with home-canned food is contamination with the spores of *C. botulinum*, which, as noted earlier, grows anaerobically and produces a toxin that is among the most poisonous substances known, the cause of botulism.

Food Additives

Chemicals are added to food to prevent bacterial proliferation, to enhance flavor or color, and to prolong shelf life. A few additives are actually or potentially toxic. Some cause food allergies. Nitrites combine with amines to produce nitrosamines, which are carcinogenic. Monosodium glutamate (MSG) is a widely used preservative that prolongs shelf life; it is very popular in Chinese cooking. Some people develop an allergy to MSG, which leads to severe and uncomfortable flushing and burning sensations, nausea, and headaches; but MSG has no known lasting adverse effects.

▶ NUTRITIONAL REQUIREMENTS

To maintain normal bodily functions, we must replenish energy we burn in the course of our activities and ingest protein, vitamins, minerals, and other substances that are essential for many enzyme systems as well as for growth, tissue repair, and regeneration. The range of dietary requirements is broad, and it broadens further when there are demands such as periods of rapid growth in childhood and adolescence, pregnancy, and when metabolic demand is enhanced by infection. Many nations including the United States, Canada, the United Kingdom, and other nations of the European Union have standing or ad hoc advisory committees that review and revise tables of Recommended Dietary Allowances (RDAs) of carbohydrates, fats, proteins, minerals, and vitamins. In the United States, this task is carried out by the Food and Nutrition Board of the National Academy of Sciences; the periodic revisions of RDAs are published in journals of nutrition and public health and are available in reference form.[8] If we habitually fall short of requirements, nutritional deficiency diseases occur; if we habitually exceed them, obesity is the commonest consequence.

► NUTRITIONAL DEFICIENCY DISEASES

Up to one third of the world's population goes hungry for much or most of the time. Most of the people who do not get enough to eat live in the dry savannah country of Africa, in the overcrowded nations of Asia, and in the urban slums of Latin America. In the 1980s, there were widespread famines in Africa, and in the 1990s, largely associated with war and genocide, further localized and regional famines have occurred again but in different regions, notably southern Sudan and in the refugee communities on the Rwanda–Burundi–Zaire borders. In the aftermath of the Gulf War and the imposition of sanctions, very severe food shortages approaching famine affected many of the people of Iraq. Also in the early 1990s, the economic and political disruption of parts of the former Soviet Union and the conflicts in the former Yugoslavia caused several very severe localized periods of food shortage. A series of natural disasters, mainly floods, probably aggravated by inefficient production and distribution, caused famine in North Korea in 1995 and 1996. At any time, small numbers of undernourished or starving people can be found almost anywhere, even in the richest cities in the affluent industrial nations. They may starve because of inadequacies in the social services. In the United States, victims of this situation include some elderly people on inadequate pensions; children of low-income parents, especially single parents; and marginally employed migratory laborers. In short, famines and food scarcities, whether natural or manmade, are a fairly permanent feature of the human condition.

In the following paragraphs, I offer a brief overview of the important varieties of nutritional deficiency; I omit details, because this is a textbook of elementary public health, not of nutritional biochemistry.

Protein-Calorie Malnutrition (PCM)

This is prevalent in many developing countries, where it mainly afflicts recently weaned children. The name *kwashiorkor,* derived from words used in Ghana for "first-second" or "displaced child," signifies its origin as the disease that affects the first child after the birth of the second child, who gets the breast milk and leaves the first one to survive on whatever else, often very little, that may be available. Weanling children with kwashiorkor may have multiple deficiency states that are responsible for a varied clinical picture, e.g., with skin lesions of pellagra and depigmented hair; but the principal manifestations are deficits of calories and protein. The bloated belly (full of gas and, often, intestinal parasites), the sticklike legs and arms, and old man's face are characteristic of the condition. The feet and other dependent parts may be edematous. These signs and others, such as keratomalacia resulting from vitamin A deficiency, are commonly seen in famine areas. The uncomplicated picture of marasmus, the result of simple deficit of caloric intake, is the childhood equivalent of starvation in adults. It is a sad comment on our times that pictures of children suffering from advanced malnutrition appear so often on television and in news magazines.

Malnutrition and Infection

Infections that produce a fever raise the metabolic demand for calories and protein. Occurrence of even a mild infection in a malnourished child can tip the balance toward lethal deficit. Moreover, a malnourished child is more vulnerable to infection, with lowered resistence and reduced immunity. Thus the vicious circle of infection and malnutrition is responsible for the high mortality rates in early childhood in developing nations and among populations affected by poverty and deprivation in affluent nations. The infection–malnutrition vicious circle can operate in adults, too, especially among the elderly, who, like the very young, easily suffer from impaired immune reactions (Fig. 5–1).

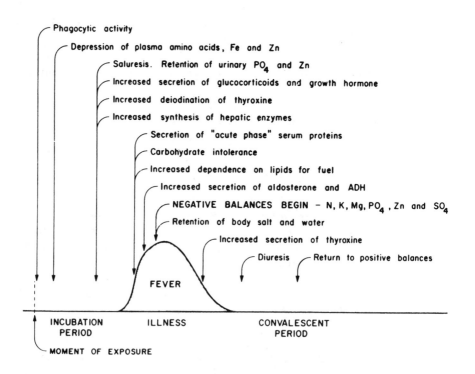

Figure 5–1. Schematic representation of the sequence of nutritional responses that evolves during the course of a "typical" generalized, febrile infectious illness. *(From Beisel WR: Magnitude of the postnutritional responses to infection. Am J Clin Nutr 30(8):1236, 1977.)*

► ROLES OF VITAMINS AND SPECIFIC DEFICIENCY DISEASES

Vitamins are essential for normal functioning of specific enzyme systems, e.g., those involved in metabolism or other bodily activities. If diets are deficient in specific vitamins, characteristic and readily recognizable diseases occur; more often, multiple deficiencies and mixed clinical pictures are seen. Some vitamin deficiency states rarely occur, but others are quite common. I will discuss only the common ones.

Vitamin A

Vitamin A (carotene) is essential for normal functioning of epithelial and glandular tissue and is needed for bone growth and for the enzyme systems involving visual purple that enhance vision in poor light. Vitamin A supplements, intended primarily to prevent xerophthalmia, have been found to significantly reduce infant and child mortality rates from infections; adequate dietary intake of vitamin A is also associated with reduced incidence and death rates from cancer.

Xerophthalmia

This condition occurs when the dietary intake of fresh fruit and vegetables containing vitamin A is inadequate. Deficiency of vitamin A leads to keratinization of secreting epithelial surfaces such as the conjunctiva. In severe forms, corneal opacities develop and the end result is blindness. This specific deficiency disease can occur in otherwise well-nourished populations—intake of proteins and calories may be adequate, but if there are no fresh fruits or vegetables, vitamin A deficiency can occur. Sometimes the right food is available but not eaten because of local custom and culture; this situation lends itself to, indeed, is ideal for nutrition education, which can successfully correct it.

Vitamin B$_1$

Vitamin B$_1$ (thiamine) is essential for certain enzyme systems involved in carbohydrate metabolism. Deficiency of thiamine leads to beriberi. This disease is due to disruption of carbohydrate metabolism consequent to breakdown of essential enzyme transformations. The effects are found in the central and peripheral nervous systems, the cardiovascular system, and the gastrointestinal tract. The principal clinical manifestations are peripheral neuropathy, tachycardia, and ultimately heart failure. Gastrointestinal atony leads to loss of appetite, which aggravates the condition. Infantile beriberi can occur in breast-fed infants whose mothers are thiamine deficient but who may themselves be asymptomatic. Beriberi commonly occurs where rice is the staple diet and milled rice, i.e., with the husks removed, is used. In these communities beriberi can be prevented by using unmilled rice; it is also possible to add thiamine to milled cereals. In industrial nations, beriberi is sometimes seen among persons with dietary deficiency associated with chronic alcoholism.

Vitamin B₃

Vitamin B_3 (Niacin, or nicotinic acid) is essential for several carbohydrate enzyme systems.

Pellagra

Deficiency of niacin results in pellagra. The full-blown case is characterized by dermatitis, diarrhea, and dementia, but mild forms with skin lesions are more common. It can occur in epidemics when there are regional deficiencies. In the early 20th century it was common in many rural areas in the southern United States, characteristically in late spring and early summer after a winter of deprivation but before the new season's food could be harvested. This pattern led to the belief that pellagra was an infectious disease caused by a microorganism. In a series of epidemiologic studies from 1914 onward, Joseph Goldberger,[9] having deduced logically from the distribution that pellagra could not possibly be due to an infection, demonstrated that it was indeed due to a dietary deficiency. Pellagra is prevented by maintaining adequate dietary intake of niacin, or its substitute, tryptophan.

Vitamin C

Ascorbic acid is also essential for carbohydrate enzyme systems.

Scurvy

This disease is due to deficiency of vitamin C. James Lind,[10] a British naval surgeon, conducted what was in effect a controlled clinical trial, which he reported in 1747, demonstrating the efficacy of fresh citrus fruits in preventing scurvy, which had formerly been a common cause of debility and death among saliors on long ocean voyages after they had run out of fresh fruit and vegetables. Scurvy can affect anyone deprived of fresh fruit and vegetables, such as persons in remote communities dependent upon imported fruit and vegetables or those unable to afford them because the price is too high. The lesions of scurvy include anemia and petechial subperiostial and intracranial hemorrhages. Infantile scurvy sometimes occurs in bottle-fed infants who are not given vitamin C supplements.

Vitamin D

One of the fat-soluble vitamins, vitamin D is essential for normal bone growth.

Rickets

This condition occurs when there is a deficiency of vitamin D. It is characterized by defective bone growth, with bone softening and skeletal deformities.

Vitamin D is synthesized in the skin by the action of ultraviolet light. Rickets can occur in high latitudes and anywhere in the world where children are deprived of access to sunlight. Among adults deprived of sunlight, an adult form, osteomalacia, can occur; this is sometimes seen among women in purdah in Moslem countries. Rickets can be prevented by a daily dose of vitamin D; this is sometimes added to milk or can be given in extracts such as cod-liver oil.

Other Deficiency Diseases

Ariboflavinosis

This causes loss of elasticity of the skin, fissuring at the corners of the mouth, and ocular lesions, progressing to interstitial keratitis; photophobia is an early symptom of this condition. Riboflavin is contained in milk and in green and yellow vegetables. Clinical deficiency states occasionally occur, e.g., among people with idiosyncratic dietary habits.

Vitamin K deficiency

Lack of vitamin K causes hemorrhagic disease of the newborn. Vitamin K is synthesized in the gut by commensal organisms, and hemorrhagic disease of the newborn may arise before this process is established; it is prevented by a single parenteral injection of vitamin K in the neonatal period.

Folic acid deficiency

In women of child-bearing age, lack of folic acid is associated with an increased risk of neural tube defects in their offspring. The pathogenic mechanism of this condition is unknown, but randomized controlled trials have established the efficacy of folic acid supplements for women in the child-bearing years, to prevent neural tube defects.[11] More severe dietary folic acid deficiency produces symptoms identical to those of iron-deficiency anemia, because folic acid is required in the synthesis of hemoglobin.

Iron deficiency

This causes a characteristic form of anemia, which is common among women in the reproductive years, especially if they suffer heavy menstrual blood loss or repeated pregnancies with excessive blood loss at childbirth; unless the iron loss is replaced by iron supplements, anemia occurs. Other causes of this form of anemia include other causes of chronic blood loss, such as infection with hookworm or schistosomiasis. If those affected subsist mainly on carbohydrates with little meat and little vitamin C (also essential for synthesis of hemoglobin), they can become severely anemic.

Iodine deficiency

This can occur in regions poor in iodine, such as some alpine areas. People who live in such regions experience difficulty in manufacturing the hormone thyroxine and become goitrous.[12] Goiter also occurs among people who subsist on vegetables such as kale and alfalfa; these contain "goitrin," a substance that blocks the uptake of iodine by the thyroid gland. Severe iodine deficiency causes not only a disfiguring goiter but, more important, metabolic and intellectual sluggishness. In infancy and childhood this is severe enough to be classified as mental retardation. About a billion people worldwide are at risk of iodine deficiency diseases.[13] It is easy to correct iodine deficiency by providing iodine supplements, usually in the form of iodized salt, ordinary table salt to which a small moiety of sodium or potassium iodide is added. Iodine deficiency diseases are targeted by the World Health Organization (WHO) for worldwide elimination by the year 2000.

Fluoride

Normally, fluoride occurs in trace amounts in water supplies. Observations of regional variation in fluoride concentration in drinking water in relation to the prevalence of dental caries led to the conclusion that fluoride concentrations of 1 to 4 parts per million are associated with lower prevalence of dental caries.[14] Deficiency of fluoride interferes with the process of enamel formation on teeth. These teeth are unusually susceptible to dental caries because they are less resistant to the action of acidophilic bacteria that normally occur in the mouth and are especially numerous when the diet is high in carbohydrates. A combination of fluoride-deficient water and high-carbohydrate diet is associated with very high prevalence of dental caries.[15] Water stored in large reservoirs is often deficient in fluoride, and this helps to account for the prevalence of dental caries in communities supplied from such sources. The best way to prevent this is to add a fluoride supplement to the drinking water to bring it up to a concentration of about 3 parts per million. But, as noted in Chapter 1, there is often political resistance to this, and there are some ethical objections, too (see Chap. 10).

Evidence on many other essential ingredients in human diets could be added to the previous account. Most, however, are of clinical rather than public health importance. Aberrations of aluminum metabolism, for example, may be associated with disease of the central nervous system, and aluminum is present in high concentration in the plaques found in the central nervous system in cases of Alzheimer's Disease; but epidemiologic studies have failed to establish an association of aluminum intake or metabolism to Alzheimer's or any other diseases of the central nervous system.[16] Vitamin E may be necessary for maintenance of vision. No significant public health problems are known to be attributable to deficits or surpluses of these or other apparently essential dietary ingredients.

▶ PREVENTION OF NUTRITIONAL DEFICIENCY DISEASES

Some allusions to prevention have been made in the preceding paragraphs. Several forms of nutritional deficiency disease can be prevented by mass medication, in which the preventive strategy is applied to the whole population. This is the method used to prevent rickets, scurvy, beriberi, endemic goiter, and dental caries. Mass medication is implemented by adding to the diet in the most expeditious manner the missing ingredient or an item of diet that contains it or a precursor. Thus iodine is added to table salt, vitamin D to milk, vitamin C as a supplement in infant feeds, and fluoride as a supplement in drinking water. All these forms of mass medication are well accepted, with the exception of fluoridation. There has been great emotional and often political resistance to the addition of fluoride to drinking water. Opponents have frequently managed to mobilize their political supporters effectively, and repeatedly have succeeded in voting down measures aimed at correcting fluoride deficiency in drinking water. Logical presentation of the scientific evidence for the efficacy of fluoride and its freedom from adverse effects on human health is ineffectual against the opponents of fluoridation. Political scientists have found this to be an interesting case study. Opponents of fluoridation tend to come from poorly educated lower socioeconomic strata of society, are politically conservative, and are intolerant in their attitudes not only to fluoride but to many other issues.[17] The only effective weapon to counter this group is political: Polemical arguments can sometimes sway voters against their position where reason and logic fail to do so. There have been many publications on the psychology of the antifluoridation movement; in many respects it resembles the extinct antivaccination movement. That said, the ethical case against fluoridation remains: It is a paternalist measure in communities that accord a high value to autonomy, and in many communities dental public health specialists nowadays often advocate oral fluoride supplements, fluoride toothpaste, or topical application of fluoride as part of regular dental health checkups.[18]

▶ OVERNUTRITION

If people consume food in excess of metabolic requirements, the surplus caloric intake is mostly stored rather than excreted. Storage is in fatty tissue, and obesity is the visible result. This is a disease of affluence and extravagance. It is widely prevalent in the United States, where rates of obesity are higher than anywhere else on earth,[19] but it is becoming more common in other rich industrial nations where more and more people not only are overeating but also taking insufficient exercise. Obese peole are rarely seen in the crowded, predominantly rural agrarian nations of the developing world.

Data from the National Health and Nutrition Examination Surveys (NHANES) reveal a rising prevalence of obesity in the United States: In 1960 to 1962, 25.4 percent of the population aged 25 to 74 years were obese; by 1971 to 1974, the proportion had risen to 26.7 percent; in 1976 to 1980, it was 27 percent; and by 1988 to 1990 it had passed 30 percent.[20] Among teenage children, the prevalence has risen more sharply, up to 40 percent in the same period; this is attributed to so much time spent watching television, and snacking while doing so. The prevalence of obesity has declined only in one age and sex group, young adult males aged 25 to 34 years—the jogging generation.

Obesity in itself harms health in several ways; the mere physical effort of moving extra weight encourages torpor, which—if the fat person continues to eat the same amount—further aggravates the obesity. In addition, the excess intake of certain dietary ingredients is a cause or determinant of important chronic conditions. Excess intake of dietary fats, especially polyunsaturated fats, is among the determinants of coronary heart disease and atherosclerosis. Adult-onset diabetes is also associated with overnutrition, probably with both high fat and high carbohydrate intake. Carcinoma of the large bowel occurs significantly more often in well-fed and overweight populations than in underfed ones.[21] Carcinoma of the breast and of the uterus also are associated with overweight.[22] Obesity is a risk factor for hypertension and for osteoarthritis. High salt intake, a custom in civilized societies, is associated with hypertension.

There can be some factors missing from the habitual diets of affluent civilized societies; dietary fiber is often deficient, and this can contribute to ailments ranging from hemorrhoids and varicose veins to chronic colitis and large-bowel cancer—although the evidence for this is debated. The relationship of dietary intake to cancer is fraught with controversy (see Chap. 7).

► A HEALTHY DIET

Good health is preserved and protected by a balanced diet. Epidemiologic and biochemical–nutritional studies have shown that the risk of certain diseases is reduced by habitual adherence to a diet that is high in fiber, low in fats; high in protein, low in salt; and that avoidance of alcohol and tobacco, and possibly caffeine, is associated with lower incidence and mortality rates from coronary heart disease and many kinds of cancer. Seventh Day Adventists, who follow strict dietary customs, demonstrate the value of these customs by more favorable health experiences than otherwise comparable individuals in the same community and socioeconomic class.[23,24] Vegetarians on the whole have more favorable health experience than meat eaters, other things being equal. These mostly empirical observations about the relationship between habitual diets and health support the view that humans evolved as hunter-gatherers mainly of fruits, vegetables, berries, and the like and were only occasionally meat eaters. The historical evidence suggests that diets rich in meat, animal fats, and dairy products have become customary only during the past 10 to 20 generations of human existence; because of our evolutionary history we may not be as well adapted to such diets as we might wish.[25] Supporting evidence comes from paleopathology: well-preserved cadavers such as the "bog man" from Denmark and the "ice-man" found in the Austrian Alps in 1989 appear to have subsisted mainly on vegetables and fruit. But our ideas about primitive diets are speculative; there is only anecdotal information, no reliable data on large population samples.

Other observations, mostly empirical, some supported by epidemiologic evidence, can be added to those previously mentioned. Comparison of populations where red meat and fish respectively are habitually eaten has shown that both coronary heart disease and large-bowel cancer occur more commonly among red-meat eaters.[26] On the other hand, cancer of the stomach appears to be more common among persons who habitually eat fish, while habitual fish-eating people have lower mortality rates from cardiovascular disease.[27] Evidence from cross-cultural studies must be interpreted with caution, however; many other variables could confound the comparison. Nonetheless, nutritionists advise moderation in red-meat intake and suggest that those who seldom or never eat fish should partake at least occasionally. Of course such advice would have to be modified if the locally available fish came from water or food chains with high mercury or PCB content.

A "high-fiber diet" is not necessarily one containing a lot of stringy fruits and vegetables or certain widely advertised breakfast cereals. Most fruits and vegetables, whether "stringy" in consistency or not, contain fiber of the sort recommended as a dietary ingredient that will encourage motility of bowel contents and the growth of intestinal commensals of a "healthy" variety. A low-fiber high-fat diet, on the other hand, may encourage intestinal stasis and perhaps also the growth of intestinal commensal organisms that metabolize sterols to precarcinogenic steroids—hence the connection with a higher incidence rate of large-bowel cancer.[28]

▶ NUTRITION IN PREGNANCY AND INFANCY

Everybody knows that nutritional requirements increase during pregnancy. The pregnant woman needs a higher calorie intake, but proportionately she needs a higher intake of protein, iron, and calcium and not such a high proportional increase of fats or carbohydrates. Some dietary ingredients, e.g., salt, may be restricted if there is a history of high blood pressure or renal disease. Vitamin supplements are often recommended, but fresh fruit and vegetables are generally better unless they cause indigestion or "heartburn" (esophageal reflux), a common complaint of women late in pregnancy. If nutrition is inadequate during pregnancy, the metabolic demands of the developing fetus are met first, so the mother's health suffers. Only in extreme starvation does the fetus's health also suffer.

The newborn infant unquestionably does better on breast milk than on any artificial formula feed. Breast milk has exactly the right composition, even to the extent of varying in consistency, flavor, and composition from the beginning to the end of each feed and during the period of lactation as the baby grows and develops. It also contains and transmits to the infant maternal anti-bodies, which enhance the infant's immunity or resistance to many infections. Breast milk does not require preparation or storage; it is already at the right temperature and, unlike artificial feeds, there is little or no risk of con-tamination with pathogenic microorganisms. It has also been observed that it comes in attractive containers. Breast milk may, however, be deficient in some vitamins, notably vitamin C. Given a normally nourished mother, breast milk is entirely adequate for the first 3 to 6 months of a baby's life, and in many cir-cumstances it remains the milk of choice for another 3 to 6 months.

Regrettably, infant food manufacture is a lucrative business that engages in high-pressure salesmanship aimed at encouraging the replacement of ma-ternal milk with artifical formula feeds. All sorts of subtle and unsubtle pres-sures are applied to mothers of newborn infants to encourage them to adopt artificial formula feeds. Infant formula manufacturers have access to mater-nity services in most hospitals, provide "free" samples and lavishly produced books on infant feeding, conveying the message that formula feeding is more convenient, "liberates" the mother, and even implying that breastfeeding is somehow "disgusting" or obscene. The obscenity is in the lies contained in such books. The proportion of women who breastfeed began to decline in the industrial nations in the 1920s and remained low until after World War II, when according to many surveys, as few as 10 percent of mothers were breastfeeding. In the 1950s, however, the proportion of mothers breastfeed-ing their infants for 3 months or longer began to rise, and by the early 1980s it had reached 60 to 70 percent; the highest rates were among the better-edu-cated mothers, often those who did not have to return to work soon after childbirth.[29] One action that many women's groups have taken has been to encourage the setting up of nurseries and quiet rooms set aside for breast-feeding in places where women who have recently had a baby are working.

In the developing nations, transnational infant formula manufacturers have actively promoted infant formula. A campaign led by UNICEF with con-siderable support from associations of pediatricians and public health spe-cialists around the world has reduced, but not entirely put a stop to this unsa-vory practice. Infant formula can do great harm in settings where there are inadequate facilities for preparing, sterilizing, and storing it. In 1979, a WHO/UNICEF conference condemned the practices of the infant formula manufacturers,[30] and in 1981, all the nations of the world, with the solitary exception of the United States, voted to restrict the activities of infant for-mula manufacturers in developing countries. The United States voted against the resolution on grounds advocated by the Reagan administration, that it was an interference with free-market competition.

Weanling infants and toddlers develop high sensitivity to taste sensa-tions. This is a period of great experimentation and exploration in the child's life. It is also a period when nutritional requirements are declining. Parents who force food on their children at this stage of their development may promote conditioned responses that lead to permanent dislike of foods that are nutritionally desirable. Another consequence is that these children may become habituated to eating more food than they need, so this practice can sow the seeds for obesity in later life.

▶ ETHNICITY, SOCIOECONOMIC STATUS, AND DIETARY HABITS

There are conspicuous ethnic and cultural differences in dietary customs, some determined by religious beliefs (e.g., Jews and Moslems do not eat pork, many Hindus are strict vegetarians); some by availability or price of certain classes of food. Coast-dwelling people eat more seafood than people who live in the middle of a continental landmass; dairy farmers consume more milk products; beef cattle farmers eat more beef, and so on. Those who migrate from one part of the world to another usually take their traditional diets and methods of preparing meals with them. Some of them open restaurants that become popular in their adopted land, so almost all large cities in industrial nations offer a variety of "ethnic" restaurants—Chinese, Italian, etc. Traditional "ethnic" diets are mostly as nutritionally rich and varied as those that are customary among those born and raised in Western industrial cities, sometimes more so.

Rich people can afford more expensive foods than poor people, but this does not necessarily mean that they eat more nourishing or "healthier" foods. Data from nationwide U.S. Food Consumption Surveys in 1965 and 1977–1978 and the 1989–1991 Continuing Survey of Food Intake have been analyzed using a 16-point Diet Quality Index. The analysis showed an overall improvement in dietary quality and also, rather surprisingly perhaps, that both whites and blacks in lower socioeconomic classes had a higher quality diet than upper-class whites; but differences narrowed over this period, and by 1991 diets were similar in all groups.[31]

▶ POPULATIONS AT NUTRITIONAL RISK

The previous paragraphs have identified several groups in society that can be at special risk of nutritional diseases. Another important group is mothers and children without adequate financial resources to pay for food, for whom the U.S. federal government program of Aid to Families with Dependent Children (AFDC) was created. This has been literally lifesaving; it was almost a victim of the Republican "revolution" of the 1994–1996 Congress, and it remains to be seen whether the nutritional well-being of many defenseless children will suffer as a result of the legislated changes to the U.S. welfare system enacted and signed into law in 1995–1996. It is more necessary than ever for voluntary bodies and food banks to reach out to members of these disadvantaged groups.

Others at high risk of nutritional deficiency states include elderly people, especially elderly house-bound people living alone. Not only may they have difficulty obtaining food supplies, they may lose interest in cooking and eating and subsist on a diet of bread and jam. They can develop vitamin deficiency states, and even starve. The Meals on Wheels programs operated by voluntary bodies in many communities are a valuable system to protect many elderly infirm people from these risks.

Food Fads

Occasionally food faddists carry their dietary customs to dangerous extremes. Vegans, extreme vegetarians who avoid milk and milk products and eggs because these foods are derived from animals, sometimes suffer protein deficiency. A few people become so obsessed by their perceived need for a high vitamin intake that they develop carotene poisoning from overdoses of vitamin A. Adolescent girls and young women (and occasionally men) who become obsessed with the quest for extreme thinness suffer from anorexia nervosa, a very serious and sometimes life-threatening psychopathologic condition. Because affluent Western culture projects an image that being thin is a desirable social attribute, enough young women have developed an obsessive desire for this fashion to have created a public health problem out of anorexia nervosa and the related condition of bulimia.

► NUTRITION EDUCATION

In societies at every level of development, and for several age epochs, certain forms of nutrition education are required. This is one of the most useful forms of health education, and often the most effective.

In developing nations, the entire population may require education to promote the use of healthier diets than have been customary or usual in the past. For example, fresh fruit containing vitamin A that would prevent xerophthalmia may rot on the trees because it has never been customary to eat it. Education to correct this practice is relatively straightforward and usually very effective. It is more difficult to change a custom that is deeply ingrained as part of the culture. For example, in many traditional African tribal societies it has been the custom for the menfolk to get the first, often the only, serving of meat, while the women and children make do with whatever else there may be, perhaps not much and not very nutritious food. A variation on this theme is to share the food unequally, with the smallest shares meted out to the least-valued members of the family or tribe, often weanling female children. In rural Indian villages, small girls are often the least-valued members of the family, and in bad times they may be left altogether without food so that a visitor to the village can see them quietly starving to death in a dark corner of the family hut. Much remains to be done to improve nutrition education for mothers and children in many developing countries. Education on the benefits of breastfeeding and on other aspects of nutrition during pregnancy and early childhood is equally necessary and requires constant reinforcement, not only in developing nations but also in the industrially developed ones.

Other forms of nutrition education are needed in affluent industrial nations. Overnutrition has had much adverse publicity in the past 15 to 20 years, but this has had little impact; obesity is still widespread and increasingly common in the United States and other rich nations. Nonetheless, the decline in the death rate from coronary heart disease in the United States, Canada, and some other countries since the late 1960s is at least partly—some assert mostly—attributble to changes in habitual diets. This change can be credited to publicity in the mass media, which is an effective form of nutrition education.

Other and more carefully designed nutrition education programs are required, beginning in grade school, where children can be taught about the nutritional values of foods, preferably in relation to the costs of these foods. It is worth emphasizing that fresh fruit is nutritionally superior to and often cheaper than popcorn. Messages such as this are part of health teaching in many schools, but reinforcement is needed, for instance when young women begin their first pregnancy, and again after childbirth when the visiting public health nurse's tasks include reminding mothers about food values.

The prevalent obesity in the United States is partly due to the habitual consumption of heavily promoted "junk foods." Junk foods include mass-produced breakfast cereals, doughnuts, precooked TV dinners, sweetened carbonated beverages, and many kinds of biscuits and pasta dishes. These are consumed especially by people on low incomes, and there is a syndrome of "obesity of poverty" among this segment of the population. The fast food catering establishments (they do not deserve to be called restaurants) mainly serve foods that fall into the junk food category. Although the food served in such places constitutes an adequate diet in the caloric sense and may taste pleasant, its nutritional value may be suspect. There is no evidence that such foods contain any actually harmful substances, but they are expensive. People on low incomes can waste their meager financial resources on such foods, while they go short of fresh fruit and vegetables and meat, with consequent nutritional imbalance, unless they receive appropriate nutrition education. Encouraging intelligent budgeting of food purchases as well as instruction in nutritional value of foods are goals of nutrition education for this financially disadvantaged group of people. Unfortunately such education is rarely readily available.

Nutrition education is useful also for old people who live alone. Elderly widows who live alone often lose interest in cooking just for themselves and are deterred from food shopping by the price and by the packaging of many supermarket foods into "family size" cartons. Their declining physical mobility also may deter them from shopping expeditions, and with fewer corner stores to choose from, they face a difficult and challenging task to find what they need and want. It is easy to fall into the habit of subsisting on bread and jam under such circumstances, and this diet can lead to nutritional deficiency diseases.

▶ **REFERENCES**

1. World Resources Institute, U.N. Environment Programme, UN Development Programme, World Bank: *World Resources: A Guide to the Global Environment 1996–97.* New York: Oxford University Press, 1996, pp. 225–246; 295–314.
2. Waltner-Toews D: *Food, Sex and Salmonella. The Risks of Environmental Intimacy.* Toronto: NC Press, 1992.
3. Rogan WJ, Bagniewska A, Damstra T: Pollutants in breast milk. *N Engl J Med* 302:1450–1453, 1980.
4. Jacobson JL, Jacobson SW: Intellectual impairment in children exposed to polychlorinated biophenyls in utero. *N Engl J Med* 335:783–789, 1996.
5. Ginsburg J: Tackling environmental endocrine disrupters. *Lancet* 347:1501–1502, 1996; see also Colborn T, Dumanoski D, Myers JP: *Our Stolen Future.* Boston: Little, Brown, 1996.
6. Toxic epidemic study group: Toxic epidemic syndrome, Spain, 1981. *Lancet* 2:697–702, 1982.
7. Baker G: *An Essay Concerning the Cause of the Endemial Colic of Devonshire.* London: J Hughes, 1767. (Reprinted, New York: Delta Omega Society, 1958.)
8. Recommended Dietary Allowances. 10th ed. Washington, DC: National Academy Press, 1989.
9. Terris M (ed): *Goldberger on Pellagra.* Baton Rouge: Louisiana State University Press, 1964.
10. Lind J: *A Treatise of the Scurvy.* Edinburgh: Sands, Murray & Cochrane, 1753. (Reprinted annotated edition, Edinburgh University Press, 1953.)
11. Wald N, Sneddon J, Densem J, et al.: MRC Vitamin Study Research Group, prevention of neural tube defects. Results of the Medical Research Council Vitamin Study. *Lancet* 338:131–137, 1991; see also Daly LE, Kirke PN, Molloy A, et al.: Folate levels and neural tube defects. Implications for prevention. *JAMA* 274: 1698–1702, 1995.
12. World Health Organization: Endemic Goitre. Geneva: WHO Monograph Series, No. 44, 1960.
13. Hetzel BS: *The Story of Iodine Deficiency; An International Challenge in Nutrition.* Oxford: Oxford University Press, 1989.
14. Dean HT: Epidemiological studies in the United States. In Moulton FR (ed): *Dental Caries and Fluorine.* Washington, DC: American Association for the Advancement of Science, 1942, pp. 5–31.
15. *Fluoride, Teeth and Health: A Report of the Royal College of Physicians of London.* London: Pitman, 1976.
16. Martyn CN, Barker DJP, Osmond C, et al.: Geographical relation between Alzheimer's disease and aluminium in drinking water. *Lancet* 1:59–62, 1989.
17. Evans CA Jr, Pickles T: Statewide antifluoridation initiatives: A new challenge to health workers. *Am J Public Health* 68:59–65, 1978.

18. Greene JC, Greene AR: Oral health. In Woolf SH, Jonas S, Lawrence RS (eds): *Health Promotion and Disease Prevention in Clinical Practice.* Baltimore: Williams & Wilkins, 1996, pp. 315–334.

19. Obesity in Perspective. Washington, DC: Fogarty International Center Series on Preventive Medicine, 1975.

20. NCHS: Advance data series: Preliminary estimates from National Health and Nutrition Examination Survey. Washington, DC: NCHS 1996.

21. Graham S: Towards a dietary prevention of cancer. *Epidemiol Rev* 5:38–50, 1983.

22. McMichael AJ, Jensen OM, Parkin DM, et al.: Dietary and endogenous cholesterol and human cancer. *Epidemiol Rev* 6:192–216, 1984.

23. Wynder EL, Lemon FR, Bross IJ: Cancer and coronary artery disease among Seventh Day Adventists. *Cancer* 12:1016–1028, 1959.

24. Phillips RL: Role of lifestyle and dietary habits in risk of cancer among Seventh Day Adventists. *Cancer Res* 35:3513–3522, 1975.

25. Brothwell D, Brothwell P: *Food in Antiquity.* New York: Praeger, 1969.

26. Diet, nutrition and cancer: Interim guidelines. *J Natl Cancer Inst* 70:1151–1170, 1983.

27. Blackburn H, Luepker R: Heart Disease. In Last JM, Wallace RB (eds): *Maxcy-Rosenau-Last Public Health and Preventive Medicine.* 13th ed. E. Norwalk, CT: Appleton & Lange, 1991, pp. 827–847.

28. Burkitt DP, Trowell HC: *Refined carbohydrate foods and disease—Some implications of dietary fibre.* New York: Academic Press, 1975.

29. Hendershot GE: Trends in breastfeeding. Washington, DC: National Center for Health Statistics, Advance Data 59:1–7, 1980.

30. World Health Organization/UNICEF: Meeting on infant and child feeding. *WHO Chronicle* 33:435–443, 1979.

31. Popkin BM, Siega-Riz AM, Haines PS: A comparison of dietary trends among racial and socioeconomic groups in the United States. *N Engl J Med* 335:716–720, 1996.

6

Social and Behavioral Determinants of Health

Despite much study, uncertainty persists about many aspects of behavior that empirical observations tell us can influence individual and community health. Knowledge of the effects on health of behavioral, social, and cultural factors is based on observations by behavioral and social scientists, medical anthropologists, and epidemiologists. Physiologists, endocrinologists, immunologists, and psychologists have related the empirical observations to underlying concepts of mind–body interactions for which there is experimental and clinical supporting evidence. But what we know raises many questions about what we do not know. Are individual and community health related to a sense of self-worth or self-esteem? What is the impact of conquest on the collective psyche of the conquered? Does this contribute to high rates of suicide and substance abuse observed in some societies and cultural groups that have been overrun by foreign invaders or marginalized by European colonization? Does a social or occupational group—the long-term unemployed—develop a collective belief that they are inferior to others, and if so, is this reflected in their experience of illness? Can something like this happen to the entire female sex in cultures where women are subjugated? How do we account for variations in immune response, the "psychosomatic" basis for many cases of asthma, the relationship of high blood pressure to occupational stress, the remissions and relapses of cancer sometimes observed in relation to emotional crises in cancer patients' lives? Such questions are endless. Neuroendocrine and neuroimmunologic study of the connections may enlighten us. Medical anthropologists approach the mind–body question from another perspective, studying the way in which the experience of illness is shaped by the mind. Interpretations of illness are deeply linked to cultural experience.[1] Differing cultural concepts about the way the body works can shape symptoms, sometimes in a dramatic fashion. Studying the way in which individuals interpret and assign meaning to their illness provides valuable insights into the rapidly emerging discipline of "mind–body medicine."[2] Turning this interpretation "inside out," so to say, might become a way to prevent the illness from occurring in the first place. For instance, by explaining how stress can contribute to hypertension, it might become possible to condition susceptible individuals so that they would not become hypertensive. But we are still a long way from possessing the necessary insights and skills to make such an approach work.

Health and the behavior of individuals and of social groups manifestly are interrelated in complex ways. The behavior of individuals is influenced by and influences their own and other people's personalities. Interactions with family members, working colleagues, neighbors, leaders and members of church, synagogue, mosque, or other place of worship all have health implications. Individuals, families, and the groups to which they belong are all part of the social and cultural environment of the community, society, and nation in which they are located, and these are shaped by geographic and other factors that make up the physical environment (Fig. 6–1).

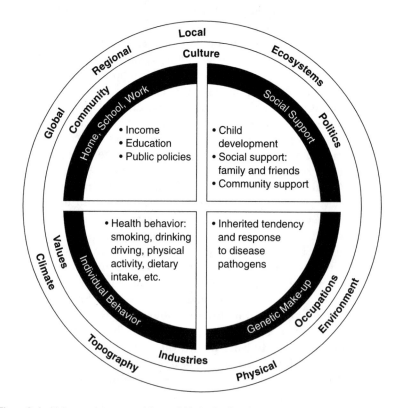

Figure 6–1. Linkages of person and the social/behavioral environment. *(Illustration by Jon W. Last.)*

► SOCIAL FACTORS

These include occupation, socioeconomic status, the cultural milieu, and the network of family, friends, and working colleagues to which individuals belong (Box 6–1).

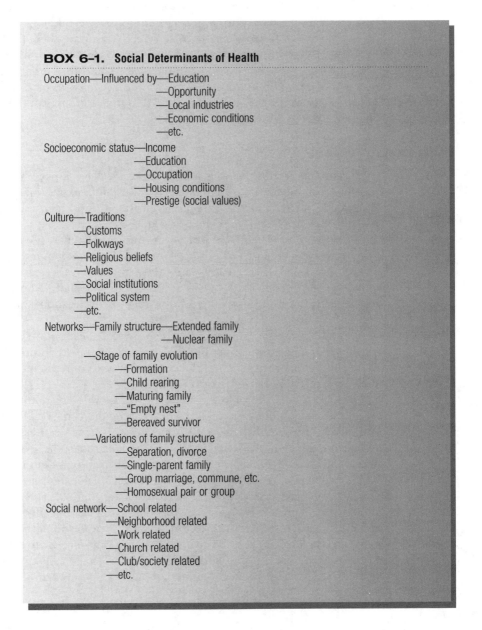

BOX 6–1. Social Determinants of Health

Occupation—Influenced by—Education
                         —Opportunity
                         —Local industries
                         —Economic conditions
                         —etc.
Socioeconomic status—Income
                        —Education
                        —Occupation
                        —Housing conditions
                        —Prestige (social values)
Culture—Traditions
        —Customs
        —Folkways
        —Religious beliefs
        —Values
        —Social institutions
        —Political system
        —etc.
Networks—Family structure—Extended family
                         —Nuclear family
      —Stage of family evolution
            —Formation
            —Child rearing
            —Maturing family
            —"Empty nest"
            —Bereaved survivor
      —Variations of family structure
            —Separation, divorce
            —Single-parent family
            —Group marriage, commune, etc.
            —Homosexual pair or group
Social network—School related
              —Neighborhood related
              —Work related
              —Church related
              —Club/society related
              —etc.

Occupation

I described and discussed risks to health associated with some occupational exposures in Chapter 4. Some occupations are well known to be hazardous, but these occupations attract people for many reasons. The pay may be high because of the known risks, or this may be the only work available. Sometimes workers resist changes that would reduce or eliminate risks if they fear their prospects of employment might be reduced. Group solidarity and pride in acceptance of hazardous working conditions are other factors. Workers who are aware of hazards and seek to reduce or remove them face resistance to change from employers, sometimes threats to close the industry and move it elsewhere or to dismiss complaining workers and hire others. The sociology, psychology, and politics of work are too complex to be discussed more fully here. Interested readers are referred to the references at the end of this chapter.

Socioeconomic Status

Socioeconomic status (SES) is a descriptive term for a person's position in society. It can be classified in many ways and is often expressed on an ordinal scale using such criteria as income, educational level, occupation, and the real estate value (based on realty taxes) of the residence.

The simplest classification of SES is into manual and nonmanual workers, or blue-collar and white-collar workers. There is generally an income diference between these groups and, more important, there are often differences in educational level and in social values or beliefs. These may affect leisure activities and habitual diets as much as occupation and income do and so may affect health.

Simple and elaborate methods of social classification are available. The most elaborate classification methods require detailed information about personal characteristics such as the number of years and the nature of education, an exact description of occupation, income from all sources, ratable value of residence, and whether the residence is owned or rented.[4,5]

Table 6–1 outlines the features of some methods of social classification. Although it is customary to "rank" persons who have been assigned to SES categories, this is misleading if it conveys the idea that some are "better" than others; SES classifications are simply that—classifications—not rank orders of social excellence or otherwise. Of course social values ensure that prestige and high income are rewards for persons in the "higher" SES categories. In this respect, high SES is clearly "better than" low SES. But income alone, for instance, is an insufficient criterion of SES: a professional sportsman can earn a great deal more than a justice of the Supreme Court, but no one would suggest that the sportsman has a higher SES. For this discussion, what matters is that there is almost always a relationship between SES and health status.

One scale that has been much used in epidemiologic studies is the

TABLE 6–1.   Summary of Some Methods of Social Classification

Scales	Comments
Occupational scales	
Manual/nonmanual work (blue-collar/white-collar)	Crude; no income data; no rating for nonworking population
Registrar-general's classification	One question gives class; inadequate for some, e.g., students, housewives
Income-based scales	
Arrange population according to income groups	Gives reproducible classes
	Resistance to revealing income
Socioeconomic scales	
Answers to questions on	More precise categories
Education	Covers most people
Occupation	Requires several questions
Income	
Value of dwelling (e.g., Hollingshead, Blishen scales)	
Status/prestige rating scales	
Based on consensus (value) judgments Occupational ranks	Highly subjective, e.g., pop singer > Supreme Court justice
Value of dwelling	
Public image	
(e.g., Congalton scale)	

United Kingdom's Registrar-General's (RG) Occupational Classification, developed in 1910. This has repeatedly demonstrated its utility, and because of this it has been adopted or adapted to suit local conditions in many other countries. Based on occupation, the population is divided into five social classes, conventionally designated by roman numerals (Table 6–2). This has the advantage that it is possible to assign many individuals to a class on the basis of information about their occupation that is available in existing vital

TABLE 6–2.   The Registrar-General's Occupational Classification

I	Leading professions and businesses	Physician, lawyer, stockbroker, bank manager
II	"Minor" professions and businesses	Schoolteacher, pharmacist, shopkeeper
III (a)	Skilled nonmanual workers	Clerk, bank teller
(b)	Skilled manual workers	Factory foreman, crane operator
IV	Semiskilled workers	Factory shop-floor worker, truck driver, salesperson
V	Unskilled workers	Porter, waiter, delivery person, tollbooth attendant

or other records or can be obtained by the answer to a single question. This has obvious advantages over methods that require several questions, or a complex questionnaire. Dependent family members are assigned to the class of the head of the household. A weakness of the RG's classification is that the single question does not tell us, for example, what sort of "engineer" someone is—a university graduate collecting large fees for consulting practice or the assistant holding an oilcan beside a moving conveyer belt in an automobile assembly plant. Despite its lack of precision, however, the RG's occupational classification is a valuable sociologic tool.

Virtually every health indicator ever examined in Britain shows a relationship to social class—infant mortality rates, leading causes of death, reasons for hospital care, use of family doctors' services, health-related behavior, etc. Table 6–3 shows some recent British social class health differentials.

Inequalities of health experience among the social classes have persisted since observations began in 1910. The United Kingdom National Health Service was created after World War II at least partly with the aim of reducing socioeconomic inequalities in health, but the inequalities remain as large as ever,[6] or larger.[7] Providing an egalitarian health service did not reduce inequalities. Similar mortality and morbidity differentials have been observed in many other countries, including socialist and Marxist states where all peo-

TABLE 6–3. Social Class, Mortality, and Health Behavior, United Kingdom, 1980, 1991–1994[a]

Registrar-General's Classification		Infant Mortality Rate	Standardized Mortality Ratio	Cigarette Smokers (%)	Physical Activity, Men[b]	Doctor Visits[c]
I	1980	10.2	77	21	44	76
	1991–1994	4.2 (7.1)[d]	65	M 14, F 13	84	9
II	1980	11.1	81	35	36	75
	1991–1994	4.5 (6.1)[d]	74	M 23, F 21	74	11
IIIa	1980	11.8	99	35	23	122
	1991–1994	5.0 (6.2)[d]	100	M 25, F 27	45	13
IIIb	1980	13.7	106	48	23	112
	1991–1994	5.3 (6.8)[d]	121	M 34, F 31	48	13
IV	1980	16.3	114	49	17	125
	1991–1994	6.5 (7.7)[d]	120	M 34, F 35	36	14
V	1980	23.0	137	57	15	146
	1991–1994	7.7 (9.3)[d]	195	M 42, F 35	26	13

M = male; F = female.
[a] Although different definitions and criteria make some data not strictly comparable between the two periods, the social class trends are generally consistent throughout.
[b] 1980s figures are annual participation rates; 1990s are for previous 4 weeks.
[c] 1980s figures are consultations per 1000 per annum; 1990s figures are percentages consulting in previous 2 weeks.
[d] Numbers in parentheses are for infant deaths outside marriage, separately tabulated in the 1990s, not in earlier periods
(UK Office of Population Censuses and Surveys, General Social Survey, various years.)

TABLE 6-4. Family Income and Health Indicators (United States, 1957–1980)

1957–1961: Four Income Classes (1, Lowest; 4, Highest)

	1	2	3	4
Disability days/person/yr				
Restricted activity	29.8	17.7	13.8	13.0
Bed disability	10.4	6.2	4.9	4.6
Physician visits/person/yr	2.8	3.1	3.4	3.8
Dentist visits/person/yr	0.7	1.0	1.5	2.3

1969: Five Income Classes (1, Lowest; 5, Highest)

	1	2	3	4	5
Disability days/person/yr					
Restricted activity	21.6	21.9	19.2	15.3	10.4
Bed disability	9.9	10.3	8.9	7.3	5.4
Physician visits/person/yr	4.2	4.6	4.5	4.5	4.4
Dentist visits/person/yr	0.9	0.9	0.8	1.1	1.7

1979–1980: Five Income Classes (1, Lowest; 5, Highest)

	1	2	3	4	5
Disability days/person/yr					
Restricted activity	22.9	26.4	22.1	18.9	12.1
Bed disability	11.0	13.4	10.7	8.7	5.6
Physician visits/person/yr	5.5	6.0	5.4	4.9	4.7
Dentist visits/person/yr	1.4	1.3	1.1	1.2	1.9

Notes: Cut-points for income classes vary; figures for 1969 and for 1979 are age adjusted; the higher rates for doctor visits for lower income classes in recent years probably reflect removal of economic barriers to care since introduction of Medicare and Medicaid programs.
(National Center for Health Statistics Data from Household Interview Surveys, various years.)

ple are supposedly equal—suggesting that intelligence, education, or health-related values play an important role.

In the United States, information about the relationships among health, use of health-care services, and income levels is collected in the ongoing household interview surveys of the National Center for Health Statistics. Table 6–4 summarizes findings since 1957 and shows that, as in Britain, the pattern is consistent over time. In the United States, the differentiation among social groups is usually based on answers to questions about income levels. The correlation to health status is sometimes closer with race than SES, suggesting that culturally determined behavioral factors may matter more than income as determinants of health status.

Analysis of mortality in relation to income in Canada shows the same

TABLE 6–5.   Income Level and Health, Canada, 1980

Income Level (1, Highest; 5, Lowest)	1	2	3	4	5
IMR (per 1000)	12.3	15.0	17.9	20.0	24.1
Life expectancy (yr)	72.5	71.1	70.1	69.2	66.3
Male death rates per 100,000, ages 35–64:					
Ischemic heart disease	259	284	316	335	407
Lung cancer	45	56	66	75	105
Cirrhosis	15	20	30	37	60
Suicide	21	26	30	28	43
No activity restriction (%)	64.3	62.6	61.1	57.9	50.0
QALY[a]	69.7	68.1	66.8	64.8	59.4

[a] For a discussion of quality-adjusted life years (QALY), see Chap. 2.
IMR = Infant Mortality Rate

consistent pattern[8] (Table 6–5). The data in Table 6–5 were derived by aggregating the mortality and morbidity rates in census tracts for which average income levels had been computed. This method of classifying health experience according to SES smoothes out disparities between the well-educated well-to-do and poorly educated, predominantly less well-off persons who live in a particular region or census tract. This can introduce fallacies in interpretation, particularly the ecologic fallacy, i.e., attributing to individuals the experience of the group. Even so, it is a good way to show how mortality rates differ according to economic conditions and can be used to advocate health policy decisions aimed at reducing the inequalities in health while elevating health levels everywhere.

The same relationship is found in developing countries, where malaria and cholera attack the poor significantly more often than the wealthy. There is an epidemiologic explanation: Nutritional status influences the risk of getting or dying of cholera, and the poorest people in developing countries are more exposed to mosquitoes and other insect vectors.

Before making policy decisions based on these facts, we must ask some questions. What do these patterns represent? Risk factors? Use of health and social services? Sociocultural differences in health-related behavior? Genetic or inherited characteristics? Other events in people's lives? Housing conditions or other factors in the physical environment? It is difficult to unravel the relationships because several mutually reinforcing vicious circles may operate, especially among the poorest people.

Poverty and Health

The poor are a mixed group, comprising persons who are unemployed or marginally employed, the working poor, persons often receiving subsistence from welfare. An important group of poor people are single-parent families and others are elderly or invalid pensioners. The support provided for such people from public funds or charities is almost never adequate to meet their needs for shelter, food, and clothing. Some are in poor health because they are poor, and others are poor because they are in poor health; but for many, there is a constantly reinforcing vicious circle:

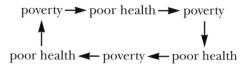

Poor people usually live in poor-quality housing, live in overcrowded conditions that favor the spread of infection, and often have inferior diets that may be nutritionally inadequate. All these factors increase the risk of infection, especially among infants and young children. Poor people are often poor because they are poorly educated (from lack of opportunity, application, ability, or all of these, and perhaps because of other factors); and because of their poor education they are unable to get well-paying jobs, or any jobs at all. Their poor education renders them less able to understand or to react appropriately to health education, which better-educated people can understand and act on; therefore they may neglect to provide their children with nutritious diets, get them immunized against communicable diseases, take precautions against the hazards of accidental injury and death in the home and in traffic. Poor education also condemns them, and often their children, to a lifetime of unequal opportunity in many other ways, unequal opportunity to share in almost all amenities to which better-off people have access. It can help if we can intervene to provide skill-enhancing opportunities for children, teaching them sports as well as work-related skills that improve their self-esteem.

The poor often have a low level of self-esteem; their experience of the world around them can help confirm their feeling that they are second-class citizens, and this in itself may be a psychologic determinant of illness and of their own reactions to illness.[9]

Some poor and poorly educated people lack much understanding of bodily functions, of how disease is caused, of what constitute "serious" symptoms.[10] In a classic study in the 1950s, Koos[11] recorded people's perceptions of illness and symptoms and what they did about it, in "Regionville," a small city in upstate New York. He divided his study population into three classes according to educational level, which correlated closely with occupation and income. Poorly educated and poorer people were less likely to seek medical care for serious or ominous symptoms and more likely to rely on popular but useless nostrums, compared to those who were better educated and better off (Table 6–6). A repeat survey in the same community a generation later[12] showed smaller health status differences, but they had not disappeared.

A further difficulty for poor people is that, compared to the well-off, they are separated by a greater social distance from providers of health care.

TABLE 6–6. Regionville Data (Class I, Highest Educational Level)

Symptoms	Percent Recognizing Need for Medical Attention		
	Class I	*Class II*	*Class III*
Continued coughing	77	78	23
Blood in stool	98	89	60
Blood in urine	100	93	69
Excessive vaginal bleeding	92	83	54
Loss of weight	80	51	21
Chronic fatigue	80	53	19
Shortness of breath	77	55	21
Persistent headaches	80	56	22
Pain in chest	80	51	31
Lump in breast	94	71	44

Remedy	Percent of Families Reporting Possession of Remedies		
	Class I	*Class II*	*Class III*
Analgesic	98	97	53
Antiseptic	91	88	52
Burn remedy	24	54	18
Laxative	89	96	88
Cough or cold remedy	96	97	70
"Kidney pills"	8	20	62
"Liver pills"	10	21	66
"Stomach medicine"	32	72	84

(Based on Koos, EL: The Health of Regionville, 1954.[11])

They have little in common with physicians and nurses, remote figures who do not "speak the same language." They may identify health workers with an authoritarian "establishment" that spies on them and does not give them their welfare support without humiliating and depersonalizing rules. For this reason, poor people are sometimes reluctant to use medical care even when it is available without charge. Another factor known to inhibit use of needed health services is shame—some poor people are ashamed to be seen in the waiting room in their shabby clothes, feeling conspicuously different alongside well-dressed and well-shod patients.[13] Shame is particularly acute for the unemployed, especially the recently unemployed, who may perceive their dismissal from the workforce as a stigma of their personal inadequacy. The unemployed have significantly elevated rates of both minor and major illness when compared to the rest of the population; they also have higher suicide rates.[14]

Physicians and other providers of health care can aggravate the sociocultural barrier between them and their poor patients if they lack perception of these factors, as may happen if there has been little or no pertinent discussion or demonstration of these relationships in programs of health professional education. Some attempts have been made to recruit health workers from such backgrounds as urban ghettos, and while this is desirable, providing the necessary insights to health workers from more fortunate backgrounds is just as important, or more so. In providing health care for people from an altogether different cultural background, a similar approach of recruiting health workers from the cultural background of the population that will be using the service is equally important.

Culture

Culture is the term that describes the socially acquired and transmitted behavior patterns of an ethnic group, community, society, or nation; it includes language, skills, beliefs, arts, sciences, laws, forms of government, religious beliefs, and moral and ethical standards. In a large and populous nation like the United States, there are many "subcultures," each differing from the others in some of the characteristics that are part of the national cultural mosaic. In almost all rich industrial nations, e.g., the European Union as well as the United States and Canada, large numbers of immigrants and guest workers from altogether different cultural backgrounds and ethnic groups have brought with them the health-related customs and folkways of their places of origin, introducing patterns of illness that health professionals would find easier to understand and manage if they had some education in medical anthropology.

Cultural milieu influences health in several ways. Customs, traditions, religious beliefs and practices, and health-related values are all important. In many countries there are large differences in values among cultural subgroups, often related to ethnic, religious, or linguistic origin, even to occupation or neighborhood. The "subculture of the poor," discussed earlier, is one component of this cultural mosaic in all industrial nations, and it is important because it is associated with high morbidity and mortality; but there are many others. Participation in or exclusion from the influence of the mass media is affected by the cultural milieu. New immigrants from other language groups may be isolated and unaware of health-protecting services such as immunizations. Some religious sects have health-related cultural characteristics. Seventh Day Adventists abstain from tobacco, alcohol, coffee, and tea, are vegetarian, and "health-conscious," practicing healthful habits of exercise, maintaining immunization schedules, etc. They have significantly lower age-adjusted mortality and incidence rates than the rest of the population from most forms of cancer and from heart disease and stroke.[15]

The culture to which we belong strongly influences our values, including our attitudes toward health. In Western societies, one value is compassion for the sick, especially for those who are mortally sick with conditions such as cancer or heart disease (but not necessarily compassion for sufferers from other conditions such as acquired immunodeficiency syndrome [AIDS] or alcohol-related cirrhosis of the liver). Some people set a higher value on care of the sick than on preserving good health. Many people show little interest in health or ways to preserve it—until their own health is damaged or threatened. This can be related to ignorance about determinants of health, or to a fatalistic attitude—that fate, rather than individual actions, affects the occurrence, progress, and outcome of illness.

Values regarding health and illness can be transmitted from one generation to the next without being formally discussed. These values not only influence the chances that we will get or die of various kinds of sickness, but also the ways we react to people who are sick. Many of our attitudes are inconsistent and thereby constrain our society's ability to make progress toward preventing certain kinds of illness. We regard it as unfortunate when someone we care about is afflicted with coronary heart disease, even if we think that two of the "seven deadly sins," gluttony and sloth, may have been causal factors. (I use these value-laden words deliberately for emphasis!) On the other hand, it is often perceived as shameful to be an alcoholic, even when we are aware that the individual may have no control over the compulsion to drink. (We have made some progress; it is considered undesirable to drive a car after drinking alcohol; in the 1940s and 1950s, many people believed it was acceptable, even praiseworthy, for a drunk driver to ferry passengers home from a party.)

When I was a medical student in the 1940s, there were about 20 to 30 cases of paralytic poliomyelitis every year, on average, in our community of about half a million; occasionally there were epidemics with a few hundred cases. At that time also there were up to 1000 infant deaths each year from diarrhea. The local campaign to raise money for research on poliomyelitis was highly successful; but there was very little public support, let alone voluntary support, for research on the prevention of infant deaths from diarrhea. The emotional appeal of the occasional paralyzed child was greater than that of the many children who sickened and died of a disease associated with a bodily function not mentioned in polite society. A contemporary parallel may be strong support for research on cystic fibrosis, contrasted with "blame the victim" attitudes to human immunodeficiency virus (HIV) and AIDS: "If they lived respectable lives, they would not get this disease." Such inconsistencies in our values and behavior are commonplace and difficult to alter.

Health-related values can and do change, as I discussed in Chapter 1. In most respects the changes are for the better, but the prevailing cultural norms in industrial nations and the values they espouse—values also aspired to by most people in emerging industrial nations—include features incompatible with long-term global ecosystem sustainability. I will return to this theme in Chapter 11 and the Epilogue.

Social Support Systems

"Networks" of family, friends, and workmates influence health—and health, especially mental health, influences networks. Another name for networks, social support systems, suggests how networks influence health—without, however, going below the surface to examine and explain mind–body interactions that are probably part of the process.

The most important part of this network for most of us is our immediate family. Evidence from vital statistics and other sources demonstrates higher death rates from all causes, and from certain causes in particular, of single, widowed, and divorced persons, in contrast to those who are married. The differences are more marked for males than for females. The relationships among marital and family status and health experience are complex. Some people are unable to marry because their health is already impaired; others are unable to remain married because they have conditions such as mental disorders that their spouse cannot tolerate; some reject their family support systems for emotional or other reasons or are obliged by economic or other circumstances to live away from family in situations where they cannot take proper care of themselves. Any of these factors can increase the risk of disease and premature death. The death of a spouse is associated with higher than expected mortality rates among surviving bereaved widows and widowers; the recently bereaved may feel that they have less to live for than before the bereavement and may not take proper care of themselves. There are other subtle psychologic factors at work; in the words of the popular song, we all need some love in our lives.

Apart from the family, individuals belong to many kinds of social networks—persons with whom they work or share leisure, neighbors, friends from schooldays, and many others. There is great variation among individuals in the number and nature of these network relationships. The relationship between social support systems and health shown in Figure 6–2 is consistent enough to have prognostic value, so questions on social as well as family networks are often included in health surveys and even in some application forms for life insurance policies.

Persons with extensive networks generally have longer life expectancy and are less likely to die from many causes, compared to persons with few family, social, or work-related connections. Men experience greater effects related to their social networks than women. Factors that may play a part in the interaction between social networks and health include coping styles and ability to socialize, and perhaps that sense of self-worth I have mentioned before. The size and complexity of social networks is determined by many factors—family size and composition, occupation, other interests, and individuals' personal makeup, likes, and dislikes are some of the more obvious. Some of these factors can alter the risk of certain diseases, and the occurrence of certain diseases can influence the size and composition of a person's social networks. Sex differences are a clue. Do men with limited networks have higher age-specific death rates than women because of greater inability to cope with isolation, or does a health impairment that limits their capacity to form networks have greater impact on men than women? Probably both. Are women emotionally more resilient than men? These observed differences

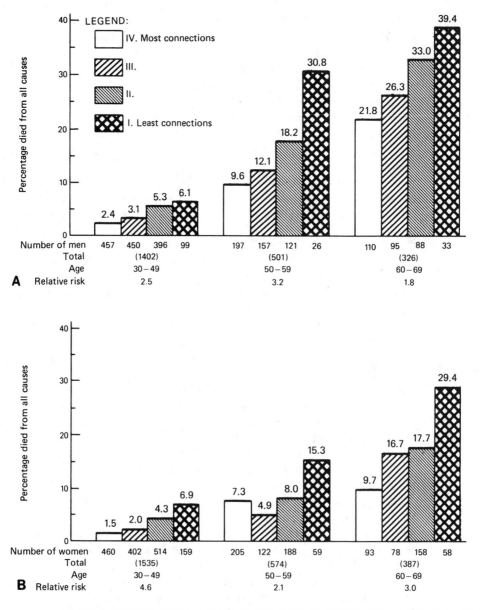

Figure 6–2. Social ties and 9-year mortality in Alameda County, California: **(A)** men; **(B)** women. *(From Berkman L, Syme SL: Social networks, host resistance, and mortality: A nine-year follow-up study of Alameda County residents. Am J Epidemiol 109:186–204, 1979.)*

are discussed in some of the monographs and journal articles listed among the references at the end of this chapter.[16-18]

Village society is believed to be a more hospitable setting for network formation than the anonymity of cities. In a village, deviant behavior, such as that of persons with mild mental retardation, is often tolerated; victims of disabling illness often are assisted by neighbors who notice when help is needed. Often in cities no one comes to the aid of those who need help. Deliberate attempts in some cities to establish neighborhoods with a sense of identity may have helped to develop social support systems, even if this was not the primary reason for this initiative. Health workers should encourage neighborhood development projects, e.g., in high-density high-rise apartment complexes that are sometimes a setting for social pathology.

Mobility

Sociologists distinguish geographic and social mobility; both influence health. Social mobility means movement from one SES group to another, e.g., from a working-class or blue-collar origin to a position in a profession such as law or medicine, or from a high SES origin to a low SES later in life, as can happen to political refugees. We can distinguish between individual social mobility and the mobility of children compared to their parents. Parents may have aspirations for their children to do better in life than they have done themselves, so they may encourage their children to get the education that will enable them to rise above their origins. Socially mobile adults may retain contact with or cast off family members such as parents or spouses when they set off to seek fame and fortune; if they shed their family on their way upward, this can be stressful to them and to those they leave behind. Social mobility can be a consequence of innate characteristics of the individual, such as ability or lack of it; or of external circumstances such as economic pressure or social upheavals. The socially mobile tend to take on the health characteristics of the SES into which they move—those who move into a higher SES tend to be healthier, those who move downward tend to be unhealthier. Sometimes those who are downwardly mobile have mental disorders or substance abuse problems, which explain their downward social drift.[19]

Geographic mobility is very common in industrial nations. Poor health inhibits geographic mobility. The relationship between migration and health is complex, related to SES and to reasons for migrating, which may be political or economic. I discuss migration as a demographic phenomenon in Chapter 9; movement within a country is much more frequent than movement across national borders; in the United States, about 25 percent of the population move in any given 5-year period. In most industrial nations the rates are similar, brought about by the same kind of changes in industrial and economic conditions.

There has been considerable rural-to-urban migration in the 20th cen-

TABLE 6-7.   **Japanese Migrant Studies; Men aged 45–64**[a]

Variable	Japan	Hawaii	California
Relative weight (%)	109	122	126
Calorie intake/wt lb	40	37	35
Saturated fat % calories	7	23	26
Carbohydrate % calories	63	46	44
Alcohol % calories	9	4	3
Serum cholesterol (mg/dL)	181	218	228
Cholesterol > 260 (%)	3	12	16
Serum triglycerides (mg/dL)	134	240	234
CHD deaths/1000	1.3	2.2	3.7

[a] Risk factor and CHD mortality differences between Japanese on the mainland, in Hawaii, and in California, showing the "effects" of migration on risk factor levels and risk.
CHD = coronary heart disease.
(From Marmot MG, et al, 1975.[21])

tury, especially in developing countries where seemingly inexorable forces are at work to impel the movement, and the consequent periurban slum development (see Chap. 9).

Migrants and the socially mobile usually adopt at least some of the cultural characteristics of the group or community into which they move, although this may take time, often more than a generation. The children of migrants come to resemble the native-born members of the society into which their parents migrated. When the changes involve cultural characteristics that the parents value highly, such as marriage customs and religious beliefs, this can cause considerable tension within families, and stress-related diseases can be a consequence.[20]

A simpler and more obvious change is in dietary customs. These have been much studied, for example among Japanese migrants to Hawaii and California, who over the two or three generations of their migration have adopted the diets of native Californians—and the diseases that go with these diets[21] (Table 6–7). Japanese-Americans have higher incidence rates of coronary heart disease and of large-bowel cancer and lower incidence rates of stomach cancer than Japanese in Japan who have maintained their traditional diets. Oriental and North African Jews who migrate to Israel experience increasing incidence of coronary heart disease.

► BEHAVIORAL FACTORS

Under this heading I consider personality-related factors and beliefs that determine or influence health-related behavior. Risk-taking behavior also fits in this category. So do stressful life events and neuroendocrine and neuroimmunologic connections (Box 6–2).

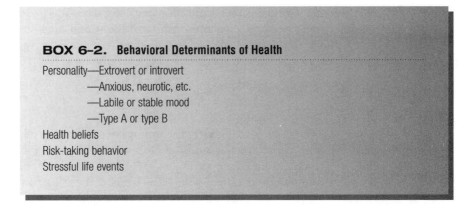

BOX 6-2. Behavioral Determinants of Health

Personality—Extrovert or introvert

      —Anxious, neurotic, etc.

      —Labile or stable mood

      —Type A or type B

Health beliefs

Risk-taking behavior

Stressful life events

Personality

Psychologists and psychiatrists have long identified varieties of personality that predispose to or protect against certain forms of mental disorder. Classifications of personality are older than modern psychiatry: They date back to the humoral theory of disease, evoked by the words choleric, melancholic, sanguine, and phlegmatic to describe four kinds of personality and, based on this, the diseases these four types were purportedly prone to develop. We rejected this ancient theory a few hundred years ago, but it has been replaced by concepts for which there is support from clinical observations and empirical research. Personality tests can distinguish introverted, extroverted, anxious, and neurotic psychologic traits; those who have volatile mood swings; and those who are habitually gloomy or cheerful. These show rather consistent relationships to susceptibility to certain forms of mental disorders and a tenuous relationship to some somatic disorders.

Friedman, Rosenman, and colleagues described type A and type B personalities and their relationship to heart disease.[22–24] Type A is characterized by aggressive, ambitious drive; time-urgent behavior; and quirks of interpersonal relationships such as a tendency to chip into conversations and complete sentences for those with whom the type A person is talking. Type A is significantly more common than type B among persons who develop coronary heart disease. The type B person is more placid, less aggressive, more relaxed about meeting deadlines. The relationship of personality type and proneness to coronary heart disease may have a simple pathophysiologic mechanism; type A is hyperresponsive to environmental stimuli, secreting catecholamines and developing elevated blood pressure when stressed. Type A may be a form of conditioned response to life in a modern competitive society (although it has been remarked that it was probably at least as stressful to be chased by a saber-toothed tiger in the Stone Age as it is to meet the chief executive officer of a corporation on a bad day). It is possible to "recondition" type A persons, e.g., those who are identified after they have had a heart attack; they can learn to become more type B in orientation and thereby reduce the risk of recurrence of heart disease.

Male and Female Sexuality

A striking aspect of personality is the emergence in adolescence of behavior patterns that are characteristic of male and female sexuality. Adolescents themselves seldom have insight into what is happening to them, and psychologists, sexologists, and others who have studied these phenomena are not much wiser: More is known about what happens than why, and (as many parents know only too well) even less is known about how to manage teenage sexuality so as to minimize unwanted pregnancies and sexually transmitted diseases, let alone the emotional crises of adolescence. Educating schoolchildren about sex and sexuality does reduce the incidence both of unwanted pregnancy and sexually transmitted diseases[25]—and does not lead to promiscuous or "immoral" behavior, as asserted by opponents of liberalized approaches to sex education.[26]

Late-20th century attitudes toward human sexuality seem to me inherently "healthier" than the attitudes that prevailed when I was a teenager and the subject was shrouded in secrecy, sex was "dirty," and masturbation was the deadliest of all sins. We are not far now from accepting that masturbation is healthier, or at any rate a great deal less risky, than promiscuous or unprotected sexual intercourse with strangers or casual acquaintances. Yet a U.S. Surgeon General was dismissed from office in 1994 for even hinting at this obvious truth. Clearly, in this respect publicly accepted values in the United States have not kept pace with understanding of human sexuality and sexually transmitted diseases.

Adult sexuality is a complex, multifaceted phenomenon. It is better understood than it was a generation ago, but we still have a lot to learn. We acknowledge that sexual behavior is astonishingly diverse, that it is healthy and life-enhancing for two people who love each other to find transcendental pleasure in lovemaking. We also recognize that sexual deviance is common and often can be harmful to others, particularly to child victims of sexual abuse. We do not have reliable ways to predict who will be perpetrators of sexual crimes or to treat potential perpetrators and prevent them from committing these heinous and harmful crimes.

Students usually are admitted to medical school shortly after the end of adolescence, when some may still be experiencing emotional instability associated with the transition from childhood to adult life. Moreover, emotionally disturbed individuals, including sexual psychopaths (who may be highly intelligent), are occasionally attracted toward a medical career, either to satisfy their prurient curiosity or even because they perceive this as an occupation that will give them opportunities to satisfy their unhealthy urges. Selection committees choosing among applicants for medical school places are not equipped to screen applicants for such potential problems, but teachers, mentors, and fellow students may observe behavior that is an early warning of trouble to come. Unfortunately, the evidence is often equivocal and little if anything can be done about it. In the 1970s, several colleagues and I were worried enough about the behavior and attitudes of a student to bring our concerns to the attention of the dean and other medical school authorities; but our evidence was too vague to be acted upon and the young man duly graduated. About 15 years later he was charged with multiple sexual offences against his female patients, served time in prison, and lost his license to practice medicine. Perhaps timely psychotherapeutic intervention might have prevented these events, but this individual was highly intelligent as well as an incorrigible sexual psychopath. Our level of knowledge, skills, and expertise was not adequate in such circumstances.

Homosexuality has come out of the closet into the mainstream of society; it is generally recognized to be an innate behavior, perhaps genetically determined, and not a learned behavior or a treatable condition that can be prevented or cured. HIV and AIDS has devastated the gay community in many Western nations because common sexual practices in this community, especially anal-receptive intercourse, favor transmission. Some homosexual men appear to have great sexual appetite and may be very promiscuous as well—extremely risky behavior in a world where HIV is so widespread.

Risk-Taking Behavior

Cohen[27] observed pedestrians crossing a busy intersection and noticed that apart from age and sex differences, there were variations in their apparent willingness to cross in front of oncoming traffic that could be explained only by the hypothesis that some were more willing to take risks than others. Cohen also studied the psychology of gamblers and identified a class who could be characterized by a predisposition for taking risks, in contrast to other persons whose behavior was more cautious. Some risk-taking behavior is age- and sex-related; in general, young adult men are more "adventurous"—more willing to take risks—than women or older persons, a phenomenon often exploited by political leaders seeking recruits in time of war. Risk-taking behavior applies to automobile drivers; it contributes to the high mortality rates of young men in traffic crashes. It may also explain the willingness to drive of persons who are aware of the danger of driving while impaired and the behavior of some tobacco addicts who expose themselves knowingly to the risks of cancer and other adverse outcomes. Some risk-taking behavior does respond to therapeutic interventions. For instance, compulsive gamblers can be helped by psychiatric treatment; mild forms of addiction to gambling (and to many legal substances) are usually regarded as normal and nothing is done about them.

Stressful Life Events

All of us from time to time experience an alteration in the even tenor of our daily lives. Our families grow as new members enter by birth or marriage or shrink as a result of deaths and departures as children grow up and leave home; or our families are disrupted by separation or divorce. Our jobs change, we take on more responsibility, or we are dismissed from the work-force. We are caught in minor or major brushes with the law-enforcement authorities. We are afflicted by natural or manmade disasters. Holmes and Rahe[29] studied the relationships between stressful life events and health and longevity. There is a close relationship between adverse health outcomes and recent occurrence of major emotional stresses such as the death of a loved one, arrest of a family member for a crime, dismissal from a long-held job, or involvement in disaster or violence and premature death. Compared to age-matched controls, Vietnam veterans have a higher risk of subsequent violent death by suicide, homicide, or fatal injury in traffic crashes, suggesting that emotional stress associated with violence might predispose to future violence.[28] The relationship of health to stressful life events is both specific for diseases associated with stress, e.g., asthma, and nonspecific, applying to all

TABLE 6–8.   Criteria Used for the Rahe–Holmes Life Events Scale

Death of spouse[a]	Change to different line of work	Trouble with boss
Divorce[a]	Change in number of arguments with spouse	Revision of personal habits
Marital separation[a]		Change in work conditions
Marriage	Pregnancy	Change in residence
Death of close family member[a]	Death of close friend[a]	Change in schools
Jail term	Change in work responsibility	Change in recreation
Personal injury or illness	Foreclosure of mortgage or loan	Change in social activities
Fired from work	Son or daughter leaving home	Change in church activities
Marital reconciliation	Trouble with in-laws	Mortgage or loan less than $10,000[b]
Retirement from work	Mortgage over $10,000[b]	
Gain of new family member	Start or end of work	Change in sleeping habits
Change in health of family member	Outstanding personal achievement	Change in family get-togethers
		Change in eating habits
Sex difficulties	Beginning or end of formal schooling	Vacation
Business adjustment		Christmas
Change of financial status	Change in living conditions	Minor violations of law

[a] "Scores" depend on emotional impact, e.g., whether grief or a happy release.
[b] In the 1990s, mortgage value could be amended to $65,000.
(From Holmes and Rahe.[29])

causes of morbidity and mortality. Some can be explained, e.g., a tendency for traffic or domestic accidents to occur while people are preoccupied by some recent stressful event.

Holmes and Rahe developed a scale to indicate the impact of life events on health experience[29] (Table 6–8). One important life event, divorce and separation, deserves further comment because of its frequent occurrence. Separation and divorce have long-term effects not only on marital partners but also on their children. The subsequent lives of children from broken homes can be affected in several ways. Intellectual development, measured by school performance, is often adversely affected for prolonged periods; these children also have higher than expected rates of stress-related diseases such as asthma; behavioral disorders are more common than in children from intact families; and they may have difficulty forming new emotional bonds, including stable marital bonds.

The preceding discussion suggests the existence of different varieties of mind–body interaction that influence health. Some interaction is at a subconscious level, or at least involves processes over which we have little if any conscious control. Risk-taking behavior may be in this category. "Stress-related" diseases like high blood pressure almost certainly are. Moreover, they sometimes respond well to nonpharmacologic interventions like meditation and yoga.[30] Allopathic physicians may be reluctant to admit it, but some will concede that yoga and meditation, long practiced in India, can work as well as or better than drugs to treat hypertension. Whether they work because training in meditation or yoga confers the ability to influence physical bodily functions like heart rate and blood pressure, or because obsessive preoccupation with personal problems is alleviated, or for some other reason, the fact is that these methods do work; and unlike many modern pharmaceutical preparations, they have no toxic adverse effects.[31] However, they are labor intensive and time consuming, which are disadvantages in a world as addicted to rushing hither and yon as ours is. Obviously more research on the underlying mechanisms of meditation and yoga is desirable.

Neuroimmune Mechanisms

Much work has been done on mind–body reactions in health and disease. Selye,[32] a pioneer in this field, published extensively in the 1930s to 1950s; he coined the term "general adaptation syndrome" to explain all stress-related disorders and postulated connections from higher cortical centers through the hypophysis-adrenal-thymus glands to circulating lymphocytes, and to electrolyte metabolism (thus affecting blood vessels, blood pressure, and various endothelial tissues). By overstating the case for "stress-related" diseases that included rheumatoid arthritis, chronic nephritis, and many other chronic diseases, he strained credulity, perhaps setting back further progress for a time. But the concept of stress-related diseases mediated through hypothalamus-hypophysis-other endocrine glands remained intact and has been reinvigorated by modern work in the field known as psychoneuroimmunology.[33] The neuroimmunologic connections are particularly interesting in offering an explanation for the often observed phenomena of remissions and relapses in the course of cancer and perhaps other conditions of unknown etiology like multiple sclerosis.[34]

Although much remains unknown about the mechanism and mode of action of mind–body interaction, effective therapeutic interventions have long existed. Some that have been used for centuries by traditional healers in India have been adopted with increasing assurance by specialist physicians trained in Western allopathic medicine. Based almost entirely on empirical observations, and initially viewed with suspicion by Western clinical scientists, techniques of transcendental meditation and yoga and, partly derived from these, biofeedback have been adopted in an increasing number of mainstream medical centers. The efficacy of these methods of treating hypertension, coronary heart disease, and anxiety disorders has been demonstrated by randomized controlled trials.[35] Immune mechanisms also are known to be affected by mental and emotional stimuli. The nature of the cortical, neural, immunologic, and endocrine pathways involved are the subject of much study by psychoneuroimmunologists. If I live long enough to produce a third edition of this book in another 10 years, doubtless there will be a great deal more to say about it.

The Health Belief Model

Health behavior is influenced by conscious thought. Several theoretical concepts have been developed to explain ways in which the process works. Mechanic and others delineated several aspects of illness-related behavior[36]; other aspects of behavior can be related to health rather than to illness.

Knowledge, attitudes, and skills play an important part in the adoption and maintenance of specific behaviors, including much consciously health-related behavior. The sociocultural environment strongly influences knowledge and attitudes. Becker developed the health belief model to explain health-related behavior[37]; this and several variations on the same theme use a cognitive approach to explain behavior as reasoned action.

The health belief model includes environmental influences such as social and ideologic factors that operate in the home, school, workplace, through the mass media, and by way of contact with health professionals or other significant persons. Individuals may perceive benefits of taking some actions and barriers to taking these actions that will influence their health; they also have perceptions about diseases that may be a threat, with respect to their own susceptibility, the seriousness of the condition, and its responsiveness to intervention.[28] The likelihood that they will take health-related action is influenced by many modifying factors, summarized in Figure 6–3. The model is useful because it shows important variables that have to be taken into account when we are attempting to influence the way people behave.

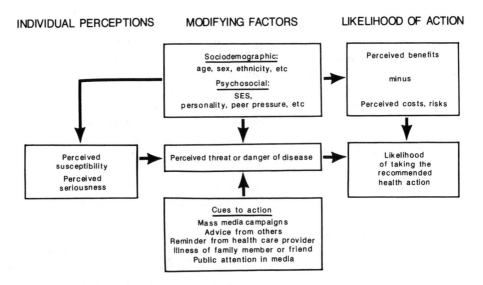

Figure 6–3. The health belief model; SES = socioeconomic status. *(Modified from Becker MH (ed):* The Health Belief Model and Personal Health Behavior. *Thorofare, NJ: Slack, 1974.[39])*

Some modifying factors are more powerful than others, and the effects of several can be influenced by reinforcement.

Sets, Settings, and Peer Pressure

Sets are the small groups to which individuals belong or with which they identify, and settings are the larger social and cultural environments, such as a school or workplace, in which the sets are located. We are all familiar with whims of fashion that determine the lengths of women's skirts, the popularity of entertainments, adherence to particular political causes. All cultures have labile fashions, as well as more fixed ways of behaving. The Opies[39] and Cole[40] described the pattern of change among schoolchildren; games, songs, even political attitudes can alter abruptly, perhaps seasonally, sometimes for no apparent reason. The tendency to change continues into adult life and on into retirement. Probably it has its most significant effects on health when it operates in childhood. One powerful influence is peer pressure within the set and setting.

Fondness for certain foods and drinks, taking up or refraining from cigarette smoking while in school, and many other behaviors, perhaps most that are learned, appear to be responses (at least in part) to peer pressure in the set and the setting. They are initiated behaviors that follow a pattern determined by opinion leaders, individuals who possess qualities that cause others in the same set to follow the lead. Following the lead is partly a response to peer pressure: Most of us find it easier to go along with the majority than to resist and be different. This is a complex process, closely linked to the efforts of young persons emerging from childhood through adolescence into adult life to find support and identity as members of a group.

To describe this complex process as an aspect of behavior that is determined by psychosocial factors begs many difficult questions; human behavior often seems to be a group process. In some respects we behave like other social animals: schools of fish, flocks of geese, herds of sheep or cattle.[41] Human groups by no means always behave rationally. Mass reactions to demagogic political leaders, popular entertainers, and to emotional stimuli of the fight–flight variety suggest that human groups often behave irrationally. As with other aspects of human behavior, there is much we do not understand; the aspect of behavioral science concerned with group processes is in its infancy.

Empirical observations over several hundred years have confirmed this. Mackay's classic work, *Extraordinary Popular Delusions and the Madness of Crowds*,[42] was a descriptive account of large group processes, i.e., the behaviors of crowds, communities, even nations, that were mostly psychopathologic. Fraudulent financial schemes, the influence of panic on prices of shares traded in stock exchanges, the maniacal witch-hunts of medieval Europe—and modern variations[43]—and the mass appeal of demagogues such as Hitler illustrate the danger that such deviant group processes can present to a well-ordered society.

Psychiatrists have studied "behavioral epidemics," which are a variation on the same theme. These are group responses to a stimulus, mediated by the power of suggestion rather than by some physical or biologic agent. Behavioral epidemics typically occur among impressionable schoolchildren who all simultaneously fall ill, e.g., from contact with an imaginary insect; but they can occur in an adult population and extend over a prolonged period, for instance when the workers in a sealed air-conditioned building believe themselves to be affected by symptoms caused by toxic fumes that circulate through the ventilation system. Such phenomena are properly described as psychosocial (although there can be a physical basis for symptoms in sealed buildings; see Chap. 4). The nature, mode of operation, and susceptibility to control of behavioral epidemics remain largely unexplored, although health educators (and politicians) have searched for ways to manipulate these processes. Health education tries to use this process for desirable ends.

► LIFESTYLE

This term refers to habits and customs that are influenced, modified, encouraged, or constrained by the lifelong process of socialization that we all undergo. Lifestyle strongly influences patterns of health and sickness. Diet, exercise, use of tobacco, alcohol, tea and coffee, safety-conscious behavior

BOX 6–3. Lifestyle

Habits and customs influenced and modified by socialization
Diet
Exercise
Games, hobbies
Other uses of leisure time
Health-related substance use
    Tea, coffee
    Alcohol
    Tobacco
    Prescribed drugs
    Self-medication
    Illicit substance use
Safety practices
    Seatbelt use
    Use of safety equipment in home and at work
Health-related values
    Immunizations
    Health maintenance procedures
        Breast self-examination
        Pap smears
        Blood pressure checks
        Occult blood test
        Etc.

such as use or nonuse of automobile seatbelts are aspects of lifestyle that demonstrably are related to health and to the risk of disease, injury, or premature death (Box 6–3).

Here I briefly discuss exercise, the use of tobacco, alcohol, and other substance abuse. Diet is discussed in Chapter 5 and violence in Chapter 7.

Exercise

Many epidemiologic studies have demonstrated lower incidence and mortality rates from coronary heart disease among persons who habitually take exercise than those who do not.[44] This evidence has become part of popular culture. It has led to the popularity of jogging and recreational forms of physical exercise among a high proportion of men and women whose work is sedentary and does not provide opportunities for exercise. People who regularly jog or take part in other physical activity say that it makes them feel good. Most people believe exercise protects them from coronary heart disease. The descriptive and analytic epidemiologic evidence is persuasive; physicians are justified in advising everyone to take regular exercise within the limits of their physiologic capability. In combination with a well-balanced diet, this is one of the most important actions we can take to preserve good health.

The facts are well enough established to justify health promotion strategies as an important component of national health policies,[45] and many countries have implemented such policies, e.g., by providing facilities for recreational exercise at public expense, encouraging work breaks for physical exercise in sedentary occupations, and including advice on the desirability of maintaining physical fitness by taking suitable exercise as part of national health education campaigns. This is a good example of synergism between individual and community responsibility for health.

Smoking and Health

Unequivocal evidence that tobacco smoke contains carcinogens was published in 1915,[46] and had made its way into textbooks of pathology and medicine by the 1930s. The first convincing evidence that cigarette tobacco smoke causes lung cancer was a case-control study published in 1939[47]; but it was in German and it passed unnoticed in the turmoil of World War II.

After the war the trickle of articles setting out the epidemiologic evidence linking cigarette smoking and lung cancer soon became a torrent.[48–50] Several studies also showed that cigarette smoking increased the risk of coronary heart disease. It had long been believed that there was a relationship between smoking and chronic bronchitis (although tobacco advertisers tried to promote the early morning cigarette as a good way to "cut the phlegm!"). Studies confirmed too that smoking causes chronic bronchitis and emphysema. All the risks have been measured. Tobacco smoke does so many other harmful things—to smokers, and to bystanders who are exposed to toxic side-stream smoke, to the infants, children, and developing fetuses of smoking mothers—that no rational society would have tolerated tobacco as we have done for so many years. Evidence on the ill effects of tobacco fills many library shelves (Table 6–9). It is the single greatest preventable cause of premature death and disability in modern times. Unfortunately tobacco is the driving force of a huge and lucrative industry[51,52] and a powerful, addictive substance, perhaps the most addictive substance known. Nicotine, the active ingredient, has both tranquilizing and stimulant properties. It is a tragic accident of history that it became so entrenched before its carcinogenic and other harmful effects were known. If tobacco had first been discovered after regulatory agencies were established to protect society from toxic products, it would never have been licensed. Tobacco companies place great emphasis on the fact that theirs is a "legal product" and sales and advertising therefore cannot be prohibited or restricted.

Its addictive nature makes tobacco smoking very difficult to stop. Many try repeatedly, only to resume again after briefly quitting. Yet many others break free from their addiction. The health belief model helps to explain why. Powerful motivation is necessary. So is social reinforcement by friends

TABLE 6–9. Some Harmful Effects of Tobacco Smoking

Condition	Risk
Coronary heart disease 45% of all U.S. deaths 35% of these deaths are attributable to smoking	Risk increases with amount smoked 80% increased risk among smokers of 20+ cigs/day
Cancer 22% of all U.S. deaths 30% of these deaths are attributable to smoking	Risk of lung cancer 20 times greater in smokers of 20+ cigs/day than in nonsmokers; many other cancers smoking-related.
Chronic obstructive lung disease 3% of all U.S. deaths 90% of these deaths are attributable to smoking	Smokers of 20+ cigs/day have 40 times higher risk than nonsmokers
Peptic ulcer disease	Smokers have 3 times greater risk than nonsmokers
Involuntary absorption of tobacco smoke	Infants and children have 2- to 3-fold increase of respiratory infections, growth retardation, higher risk of sudden infant death syndrome Adults have increased risk of angina, lung cancer, conjunctivitis, asthma, bronchitis
Effects on fetus	Growth retardation, impaired postpartum respiratory function Suspected increased risk of birth defects and childhood cancer

Smoking causes or contributes to many other conditions, e.g., peripheral vascular disease, periodontal disease, tobacco
amblyopia, facial "aging," impaired sexual function

Smoking costs the smoker many thousands of dollars in direct costs and probably more in indirect costs over a lifetime,
to say nothing of lost productivity from smoking-related disease and premature death

Smoking is often implicated in domestic fires, fires in restaurants, and other public buildings, and was the cause of at
least one major airline disaster

and family who can provide encouragement and emotional rewards for ab-
staining.

Until the 1960s, innumerable social reinforcing factors encouraged
smoking. Offering a cigarette was the preferred opening ritual in social intercourse, a custom derived from the peace pipe of pre-Columbian Indians; ash-
trays were displayed and used in all public places and smoking was permitted
almost everywhere. Although adults usually discouraged children from smoking, the sanctions were not severe; by late adolescence, up to 80 percent of
boys and 30 percent of girls were addicted. The change in attitudes toward
smoking since the 1960s has been remarkable. It has become socially unacceptable to smoke in restaurants and many other public spaces where it is legal to smoke, and in an ever-increasing number and variety of public places it
is illegal. The change is undoubtedly due in part at least to reports released
in the early 1960s by the U.S. surgeon general and the Royal College of Physi-

cians of London, with constant reinforcement ever since. In addition to increasingly strong social sanctions against smoking and greater militancy of nonsmokers seeking cleaner indoor air, governments have provided support by raising taxes on tobacco and by enacting local ordinances that prohibit smoking in many public places.

Few people are unaware of the health hazards of smoking, and powerful social reinforcement is available to the smoker who is trying to quit, as well as deterrents to young starting smokers. Nevertheless a message is communicated to many schoolchildren that smoking is "cool," a sign of the young person's eagerness to take risks or defy authority. This explains why up to 30 percent of boys and girls in most Western nations become regular smokers by the time they are in their mid- to late teens. In developing nations, rates are much higher among children, and is over 60 percent of both boys and girls in several Latin American countries (Table 6–10).

Schoolchildren who start to smoke are often poor achievers and are at odds with authority figures—but unfortunately also are often opinion leaders among their peers, and in this way, they are responsible for spreading the smoking habit. There is much not yet understood about motives for beginning to smoke; desire to defy authority figures (parents, schoolteachers) is a

TABLE 6–10. Estimated Smoking Prevalence Rates at Ages 15 Years and Over, Various Countries, Various Years, Since Mid-1980s (%)

Country	(Year of Survey)	Males	Females
Russian Federation	(1993)	67.0	30.0
China	(1984)	61.0	7.0
Japan	(1994)	59.0	14.8
Sri Lanka	(1988)	54.8	0.8
Indonesia	(1986)	53.0	4.0
Thailand	(1995)	49.0	4.0
Israel	(1989)	45.0	30.0
France	(1993)	40.0	27.0
India	(1980s)	40.0	3.0
Brazil	(1989)	39.9	25.4
Mexico	(1990)	38.0	12.0
Germany	(1992)	36.8	21.5
Switzerland	(1992)	36.0	26.0
Canada	(1991)	31.0	28.0
Australia	(1993)	29.0	21.0
United Kingdom	(1994)	28.0	26.0
United States	(1991)	28.1	23.5
New Zealand	(1992)	24.0	22.0
Sweden	(1994)	22.0	24.0

Source: WHO (http://www.who.ch/programmes/psa/toh/Alert/apr96/gifs/table3.gif)

factor. Perhaps another factor is to use the smoke as an aggressive or protective screen against perceived oppression. This may explain why smoking is common among groups who perceive themselves to be oppressed or subservient to others. A rational smoking prevention program should study and apply these factors. Some success has been achieved in school programs by identifying popular peer group leaders in classes and enlisting them as role models; but this mostly works well with children who aspire to resemble the role models and is often rejected by underachievers.

More can be done at many levels of society to control the smoking epidemic. Practicing physicians can help by reinforcing the message that tobacco in any form is harmful to health and safety. They can advise pregnant women and parents of infants and young children that their smoking will harm these innocent young lives, can cause sudden infant death syndrome, impairs their children's respiratory function, and greatly increases the risk of house fires; they can teach smoking patients about health problems attributable to tobacco addiction; and when patients die of smoking-related diseases, physicians can use the International Statistical Classification of Diseases and Related Health Problems, 10th Revision (ICD-10) coding rules (see Chap. 2) to certify that the death was caused by tobacco addiction.[53] Lung cancer or coronary heart disease may have been the immediate cause, but the addiction to tobacco was the underlying cause. If mortality statistics show increasing numbers of deaths attributable to tobacco addiction, rather than to lung cancer or coronary heart disease, this should have considerable emotional and political impact.

Physicians and other health workers should take leadership in political movements aimed at controlling the smoking epidemic,[54,55] allying themselves with others in the lobby groups that oppose the tobacco and advertising industries. Tobacco advertising is an example of the pernicious practices of commercial societies gone wrong. There is nothing wrong or evil about advertising as such. But advertising when it is aimed at children and youths with the specific aim of encouraging them to adopt a life-threatening addictive behavior is evil and should be opposed. This happens overtly in many developing countries and (despite pious claims to the contrary) covertly in the United States and other nations where the tobacco advertisers have adopted what they describe as a voluntary code of good behavior.

Alcohol Abuse

Alcohol has been used by almost all human societies. It has both stimulant and sedative properties, which might explain why some people become dependent on it. The degree of dependency is variable; sometimes it may be genetically determined. A few people are unable to control their drinking and destroy themselves by succumbing to an alcohol-related disease[56]—or destroy themselves, and often others, too, in traffic crashes caused by driving while impaired. Alcohol-related problems are summarized in Table 6–11, and information about alcohol consumption worldwide is summarized in Table 6–12.

TABLE 6–11. A Summary of Alcohol-Related Physical, Psychologic, and Behavioral Problems

Psychologic and behavioral
  Acute alcohol intoxication
  Acute alcohol poisoning
  Hangover
  Blackouts
  Alcohol dependence
Acute alcohol withdrawal syndromes and
  alcoholic psychoses
Acute alcohol withdrawal syndrome
  Delirium tremens
  Acute auditory hallucinosis
  Depression
  Attempted suicide
  Suicide
Neurologic
  Subclinical neuropsychologic impairment
  Epilepsy
  Peripheral neuropathy
  Cerebral atrophy
  Cerebellar atrophy
  Wernicke-Korsakoff syndrome
  Traumatic head injury
  Death from cerebrovascular disease
Gastrointestinal
  Oropharyngeal carcinoma
  Acute esophageal dysfunction
  Mallory–Weiss syndrome
  Esophageal varices
  Esophageal carcinoma
  Erosive gastritis
  Acute gastroduodenal ulceration
  Atrophic gastritis
  Gastric carcinoma
  Disturbed small-bowel motility
  Intestinal malabsorption
  Large-bowel carcinoma
  Subclinical pancreatic dysfunction
  Chronic pancreatitis
  Pancreatic carcinoma
  Fatty liver
  Alcoholic hepatitis
  Cirrhosis
  Hepatocellular carcinoma
Cardiovascular
  Cardiac arrhythmias
  Alcoholic cardiomyopathy
  Cardiac beriberi
  Hypertension
  Ischemic heart disease

Respiratory
  Obstructive sleep apnea
  Chronic obstructive lung disease
  Pneumonia
  Lung abscess
  Pulmonary tuberculosis
  Laryngeal carcinoma
  Carcinoma of the lung
Endocrine and metabolic
  Hypoglycemia
  Hyperglycemia
  Diabetes
  Gout
  Lactic acidosis
  Derangements of mineral metabolism
Reproductive
  Depressed testicular function
  Depressed ovarian function
  Carcinoma of the breast
Musculoskeletal
  Acute and chronic myopathy
  Ischemic necrosis of the head of femur
  Osteoporosis
Hematologic
  Anemia
  Impaired leukocyte response to infection
  Thrombocytopenia
Traumatic injuries
Ethanol–drug interactions
Nutritional deficiencies
Pregnancy outcome and developmental disorders
  Spontaneous abortion
  Perinatal mortality
  Low birth weight
  Impaired development (physical, behavioral,
    intellectual)
  Congenital birth defects
  Fetal alcohol syndrome
  Pseudo-Cushing's syndrome in breast-fed infants
  Alcohol withdrawal in newborn

(From Rankin JG, Ashley MJ: Alcohol-related health problems and their prevention. In Last JM (ed): Maxcy-Rosenau Public Health and Preventive Medicine. 12th ed. E. Norwalk, CT: Appleton-Century-Crofts, 1986, p. 1041.)

TABLE 6–12. Prevalence of Substance Use by Children in the United States, 1991 and 1995 (%)

Substance	Grade	1991	1995
Any illicit drug			
	8	18.7	28.5
	10	30.6	40.9
	12	44.1	48.4
Marijuana			
	8	10.2	19.9
	10	23.4	34.1
	12	36.7	41.7
Inhalants			
	8	17.6	21.6
	10	15.7	19.1
	12	17.6	17.4
Hallucinogens			
	8	3.2	5.2
	10	6.1	9.3
	12	9.6	12.7
Cocaine			
	8	2.3	4.2
	10	4.1	5.0
	12	7.8	6.0
Alcohol—been drunk			
	8	26.7	25.3
	10	50.0	46.9
	12	65.4	63.2
Cigarette smoking (ever smoked)			
	8	44.0	46.4
	10	55.1	57.6
	12	63.1	64.2

Source: http://www.health.org/pubs/monitor/mtf95tla.htm. More detail on use of these and other substances is available at this URL.

The control of alcohol abuse[57] requires a synergistic effort by affected individuals, their families, community leaders, the laws and regulations of the community or nation, and frequently a special effort by peers, alcoholics who have already controlled their alcohol problem and are able to help and counsel others through the worldwide organization, Alcoholics Anonymous (AA). AA meetings resemble evangelistic religious gatherings, with soul-baring confessions and strong reinforcement of recruits who are recently enough weaned from their bottles to require a great deal of social and emotional support. Medical and psychiatric management of alcohol-related disorders is described in some of the references at the end of this chapter.

Other Substance Abuse

Many users of psychoactive drugs obtain their supplies legally on physicians' prescriptions; these are patients who can easily become habituated or addicted. Physicians are sometimes responsible for initiating legal drug use, which evolves via habituation to addiction to mood-modifying drugs such as tranquilizers and antidepressants.

Other substances favored by youths and those against which there are legal sanctions, e.g., marijuana, cocaine, and heroin, have been publicized and perhaps sensationalized. Illegality gives them a peculiar power of attraction to impressionable and alienated young people who derive excitement from flouting laws and conventions.[58]

Psychoactive drugs fall into several pharmacologic groups: stimulants, sedatives, and hallucinogens. These alter perceptions of reality; if reality is unpleasant, alteration by psychoactive drugs is perceived as desirable—another reason why youths who live in urban slums, who are deprived or oppressed or in trouble with schools or the law are attracted to substance abuse.

The pattern of illegal substance abuse can change rapidly. The high prevalence of heroin addiction observed in the 1960s was replaced in the mid-1980s by addiction to cocaine. Marijuana use remains about the same. Cocaine addiction is more serious than heroin because cocaine is more addictive; cocaine addicts have greater difficulty breaking the habit. Cocaine may also do more lasting and serious damage both to the central nervous system and to other body functions.

Abuse of alcohol and drugs occurs at much higher rates than in the general population among several social groups. One group is members of ethnic communities that have been overwhelmed by another culture—e.g., Native Americans, Australian aborigines. Another, less clearly defined, is people who are unsuccessful in the competition for advancement, whether because of language differences, as are some immigrant groups, or because of limited ability. A miscellaneous group is made up of rebels, the unconventional, the socially deviant. These generalizations, while helpful to identify vulnerable groups at whom to direct health education, are potentially dangerous if they lead to stereotyping and stigmatizing. Educational messages, whether aimed at prevention or at rehabilitation, should focus on ways to encourage integration into conventional society of people in these and other groups of substance abusers.

Control of substance abuse is difficult. Health education in schools, applying similar approaches to those that have been successful in reducing cigarette smoking, sometimes helps. Law enforcement agencies can help by reducing if not eliminating illegal drug trafficking and by identifying drug abusers and helping to ensure that they get adequate support and treatment.

► BEHAVIORAL APPROACHES TO HEALTH PROMOTION

Health education has become increasingly sophisticated by applying theoretical concepts such as the health belief model and its variants.

Health education must deal with beliefs, motives, behaviors, and habits and the social environment (the set and setting) to which people belong. The emphasis of health education is on self-care and self-help as essential steps toward health promotion. Often beliefs have to be changed as a step toward providing a rationale for motivation to change health-related behavior. For example, it is necessary to inform teenaged girls about how they become pregnant in order to explain why they should be chaste, or if they are sexually active, why they must use effective contraception if they do not want to become pregnant. The behavior and habits of the group or set to which people belong are powerful determinants of individual behavior as well as of values and beliefs. In seeking to influence individual behavior by health education, it is important to identify the sets as well as the larger social setting in which these are located, such as the school that children attend.

One effective approach is to find peers who can influence the behavior of sets by providing leadership and role models, as described previously for smoking prevention programs. This can be done by "remote control"—if a film star or sports champion who is idolized by young people behaves in a certain way, e.g., declining cigarettes when they are offered, this can lead impressionable teenagers to copy the behavior. This works well when opinion leaders provide the example in the setting of schools and among sets of schoolchildren. It has proved efficacious in randomized trials in Norway, California, and Finland, and has been replicated in other countries.

The influence of the media, especially television, has been demonstrated in controlled trials, of which those in North Karelia, Finland,[59] are the best known. In some of this work, adults were the study population and, although smoking was the primary target behavior, other risk factors for coronary heart disease were also attacked. These studies showed how television can be used for desirable social purposes. They raise important questions about the influence of television on undesirable forms of behavior, such as attitudes toward violence.

Practicing physicians often encounter situations in which patients' health is adversely affected by their behavior. The proper management of this situation is a sine qua non of good medical practice. Unfortunately, it is an aspect of medical work that physicians seldom do well. Unless they are properly trained, no other health workers—nurses, for instance—do much better. Proper management requires first a diagnosis—identification of the nature and causes of the behavior problem—then treatment, which has to be directed specifically at the underlying causes. Treatment is time consuming; unfortunately is not recognized as essential and therefore is not adequately paid for in many health insurance programs.

Diagnosis requires a detailed description of the behavior, a history of its duration and associated facts, and psychosocial inquiry about the dynamics of the health-related behavior (e.g., is it related to tensions between spouses?). These steps lead to a behavioral diagnosis, which makes it possible to formulate a treatment plan in collaboration with the patient and preferably the patient's family.

Treatment requires similar attention to detail. Continuity of personal care, response to the patient's expectations, provision of necessary knowledge, simplified methods wherever possible, provision of rewards for effort, minimal arduous limitations or "costs," and instilling a sense of personal responsibility are all important. If behavior change requires complex and prolonged efforts, working into it gradually and setting limited goals, each of which is to be achieved in sequence, are sensible approaches. Constant support and reinforcement are necessary.

Health care providers can use a simple checklist to go over the points that matter when they attempt behavior change. The points to be covered include the time, effort, complexity, inconvenience, or discomfort of the regimen; and the impact on the regimen of fear, insecurity, or discouragement that the patient or client may encounter. The cost of the program is an important consideration; physicians criticize public health authorities who exhort them to counsel their patients on health-enhancing behavior, saying that they cannot afford to spend the time that this requires or their patients cannot afford to pay for the time. On the other hand, successful participation in a program of health behavior change brings other rewards: feeling good, gratifying the sense of having achieved something worthwhile, the satisfaction of being cared for, and social approval all are sources of satisfaction for clients or patients.

► CONCLUSION

As intimated at the beginning of this chapter, many concepts that remain largely theoretical have been developed by behavioral and biomedical scientists to explain and thus to control more effectively the health problems that result from unsatisfactory social and behavioral circumstances.[60] Objective scientific evidence is increasing. The emerging specialty of behavioral medicine is searching for ways in which stressful life events and the presence or absence of social support systems influence morbidity and mortality and for links between personality and physiologic reactivity. Medical anthropologists have developed both a theoretical and an applied focus in their study of the cultural context of health.[61,62] These concepts can be put to practical use in improving people's health both in a national and an international context. Indeed, a specialist in international health cannot be called truly proficient if she or he lacks insights into medical anthropology, as my comments in chapters 9 and 10 may help to underscore.

This chapter contains some ideas that are not firmly established as components of public health or medical practice. We know that behavior influences health and that health influences behavior; but many of us become uneasy at the thought of taking actions that might influence behavior, even if there are proved health benefits likely to follow. Our attitudes and part of our cultural heritage, have been influenced by recent history, the evidence from Nazi Germany in particular, of the terrible harm that can be done when actions to influence human behavior are undertaken by agents of the state. The writings of George Orwell, particularly in *1984,* added fuel to this fire. We do not want "thought police" in our society. This might explain why we have allowed television advertising and the mass culture it perpetuates an unfettered grasp on the minds of impressionable youngsters.

For similar reasons there is a pejorative ring to the term "social engineering." We are reluctant to change the way society is structured, let alone the way it functions. Our reluctance is related to ignorance, too; we lack much-needed information as well as firmly established underlying theories and concepts that have been demonstrated to work in the real world. Nonetheless, there is evidence that some approaches work. For example, poor children lack opportunities for skill development that are available to children whose parents are affluent[63]; interventions can help these children to acquire life-enhancing skills. As we learn more, we will find other situations where we can intervene effectively.

▶ REFERENCES

1. Helman C: *Culture, Health and Illness,* 2nd ed. New York: Butterworth-Heinemann, 1990.
2. Kleinman A: *Writing at the Margin; Discourse Between Anthropology and Medicine.* Berkeley: University of California Press, 1995.
3. The huge literature on this topic can be approached from the following, among many others: (1) Veblen T: *The Theory of the Leisure Class.* New York: Modern Library, 1934 1st ed. Macmillan, 1899; (2) Skinner BF: *Beyond Freedom and Dignity.* New York: Knopf, 1971; (3) Moore B Jr: *Social Origins of Dictatorship and Democracy.* New York: Carnegie Corporation, 1966; (4) Terkel S: *Working.* New York: Pantheon, 1972.
4. Benjamin B: *Social and Economic Factors Affecting Mortality.* The Hague: UNESCO, 1965.* Vol. 5 in Surveys of Research in the Social Sciences.
5. Mitchell GD, Hewitt M: Social stratification. In Mitchell GD (ed): *A Dictionary of Sociology.* Chicago: Aldine, 1968.
6. Townsend P, Davidson N: *Inequalities in Health.* Harmondsworth, England: Penguin, 1982.* [A revised version of the *Black Report.*]
7. Whitehead M: *The Health Divide.* Harmondsworth, England: Penguin, 1990.
8. Wigle DT, Mao Y: *Mortality by Income Level in Urban Canada.* Ottawa: Laboratory Centre for Disease Control, 1980.

* These are general as well as specific reference sources or are seminal papers of great interest and importance.

9. Westcott G, Svensson P-G, Zollner HFK: *Health Policy Implications of Unemployment.* Copenhagen: World Health Organization, 1985.*

10. Rainwater L: The lower class. Health, illness and medical institutions. In Deutscher I, Thompson EJ (eds): *Among the People.* New York: Basic Books, 1968, pp. 259–278.

11. Koos EL: *The Health of Regionville.* New York: Hafner, 1954.*

12. Kunitz SJ, Sorensen AA: The changing distribution of disease in Regionville. *Int J Epidemiol* 4:105–112, 1975.

13. Beck RG: Economic class and access to physicians' services. *Int J Health Serv* 3:341–355, 1973.

14. Smith R: *Unemployment and Health.* Oxford: Oxford University Press, 1987.

15. Philips RL: Role of lifestyle and dietary habits in risk of cancer among Seventh Day Adventists. *Cancer Res* 35:3513–3522, 1975. See also Fraser GE, Lindsted KD, Beeson WL: Effect of risk factor values on lifetime risk of and age at first coronary event. *Am J Epidemiol* 142:746–758, 1995.

16. Berkman LF, Breslow L: *Health and Ways of Living; The Alameda County Study.* New York: Oxford University Press, 1983.*

17. Cohen S, Syme SL: *Social Support and Health.* Orlando, Fla: Academic Press, 1985.*

18. Cassel J, Tyroler HA: Epidemiological studies of cultural change; I: Health status and recency of industrialization. *Arch Environ Health* 3:25–33, 1961.

19. Susser MW, Watson W, Hopper, K: Social mobility, stress and disorders of health. In *Sociology in Medicine.* 3rd ed. New York: Oxford University Press, 1985, pp. 316–356.*

20. Kaplan BH, Cassel JC, Tyroler HA, et al.: Occupational mobility and coronary heart disease. *Arch Intern Med* 128:938–942, 1971.

21. Marmot MG, Syme SL, Kagan A, et al.: Epidemiologic studies of coronary heart disease and stroke in Japanese men living in Japan, Hawaii and California. *Int J Epidemiol* 102:477–480, 1975.

22. Jenkins CD: Recent evidence supporting psychologic and social risk factors for coronary disease. *N Engl J Med* 294:987–994; 1033–1038, 1976.*

23. Rosenman RH, Brand RJ, Jenkins CD, et al.: Coronary heart disease in the Western Collaborative Group study. Final follow-up experience. *JAMA,* 233:872–877, 1975.

24. Mathews KA, Haynes SG: Type A behavior patterns and coronary disease risk— update and critical evaluation. *Am J Epidemiol* 123:923–960, 1986.

25. Jones EF, Forrest JD, Goldman N, et al.: Teenage pregnancy in developed countries; determinants and policy implications. *Fam Plann Perspec* 17:53–63, 1985.

26. Luker K: *Dubious Conceptions; The Politics of Teenage Pregnancy.* Cambridge, MA: Harvard University Press, 1996.

27. Cohen J, Dearnley EJ, Hansel CEM: The risk taken in crossing a road. *Oper Res Q* 6:120–127, 1955.

28. Hearst N, Newman TB, Hulley SB: Delayed effects of the military draft on mortality; a randomized natural experiment. *N Engl J Med* 314:620–624, 1986.

29. Holmes TH, Rahe RH: The social readjustment rating scale. *J Psychosomatic Res* 11:213–218, 1967.

30. Schneider RA, Staggers F, Alexander CN, et al.: A randomized controlled trial of stress reduction for hypertension in older African Americans. *Hypertension* 26:820–827, 1995.

31. Zamarra JW, Schneider RH, Besseghini I, et al.: Usefulness of the transcendental meditation program in the treatment of patients with coronary artery disease. *Am J Cardiol* 77:867–870, 1996.

32. Selye H: Stress and disease. *Science* 122:625–631, 1955; see also Selye H: The general adaptation syndrome and the diseases of adaptation. *J Clin Endocrinol* 6:117–230, 1946.

33. Berczi I, Szelenyi J (eds): *Advances in Psychoneuroimmunology.* New York: Plenum, 1994.

34. Anisman H, Baines MG, Berczi I, et al.: Neuroimmune mechanisms in health and disease; 1: Health. *Can Med Assoc J* 155:867–874, 1996.

35. Kabat-Zinn J, Massion AO, Kristeller J, et al.: Effectiveness of a meditation-based stress reduction program in the treatment of anxiety disorders. *Am J Psychiatry* 149:936–943, 1992.

36. Mechanic D: Health and illness behavior. In Last JM (ed): *Maxcy-Rosenau Public Health and Preventive Medicine.* 12th ed. E. Norwalk, CT: Appleton-Century-Crofts, 1986.

37. Becker MH (ed): *The Health Belief Model and Personal Health Behavior.* Thorofare, NJ: Slack, 1974.

38. Jenkins CD: Diagnosis and treatment of behavioral barriers to good health. In Last JM (ed): *Maxcy-Rosenau Public Health and Preventive Medicine.* 12th ed. E. Norwalk, CT: Appleton-Century-Crofts, 1986.

39. Opie I, Opie P: *Children's Games in Street and Playground.* Oxford: Oxford University Press, 1969.*

40. Cole R: *The Political Life of Children.* Boston: Atlantic, 1986.

41. Thomas L: On Societies as Organisms. In *The Lives of a Cell; Notes of a Biology Watcher.* New York: Viking, 1974, pp. 11–15.*

42. Mackay C: *Extraordinary Popular Delusions and the Madness of Crowds.* Boston: Page, 1932.* [Reprinted; original edition, London 1841.]

43. Cantril H: *The Invasion from Mars. A Study in the Psychology of Panic.* Princeton: Princeton University Press, 1940.

44. Paffenbarger RS Jr, Hyde RT, Wing AL, et al.: Physical activity, all-cause mortality and longevity of college alumni. *N Engl J Med* 314:605–613, 1986.

45. Public health aspects of physical activity and exercise. *Public Health Rep* 100:118–224, 1985.

46. Yamagawa K, Ichikawa K: Experimentelle Studie über die Pathogenese der Epithelial Geschwülste. *Mitta d Med Fakult d k Univ zu Tokyo* 25:295–344, 1915–16.

47. Muller FW: Tobaccomissbrauch und Lungencarcinom. *Krebsforschung* 49:57–84, 1939.

48. Doll R, Hill AB: Smoking and carcinoma of the lung. *Br Med J* 2:739–748, 1950.

49. Wynder EL, Graham EA: Tobacco smoking as a possible etiologic factor in bronchogenic carcinoma. A study of 684 proved cases. *JAMA* 143:329–336, 1950.

50. Report of the Surgeon General: *The Health Consequences of Smoking.* Washington, DC: U.S. Public Health Service, D, 1964.*

51. Kluger R: *Ashes to Ashes; America's Hundred-Year Cigarette War, the Public Health and the Unabashed Triumph of Philip Morris.* New York: Knopf, 1996.

52. Glantz SA, Salde J, Bero LA, et al.: *The Cigarette Papers.* Berkeley: University of California Press, 1996.

53. Bailey BJ: Tobaccoism is the disease—cancer is the sequela. *JAMA* 255:1923, 1986.

54. Bjartveit K, Lochsen PM, Aaro LE: Controlling the epidemic. Legislation and restrictive measures. *Can J Public Health* 72:406–412, 1981.

55. Farquhar JW, Magnus PF, Maccoby N: The role of public information and education in cigarette smoking controls. *Can J Public Health* 72:412–420, 1981.

56. Keller M: A lexicon of disablements related to alcohol consumption. In Edwards G, Gross MM, Moser J, et al. (eds): *Alcohol-Related Disabilities.* Geneva: WHO, 1977.

57. Moser J: *Prevention of Alcohol-Related Problems. An International Review of Preventive Measures, Policies and Programmes.* Toronto: Addiction Research Foundation and WHO, 1980.

58. Data from the National Institute Alcohol and Drug Abuse Website. http://www.health.org/pubs/monitor/mtf95tla.htm

59. Puska P, Wiio J, McAlister A, et al.: Planned use of mass media in national health promotion: The "Keys to Health" TV program in 1982 in Finland. *Can J Public Health* 76:336–342, 1985.

60. Susser MW, Watson W, Hopper K: *Sociology in Medicine.* 3rd ed. New York: Oxford University Press, 1985.*

61. Lock M, Gordon D (eds): *Biomedicine Reexamined.* Hingham, MA: Kluwer, 1988.

62. Nichter M: *Anthropology and International Health.* Boston: Kluwer, 1989.

63. Offord DR, Last JM, Barrette PA: A comparison of the school performance, emotional adjustment and skill development of poor and middle-class children. *Can J Public Health* 76:174–178, 1985.

7

Control of
Noncommunicable
Conditions

There have been some remarkable changes in the pattern of disease in the rich industrial nations in the 20th century. Many infectious diseases, which throughout previous history were the principal causes of premature death and much chronic disability, rapidly declined in incidence in the middle third of the century. Over the same period there was a sharp increase in the incidence of coronary heart disease, several kinds of cancer, and traffic-related death and serious injury, mostly affecting young people. In the final third of the century, some new and deadly infectious diseases have emerged and several old ones have reemerged. Meanwhile, most of the disorders of the middle third of the century remained prominent. This chapter is about the causes and control of those conditions that have become prominent in the 20th century that are not caused by infectious pathogens.

A simple working classification of these conditions has eluded taxono-mists and nosologists. For want of a better term, they are often called "non-communicable," but no single phrase adequately describes them. Some are "communicated" to definable social groups by poorly understood behavioral mechanisms, not by infectious pathogens. We call some of them "chronic dis-eases," but this is hardly a suitable term for a disease that can strike a person dead without warning or premonitory signs, as acute myocardial infarction can do—although there may have been precursors if we had had the oppor-tunity to search for them. Adding to the terminological confusion, some in-fectious diseases are chronic; tuberculosis and human immunodeficiency virus (HIV) and acquired immunodeficiency syndrome (AIDS), among oth-ers, are in that group. Depression and other emotional disturbances do not fit neatly into a class called "chronic diseases"; these conditions may be chronic, even lifelong, but they can also be acute. Injury as a result of traffic crashes or industrial mishaps occurs suddenly and usually without warning and is not called a disease, but it can cause chronic disability. These caveats notwithstanding, it is convenient to consider this miscellaneous group of conditions that afflict so many people in modern industrial civilization under the vague and roughly accurate heading of noncommunicable conditions. One feature they have in common is that when they do not kill outright they can cause prolonged impairment, disability, or handicap, requiring care perhaps for the remainder of the affected person's lifetime. Their prevention and control therefore have high priority.

We can assess their impact by studying vital and health statistics.[1] When we examine mortality statistics (Table 7–1), hospital separations (Table 7–2), causes of activity limitation (Table 7–3), or what people report in interviews about their symptoms and complaints (Table 7–4), we find in all these sources of data the evidence of a heavy burden of premature death and long-term disability. We get some insights into the economic and social impact of illness and injury from statistics on prescribed and over-the-counter medications, sickness and disability insurance statistics, and in various other ways, but mortality statistics, hospital separations, and responses in interview surveys are often our best sources.

The evidence is incomplete and in some ways misleading, but it does offer a reasonably consistent picture. In the second half of the 20th century, heart disease, especially coronary heart disease, has been the biggest killer and among the commonest reasons for admissions and episodes of illness in acute short-stay hospital beds; it is also a reason for a considerable proportion of encounters in doctors' offices. Malignant disease ranks second. Other conditions I discuss in this chapter and their contribution to the burden of mortality appear in Figure 7–1.

► IMPAIRMENT, DISABILITY, AND HANDICAP

Besides causing premature death, this group of conditions is responsible for a heavy burden of impairments, disabilities, and handicaps. These three words describe important concepts and should be used with precision.[2] An *impairment* is defined as any loss or abnormality of anatomic, physiologic or psychologic structure or function. Impairments result from abnormalities of body structure or appearance or organ or system function; generally, impairments represent disturbances at the organ level. A *disability* is defined as any restriction or lack of ability to perform an activity within the range considered normal; disability is the result of an impairment and affects the person rather than the organ. A *handicap* is defined as a disadvantage that results from an impairment or disability that limits or prevents the fulfillment of a role that is normal for the individual. Handicaps thus influence interaction between people and their social environment. The International Classification

TABLE 7-1. Deaths and Death Rates for the 10 Leading Causes of Death in Specified Age Groups: United States, Preliminary 1995[a]

Rank	Cause of Death (Based on Ninth Revision, International Classification of Diseases, 1975)	Number	Rate per 100,000 Population
	All Ages		
. . .	All causes	2,312,203	880.0
1	Diseases of heart	738,781	281.2
2	Malignant neoplasms, including neoplasms of lymphatic and hematopoietic tissues	537,969	204.7
3	Cerebrovascular diseases	158,061	60.2
4	Chronic obstructive pulmonary diseases and allied conditions	104,756	39.9
5	Accidents and adverse effects	89,703	34.1
. . .	Motor vehicle accidents	41,786	15.9
. . .	All other accidents and adverse effects	47,916	18.2
6	Pneumonia and influenza	83,528	31.8
7	Diabetes mellitus	59,085	22.5
8	HIV infection	42,506	16.2
9	Suicide	30,893	11.8
10	Chronic liver disease and cirrhosis	24,848	9.5
. . .	All other causes	442,073	168.2
	1–4 Years		
. . .	All causes	6355	40.4
1	Accidents and adverse effects	2277	14.5
. . .	Motor vehicle accidents	814	5.2
. . .	All other accidents and adverse effects	1463	9.3
2	Congenital anomalies	692	4.4
3	Malignant neoplasms, including neoplasms of lymphatic and hematopoietic tissues	487	3.1
4	Homicide and legal intervention	414	2.6
5	Diseases of heart	256	1.6
6	HIV infection	205	1.3
7	Pneumonia and influenza	138	0.9
8	Certain conditions originating in the perinatal period	96	0.6
9	Septicemia	67	0.4
10	Benign neoplasms, carcinoma in situ, and neoplasms of uncertain behavior and of unspecified nature	60	0.4
. . .	All other causes	1663	10.6
	5–14 Years		
. . .	All causes	8412	22.1
1	Accidents and adverse effects	3481	9.1
. . .	Motor vehicle accidents	1997	5.2
. . .	All other accidents and adverse effects	1484	3.9
2	Malignant neoplasms, including neoplasms of lymphatic and hematopoietic tissues	999	2.6
3	Homicide and legal intervention	494	1.3
4	Congenital anomalies	457	1.2
5	Suicide	329	0.9

(continued)

TABLE 7-1.   *(continued)*

Rank	Cause of Death (Based on Ninth Revision, International Classification of Diseases, 1975)	Number	Rate per 100,000 population
6	Diseases of heart	269	0.7
7	HIV infection	174	0.5
8	Chronic obstructive pulmonary diseases and allied conditions	137	0.4
9	Benign neoplasms, carcinoma in situ, and neoplasms of uncertain behavior and of unspecified nature	120	0.3
10	Pneumonia and influenza	115	0.3
. . .	All other causes	1837	4.8
	15–24 Years		
. . .	All causes	33,569	93.4
1	Accidents and adverse effects	13,532	37.6
. . .	Motor vehicle accidents	10,354	28.8
. . .	All other accidents and adverse effects	3179	8.8
2	Homicide and legal intervention	6827	19.0
3	Suicide	4789	13.3
4	Malignant neoplasms, including neoplasms of lymphatic and hematopoietic tissues	1599	4.4
5	Diseases of heart	964	2.7
6	HIV infection	643	1.8
7	Congenital anomalies	425	1.2
8	Chronic obstructive pulmonary diseases and allied conditions	220	0.6
9	Pneumonia and influenza	193	0.5
10	Cerebrovascular diseases	166	0.5
. . .	All other causes	4211	11.7
	25–44 Years		
. . .	All causes	157,971	189.5
1	HIV infection	30,465	36.6
2	Accidents and adverse effects	25,995	31.2
. . .	Motor vehicle accidents	14,087	16.9
. . .	All other accidents and adverse effects	11,909	14.3
3	Malignant neoplasms, including neoplasms of lymphatic and hematopoietic tissues	21,983	26.4
4	Diseases of heart	16,719	20.1
5	Suicide	12,518	15.0
6	Homicide and legal intervention	9693	11.6
7	Chronic liver disease and cirrhosis	4146	5.0
8	Cerebrovascular diseases	3407	4.1
9	Diabetes mellitus	2417	2.9
10	Pneumonia and influenza	2076	2.5
. . .	All other causes	28,552	34.3
	45–64 Years		
. . .	All causes	376,337	720.8
1	Malignant neoplasms, including neoplasms of lymphatic and hematopoietic tissues	131,808	252.5

(continued)

TABLE 7-1. *(continued)*

Rank	Cause of Death (Based on Ninth Revision, International Classification of Diseases, 1975)	Number	Rate per 100,000 population
2	Diseases of heart	101,975	195.3
3	Accidents and adverse effects	15,021	28.8
. . .	Motor vehicle accidents	7004	13.4
. . .	All other accidents and adverse effects	8016	15.4
4	Cerebrovascular diseases	15,015	28.8
5	Chronic obstructive pulmonary diseases and allied conditions	12,889	24.7
6	Diabetes mellitus	12,039	23.1
7	Chronic liver disease and cirrhosis	10,310	19.7
8	HIV infection	10,202	19.5
9	Suicide	7175	13.7
10	Pneumonia and influenza	5528	10.6
. . .	All other causes	54,375	104.1
	65 Years and Over		
. . .	All causes	1,699,752	5069.0
1	Diseases of heart	617,844	1842.5
2	Malignant neoplasms, including neoplasms of lymphatic and hematopoietic tissues	381,004	1136.2
3	Cerebrovascular diseases	139,134	414.9
4	Chronic obstructive pulmonary diseases and allied conditions	90,299	269.3
5	Pneumonia and influenza	74,995	223.7
6	Diabetes mellitus	44,472	132.6
7	Accidents and adverse effects	28,545	85.1
. . .	Motor vehicle accidents	7327	21.9
. . .	All other accidents and adverse effects	21,218	63.3
8	Nephritis, nephrotic syndrome, and nephrosis	20,325	60.6
9	Alzheimer's disease	20,042	59.8
10	Septicemia	17,035	50.8
. . .	All other causes	266,057	793.4

[a] Data are subject to sampling and random variation.
(From Rosenberg HM, Ventura SJ, Maurer JD, et al: Births and deaths: United States, 1995. Monthly Vital Statistics Report; vol 45 no 3, supp 2, p 31. Hyattsville, Maryland: National Center for Health Statistics, 1996. http://www.cdc.gov/nchswww/datawh/statab/pubd/453s216h.htm)

TABLE 7–2. Discharges from Short-Stay Hospitals by First-Listed Diagnosis and Sex, United States 1994

Diagnostic Group	Total	Male (thousands)	Female (thousands)
All conditions[a]	30,843	12,293	18,550
Infectious and parasitic conditions	809	381	428
Malignant neoplasms	1443	667	776
Diabetes	502	223	279
Blood disorders	341	147	194
Mental disorders	2112	1123	989
Nervous system and sense organs	577	255	322
Heart disease	4058	2100	1958
Respiratory system	3124	1531	1593
Digestive system	3077	1376	1701
Genitourinary system	1816	607	1209
Complications of Pregnancy	574	—	574
Skin	460	239	221
Musculoskeletal conditions	1515	672	843
Injury and poisoning	2605	1309	1296
Females with deliveries	3901	—	3901

[a] All conditions include others plus ones listed below.
(Source: National Center for Health Statistics Advance Data No. 278, Oct. 3, 1996.)

of Impairments, Disabilities, and Handicaps (ICIDH) assigns numerical codes to precisely defined categories of all forms of these conditions, and the codes can be used as the basis for computer-assisted charting of progress, for instance as persons are rehabilitated or as patients with progressive disabling diseases such as multiple sclerosis deteriorate (Box 7–1). Attending staff can record information about each patient's level of organ or system function, ability to perform standard tasks or activities of daily living, and integration into the community or group to which these patients belong; all such facts can be expressed in numerical ICIDH codes, a procedure that takes a few minutes to complete for each patient; the codes then become an objective computer-based record of progress or deterioration.[3]

It is important to distinguish among impairments, disabilities, and handicaps. It is possible to have a severe impairment such as deafness or loss of a limb without being disabled by this impairment or being handicapped. However, handicap, which by definition involves limitation of one's social role, often requires support by the medical care or social services systems, sometimes both.

The most important indicators of health status are those relating to functional status. Persons who are impaired in any way, whether in physical mobility, sensory perceptions, or emotional state, may be disabled, and their disability can cause handicap. Several scales have been developed to record

TABLE 7–3. Symptoms and Complaints, and Common Diagnoses, United States, 1980–1981

Number and Percent of Office Visits to General and Family Practitioners, by 20 Most Frequent Principal Reasons for Visit and Principal Diagnoses: United States, January 1980–December 1981

Principal Reason for Visit	Number of Visits (thousands)	Percent
All visits	381,710	100.0
General medical examination	20,687	5.4
Symptoms referable to throat	16,688	4.4
Blood pressure test	12,468	3.3
Cough	11,516	3.0
Head cold, upper respiratory infection (coryza)	10,764	2.8
Prenatal examination, routine	9641	2.5
Back symptoms	9015	2.4
Chest pain and related symptoms (not referable to body system)	7507	2.0
Progress visit, not otherwise specified	7347	1.9
Headache, pain in head	7163	1.9
Hypertension	6925	1.8
Abdominal pain, cramps, spasms	6418	1.7
Skin rash	6323	1.7
Earache or ear infection	6147	1.6
Vertigo-dizziness	5558	1.5
Fever	5224	1.4
Weight gain	4497	1.2
Well-baby examination	4228	1.1
Low back symptoms	4176	1.1
Leg symptoms	4155	1.1

Principal Diagnosis	Number of Visits (thousands)	Percent
All visits	381,710	100.0
Essential hypertension	28,612	7.5
Acute upper respiratory infection of multiple or unspecified sites	15,013	3.9
General medical examination	14,061	3.7
Normal pregnancy	10,606	2.8
Diabetes mellitus	10,137	2.7
Obesity and other hyperalimentation	8922	2.3
Acute pharyngitis	8831	2.3
Bronchitis, not specified as acute or chronic	6718	1.8
Suppurative and unspecified otitis media	6445	1.7
Health supervision of infant or child	6060	1.6
Neurotic disorders	4758	1.2
Chronic sinusitis	4751	1.2

(continued)

TABLE 7-3.   *(continued)*

Principal Diagnosis	Number of Visits (thousands)	Percent
Other and unspecified arthropathies	4571	1.2
Certain adverse effects, not elsewhere classified	4504	1.2
Sprains and strains of other and unspecified parts of back	4499	1.2
Other forms of chronic ischemic heart disease	4474	1.2
Other noninfectious gastroenteritis and colitis	4455	1.2
Acute tonsilitis	4395	1.2
Other disorders of soft tissue	4345	1.1
Allergic rhinitis (hay fever)	4162	1.1

(From National Center for Health Statistics, Series 13, No 73, DHHS Public No (PHS) 83-1734.)

degrees of activity limitation (disability) and associated handicap; one that is widely used is the Activities of Daily Living (ADL) scale, developed by Katz and others[4]; Table 7–5 shows data from the National Center for Health Statistics (NCHS) on activity limitation, using some of the criteria of the ADL scale. Note the striking relationship to age.

TABLE 7-4.   Activity Limitation—Selected Reported Chronic Conditions, United States 1979–1981

Condition	Rank	Number (Thousands)	Rate per Thousand	Rank by Sex		Rank by Age	
				Male	*Female*	*45–64*	*65+*
Chronic sinusitis	1	30,227	137.7	1	1	3	5
Arthritis	2	26,958	122.8	4	2	1	1
Hypertension	3	24,728	112.6	2	3	2	2
Deformities, or-thopedic impairments	4	18,427	83.9	5	4	6	6
Hearing impairments	5	17,565	80.0	3	7	4	3
Hay fever	6	16,975	77.3	6	6	7	—[a]
Heart disease	7	16,682	76.0	7	5	5	4
Hemorrhoids	8	8759	39.9	9	10	8	—[a]
Visual impairments	9	8545	38.9	8	—[a]	10	8
Dermatitis	10	8107	36.9	—[a]	8	—[a]	—[a]

[a] Rank is not in top ten in this section of the population; table shows condition prevalence, not person prevalence, as persons may have more than one condition. Other conditions that appear among top ten in certain age or sex classes include asthma, varicose veins, diabetes, chronic bronchitis, hypertrophy of tonsils and adenoids, acne, cataract, arteriosclerosis, tenosynovitis, bursitis.
(From NCHS Data Series 10, No. 155, Hyattsville, MD: U.S. DHHS, July 1986.)

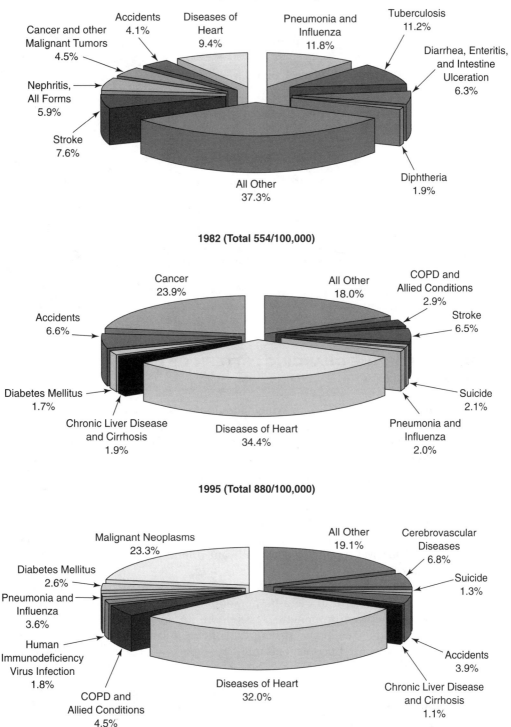

Figure 7–1. Age adjusted rates per 100,000; major causes of death, United States, 1900, 1982, and 1995. *(Illustration by Jon W. Last.)*

> **BOX 7–1. Impairment, Disability, Handicap**
>
> **Impairment**
> Loss of structure or function (organ or system level)
>
> **Disability**
> Restriction or lack of ability to perform a function
> Consequence of an impairment
> Affects function of the person but does not necessarily lead to handicap
>
> **Handicap**
> Disadvantage resulting from impairment or disability
> Limits or prevents fulfillment of role in society
> ICIDH code numbers for all categories permit computer-based charting progress of
>   individuals and of groups, e.g., in rehabilitation programs (tertiary prevention
>   programs)

► REASONS FOR THE CHANGING PATTERN OF DISEASE AND DISABILITY

In chapters 1 and 3, I described and discussed the decline of infections as a cause of premature death. In the affluent industrial nations, the reasons have been primarily ecologic. Improved environmental and housing conditions, improved nutrition, and smaller family size that reduced the probability of exposure to infection of younger siblings by older ones probably have played a more important role than advances in medical science and technology such as the development of antibiotics, which came after, not before, the period of greatest decline in death rates from infectious diseases. Vaccines, oral rehydration therapy, and other measures to enhance child survival have played a significant role in the developing nations (see Chap. 9).

Why have the "new" conditions—coronary heart disease, several varieties of cancer, traffic crashes, emotional disorders, and diseases of senescence—become prominent? The reasons are in part self-evident, related to obvious changes in the structure of the population and the way of life of modern civilized people, and in other respects are complex and not all fully understood.

Demographic Transitions: Aging of the Population

One obvious change in the population of the rich industrial nations is its age composition. There is bound to be a higher prevalence of conditions associated

TABLE 7-5. Rate per 1000 Adults[a] Requiring Assistance with Basic Physical Activities Because of a Chronic Health Problem by Type of Activity and Age in the United States (1979)

Age (Yr)	Needs Help in One or More Basic Activities	Walking Outside	Going Outside	Bathing	Dressing	Using the Toilet	Getting In or Out of Bed or Chair	Eating
Total	22.5	16.1	13.7	9.1	7.1	5.5	4.9	2.0
18–44	5.1	3.6	2.6	1.7	1.8	1.4	1.3	0.6
45–64:	20.6	13.7	10.2	7.3	7.2	4.3	4.8	1.8
45–54	13.3	8.9	6.6	4.0	5.8	2.8	3.7	1.0
55–64	28.6	19.0	14.1	11.1	8.8	6.0	6.0	2.8
65–74	52.6	39.2	34.2	20.4	14.4	11.6	9.0	3.9
75 and over:	157.0	115.9	109.3	73.1	48.3	42.3	34.5	13.8
75–84	114.0	83.6	73.5	50.7	32.9	28.4	25.8	8.4
85 and over	348.4	259.7	268.8	172.9	116.6	104.9	72.5	37.6

[a] Both sexes.

with senescence in an aging population, i.e., in a population with a higher proportion of older persons, than in a population consisting mainly of children and young adults. This is one of the basic differences between the population structure of industrial nations at the beginning of the 20th century and as we approach the end (Fig. 7–2). The age structure of the population in most developing nations resembles that of the industrial nations at the beginning of the 20th century, and as these populations undergo a similar age transformation, the pattern of disease and disability will move in the same direction—as it is already doing in India and China.[5] Difficult social and economic (and probable cultural and emotional) problems in caring for older people will arise in China when the cohorts of "one-child" families grow old in the middle third of the 21st century. Conditions associated with senescence, however, are not the most important of the new public health problems that have arisen since the mid 20th century, although they will continue to increase in prevalence because of the rising proportion of older persons in the population.

The proportion of persons aged 65 and over has risen mainly because birth rates have declined; fewer children are being born, but more of those born are surviving to reach old age. As recently as 1900, up to a fifth of children in industrial nations died before they finished school, many more in the 1800s. (Mark Twain's account of Tom Sawyer's life is unrealistic in failing to mention the empty desks that Tom might have seen as the school year progressed; Jane Eyre's time at Lowood School and her best friend's death from tuberculosis were portrayed more accurately by Charlotte Brontë.) In the least developed countries today, as many as 50 percent of all live-born infants may die before reaching reproductive age, and only a small proportion, 5 percent or less, survive to age 65 or over; in the most favored nations of the industrial world, less than 5 percent die before the age of 65. Consequently the proportion of older people has risen already to over 15 percent in some European nations; it will continue to rise as the members of the "baby boom" generation grow older, reaching or exceeding 20 percent by the early 21st century.[6] The prevalence of diseases of older people inevitably rises in step with aging of the population.

Impact of Automobiles

It is equally obvious that the increased incidence of traffic-related injury, disability, and premature death is a consequence of the use of private cars as the principal means of transport for work and recreation. The recent leveling off, and in many countries the decline, of death rates from traffic-related injury is a result of improved car and highway design, enforcement of speed limits, mandatory seatbelt laws, and stronger sanctions against alcohol-impaired drivers. Other factors include improved roads with controlled access, improved driver education, and possibly reduced driving distances because of rising fuel prices.

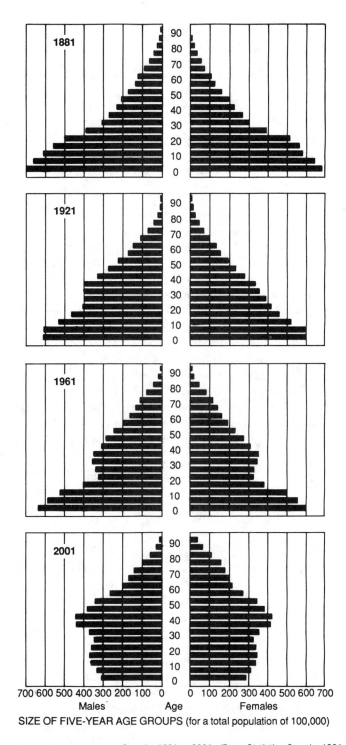

Figure 7–2. Changes in age structure, Canada, 1881 to 2001. *(From Statistics Canada, 1881, 1921, and 1961 Censuses of Canada, and projection 4 [catalogue 91-520]. Reproduced with permission of the Minister of Supply and Services Canada.)*

Lifestyle Changes

The causal factors for coronary heart disease and many kinds of cancer that have increased in incidence appear to be related mostly to changes in lifestyle.[7] It is more accurate to refer to these as risk factors than causal factors, although some, notably tobacco addiction, are directly causal. These and other factors associated with coronary heart disease and cancer respectively are further discussed in the following sections.

Tobacco Addiction

Cigarette smoking has contributed powerfully to the changing pattern of disease. Tobacco smoking is the single greatest cause of preventable premature death and disability from several of the commonest causes affecting both men and women in the middle-age group, that is ages 45 to 64, as well as in persons in the age range of 65 years and over. About 30 percent of all cancers are attributable to tobacco addiction,[8] and smoking is a major risk factor for coronary heart disease and chronic obstructive pulmonary disease (COPD). The surgeon general's *Report on the Health Consequences of Smoking* in 1983 attributed 30 percent of coronary heart disease deaths to smoking,[9] and the *Report* for 1984 attributed 80 to 90 percent of COPD deaths to smoking.[10] Coronary heart disease is much more common than lung cancer, so the number of deaths attributable to smoking is considerably greater for coronary heart disease than it is for lung cancer. The relatively more recent adoption by women than men of cigarette smoking and the decline in the prevalence of cigarette smoking among men has begun to change the distribution of several of the conditions discussed here. The incidence and mortality rates of respiratory cancer have sharply increased among women since the 1970s; lung cancer now ranks above breast cancer in many jurisdictions (see Fig. 2–4, Chap. 2). The female death rate from COPD has also sharply increased. While relatively rare, thromboembolic disorders, including coronary heart disease and cerebral hemorrhage, occur at significantly higher rates among young women who smoke and use the oral contraceptive pill.[11]

Physical Activity

Another striking characteristic of affluent industrial nations, particularly obvious in the United States, is the high prevalence of obesity. (NCHS data for 1996 give the prevalence of obesity in adult Americans as 40 percent or greater in every age and sex class.[12]) People in all industrial nations have become less physically active and more obese, with a higher proportion of body mass made up of fat and less of muscle, compared to their grandparents. The prevalence of obesity among American teenagers has risen about 40 percent since the late 1970s, a trend attributable to many hours spent watching television and snacking while doing so.[13] The obesity that some older Americans are trying to reduce by jogging and similar forms of physical activity is reappearing among members of the next generation. The high fat intake in the diet of modern Americans and Europeans may be associated also with the rising incidence of certain cancers, notably of the large bowel,[14] perhaps also of the uterus and breast.[15] Obesity is also a risk factor for hypertension and stroke and for osteoarthritis of weight-bearing joints.

Social and Behavioral Factors

Changes in the pattern of incidence and prevalence of mental, emotional, and personality disorders are harder to explain and less well understood— much about the mind remains mysterious. Cultural factors are suggested, and some critics of the human condition believe that crowding and encroachment on personal space (the "territorial instinct") may play a role.[16] This would be hard to demonstrate empirically, but it is intuitively plausible and is analogous to the social breakdown, aggression, and destructive behavior observed in colonies of rats under conditions of extreme overcrowding.[17]

Attitudes toward aggressive and violent behavior vary greatly among countries and cultures, if gun laws and overt acts of violence are reliable indicators. In the United States more than in any other rich and orderly industrial nation, there is a widely held view that disputes can be settled by force, that citizens should protect themselves by possessing lethal weapons, and that criminal and antisocial behavior are best dealt with by harsh punishment after they occur, rather than by preventive measures such as provision of improved opportunities for socioeconomically deprived communities. This attitude is clearly demonstrated by lax gun laws in many states and is reinforced by the media and demonstrated by the popularity of entertainments that glorify violence. There is a serious dissonance in a society that regards gentle erotic art as pornography while actively supporting forms of mass culture such as movies and television plays in which the theme is that "good" prevails over "evil" by means that are aggressive and often extremely and even obscenely violent.

More information about some of the generalizations in the previous paragraphs is given in subsequent sections of this chapter, in which I consider several "noncommunicable" disorders individually. One further comment: few of them are truly noncommunicable. Their enabling causes often are determined by cultural conditioning and transmitted by the media, especially television. This applies particularly to health-related behaviors such as diet, the use of legal stimulants and sedatives, and aggressive and violent behavior.

▶ SPECIFIC NONCOMMUNICABLE DISORDERS

A popular convention is to consider chronic conditions according to the chapter headings of the International Classification of Disease (ICD). Since the ICD is to some extent both topographic and etiologic, this makes some sense. However, as the preceding paragraphs make clear, the ICD chapters have not kept pace with expanding knowledge of etiology and risk factors for several conditions in the group we are considering here. Arranging preventable conditions according to chapter headings of the ICD, therefore, is not always helpful, because preventable etiologic factors such as smoking overlap several chapters (Box 7–2). Although our understanding remains incomplete, we know enough to be able to take general and specific steps to reduce risks if not to control or prevent altogether certain classes of disabling, life-shortening noncommunicable conditions.[18]

Heart Disease

As a medical student in the early and mid-1940s, I saw many patients with congestive heart failure resulting from valvular disease, a late effect of rheumatic fever; this disabled and shortened the lives of innumerable young people. Another common cause of valvular heart disease, mainly among older men, was tertiary syphilis. Coronary heart disease was rarely diagnosed, although we occasionally saw patients with angina pectoris. Rheumatic and syphilitic valvular heart disease are now rare in the affluent nations, but beginning in the late 1940s and early 1950s, coronary heart disease soon became the leading cause of death, accounting by the early 1960s for up to a third of all deaths among middle-aged men and a considerable proportion of deaths among women.

Epidemiologic studies have clarified our understanding and control of heart disease. Descriptive epidemiologic studies reveal how coronary heart disease has varied over time, in different places, and among different classes of persons.[19] Cohort and case-control studies have enabled us to measure and assess risk factors, if not to identify underlying causes. Randomized controlled trials have demonstrated the efficacy of some preventive and therapeutic regimens and the lack of benefit of others.[20]

The death rate from coronary heart disease began to decline in the United States, Canada, Australia, and some other countries around the mid-1960s; by 1995 it had fallen by 40 to 50 percent from its peak, to reach rates about the same as those of the early 1950s. But the trend differs sharply among the nations for which reliable mortality data are available, and the pattern also differs between the sexes. In some nations the men's rates have risen while women's rates have fallen, and in all the nations for which data are available, women's rates have always been well below those of men.[21] No good explanation for these trends is immediately obvious; competing causes of mortality, fashions in death certification, and differing exposure to certain risk factors cannot easily be reconciled with this pattern. There is a challenging conundrum here, awaiting solution, perhaps by some of the students who read this book. It would be encouraging to those of us who believe in preventive medicine if we could identify why mortality has declined, but the fact that

**BOX 7-2. Risk Reduction Strategies and Preventable Health Problems,
Arranged by ICD Chapters—Sensible Behavior Is the Best Way to
Reduce Risks!**

Safe Environment

I	Infectious and parasitic diseases
II	Neoplasms
V	Mental disorders
VIII	Respiratory diseases
XII	Skin diseases
XIV	Congenital anomalies
XVI	Injury and poisoning

Enhanced Immunity

I	Infectious and parasitic diseases

Good Nutrition

I	Infectious and parasitic diseases
II	Neoplasms
III	Endocrine, nutritional, and metabolic diseases
IV	Diseases of blood
V	Mental disorders
VI	Diseases of nervous system and sense organs
VII	Diseases of circulatory system
IX	Diseases of digestive system
XI	Complications of pregnancy and puerperium

Sensible Behavior

I	Infectious and parasitic diseases
II	Neoplasms
III	Endocrine, nutritional, and metabolic diseases
V	Mental disorders
VI	Diseases of nervous system and sense organs
VII	Diseases of circulatory system
VIII	Diseases of respiratory system
IX	Diseases of digestive system
X	Diseases of genitourinary system
XI	Complications of pregnancy
XII	Diseases of skin
XIII	Diseases of musculoskeletal system
XIV	Congenital anomalies
XVII	Injury and poisoning

Wellborn Children

XI	Complications of pregnancy, childbirth, and puerperium
XIV	Congenital anomalies
XV	Certain conditions originating in the perinatal period

(continued)

BOX 7-2.   Risk Reduction Strategies and Preventable Health Problems, Arranged by ICD Chapters—Sensible Behavior Is the Best Way to Reduce Risks! *(continued)*

Prudent Health Care

II	Neoplasms
III	Endocrine, nutritional, metabolic, and immunity disorders
IV	Diseases of blood and blood-forming organs
V	Mental disorders
VI	Diseases of nervous system and sense organs
VII	Diseases of circulatory system
IX	Diseases of digestive system
XII	Diseases of skin
XIII	Diseases of musculoskeletal system and connective tissue
XIV	Congenital anomalies
XVII	Injury and poisoning

it did not begin to decline until very recently in the United Kingdom, Norway, and Switzerland, which seem closely similar in exposure to known risk factors to the United States, Canada, and Australia, suggests that though some of us must be doing something right, we do not know exactly what it is.

The most important known risk factors are elevated serum cholesterol, smoking, and high blood pressure. Elevated serum cholesterol is related to dietary intake of fats, and to some extent also to lack of physical exercise.[22] Cigarette smoking contributes directly to coronary heart disease both by causing coronary vasoconstriction and by enhancing the tendency to blood clotting. High blood pressure causes left ventricular hypertrophy, which in the presence of coronary arterial occlusion or narrowing leads to myocardial infarction.

Behavioral factors and in particular the set of behaviors known as "type A" personality (see Chap. 6) also contribute to the risk, probably because certain behaviors are associated with adverse physiologic responses to stress, notably catecholamine release and labile hypertension.[23] Environmental factors may include drinking water quality. Age-adjusted coronary heart disease and stroke mortality rates are lower in communities supplied by water that is "hard"—i.e., containing dissolved salts—than in those supplied by "soft" water[24]; but the evidence for this is disputed.[25] Hereditary factors may play a part, too; some cardiologists assert that if there is a family history of long life and freedom from heart disease, this alone may be worth more than attention to all the controllable risk factors put together in protecting against premature death from coronary heart disease. The epidemiologic evidence, however, is less persuasive on this point than clinical impressions (Box 7–3).

BOX 7-3. Risk and Protective Factors, Coronary Heart Disease

Risk Factors—The Seven Deadly Sins
Lust, avarice: For cigarettes
Gluttony: High animal fat diet; perhaps meat and sugars, too
Sloth: Lack of regular, systematic physical exercise
Pride, wrath: Type A personality
Envy: Middle and lower management envious of higher ranks

Protective Factors—The Four Cardinal Virtues
Choosing the right parents—family history free of early death
Spare (preferably vegetarian?) diet
Regular, systematic exercise
Equanimity?

Some behaviors undoubtedly increase the risk of getting or dying of coronary heart disease. Our evidence comes from several famous cohort studies, such as the Framingham Heart Study,[26] and from a number of population laboratories such as North Karelia, Finland,[27] and several Californian communities,[28] where other kinds of epidemiologic investigation have been conducted. The multiple risk factor intervention trial (MRFIT) disappointed many cardiologists and epidemiologists because early results showed no significant difference in death rates between the group subjected to maximum interventions and the control group that had no interventions.[29] Further examination of the results revealed several interesting details. Violent deaths (homicide, traffic fatalities, etc.) occurred more often among men whose serum cholesterol levels were reduced by intervention, suggesting that elevated serum cholesterol might possibly be associated with greater equanimity or reduction of serum cholesterol levels might make men more inclined to get involved in violence.[30] Another problem of MRFIT was confounding of the results by "contamination" of the control group, which could hardly avoid being influenced by widely publicized health-promoting behaviors (diet, exercise, cessation of smoking); death rates from coronary heart disease in the control group were reduced because of this, in the same way as they were in the general population during the period of study.

A more serious criticism of MRFIT was that it dealt only with "misters" and not with "missuses"—the investigators and the granting agencies that supported them were concerned only about coronary heart disease in men, although the high death rates among women would have justified investigation and intervention trials far sooner than these actually began.[31] Inclusion of women in epidemiologic and other studies of heart disease did not begin seriously until the late 1980s; as a card-carrying feminist I deplore this. Studies so far reported show essentially the same spectrum of risk factors for women as for men, although hypertension probably plays a more prominent role among women.

High Blood Pressure (Hypertension)

What is hypertension? The common form of so-called essential hypertension, i.e., the kind that is not secondary to some other condition such as renal disease, can only be diagnosed on the basis of a physiologic measurement, the level of arterial blood pressure. The level that is called hypertension is arbitrarily set: Blood pressure has a slightly skewed distribution in the population (Fig. 7–3) and the decision as to what constitutes high blood pressure is arbitrary. Usually a reading above 95 mm Hg diastolic and 145 mm Hg systolic is defined as hypertension. Empirical support for this is derived from many observations that persons with higher blood pressures than these arbitrary levels have higher incidence and mortality rates from complications such as stroke and heart failure when compared to persons whose blood pressure is lower. There is, however, no sharp distinction in prognosis between persons with slightly elevated and "normal" blood pressure. Epidemiologic studies

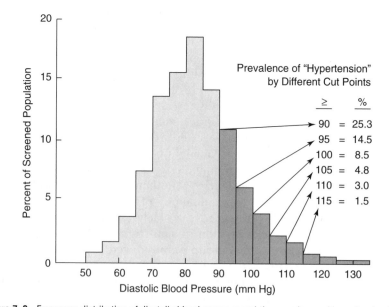

Figure 7–3. Frequency distribution of diastolic blood pressure and the prevalence of hypertension by different cut points. *(From Tyroler HA: Hypertension. In Last JM (ed):* Maxcy-Rosenau Public Health and Preventive Medicine. *12th ed. E. Norwalk, CT: Appleton-Century-Crofts, 1986, p. 1196; after Hypertension Detection and Follow-Up Program Cooperative Group: The hypertension detection and follow-up program: A progress report.* Cir Res *40 (suppl 1):106–109, 1977.)*

have helped to clarify the nature and risk factors for hypertension, although more uncertainty remains than does regarding coronary heart disease.

The prevalence of hypertension is higher among women than men and among blacks than whites, and a family history of hypertension increases the risk of an individual becoming hypertensive. Obesity is an important risk factor. Salt intake (more precisely, sodium intake) is related to the risk of hypertension—restricted salt intake is part of an effective medical regimen for reduction of high blood pressure. Heavy alcohol consumption also increases the risk of high blood pressure. There are striking geographic, cultural, and ethnic variations: among blacks, high blood pressure is commoner among those in the United States than genetically similar blacks in Africa. Some of the variation among African blacks may be a consequence of generations of selection in populations that traditionally had low salt intake.[32] Among Pacific Islanders, high blood pressure is absent altogether in some groups that have had very limited contact with Western civilization.[33] These observations fit either of two hypotheses: First, that dietary factors related to civilization, notably salt intake, could be responsible; or second, that the stress of civilized life is conducive to development of high blood pressure—but no one has been able to prove that civilized life is more stressful than life in primitive societies. What is "stress," anyway? Finally, while cigarette smoking leads to transient elevation of blood pressure, smoking per se is not an important risk factor for hypertension.

The hypertension detection and follow-up program in the United States has demonstrated convincingly that active searching for and intensive management of patients with high blood pressure leads to considerable reduction in the rates of premature death and disability from the commonest end result of hypertension, i.e., stroke. Mortality rates from stroke have declined sharply since control of hypertension became a priority for practicing physicians, although it is possible that other factors besides effective medical care have played a part in this reduction.[34]

Cancer

The word *cancer* describes a large and complex family of neoplastic diseases characterized by aberrations of cellular growth that cause abnormally proliferating cells to invade and destroy normal tissues. This can happen to the cells of every organ and tissue in the body; the rate of progression is very variable. Because of the variation in many other characteristics of malignant change in body cells, it is not easy to formulate general rules about neoplasia.[35] The causative factors are extraordinarily variable (Box 7–4). Eating food containing nitrosamines, drinking certain forms of alcohol, breathing air contaminated by tobacco smoke or asbestos fibers, working in radioactive mines, iron foundries, or many other settings, basking too long in the ultraviolet light of the sun, having sex with too many or the wrong sort of partners, or having doctors who prescribe certain drugs or order too many

BOX 7–4. Causes of Cancer

Eating
Nitrosamines, aflatoxins, too much fat, ?red meat
Chewing betel nut

Drinking
Alcohol, perhaps coffee

Breathing
Air containing tobacco smoke, asbestos fibers

Living
In the wrong place, e.g., where exposed to nuclear fallout or to schistosomiasis

Working
Occupational exposures too numerous to mention

Sunshine
Sunbathing and fair complexion are a bad combination

Sex
Too many or the wrong kind of partners

Doctors
May order too many x-rays or cancer-causing drugs

x-ray examinations all increase the risk of getting or dying of cancer. So may poor choice of one's parents: Several familial factors, including specific cancer genes, have been identified.[36]

There has been an absolute as well as a relative increase in the age-adjusted mortality (and incidence) rates from all forms of cancer combined since the mid-1940s in the United States and similar countries. Some varieties, notably cancer of the stomach and of the oral cavity and tongue, have declined during this period, but these gains are more than offset by the rising incidence and mortality rates from cancer of all parts of the respiratory system and smaller increases in cancer of the breast, prostate, testis, and malignant melanoma and several forms of lymphoma and leukemia. There have been small gains in the relative survival rates from some of the common forms of cancer. In the United States, an analysis of data from the Surveillance, Epidemiology and End Results (SEER) program of the National Cancer Institute showed a gain in 5-year survival rates for all forms of cancer from 46.8 percent in 1973 to 49.1 percent in 1978. The largest improvements were from 60.7 percent to 69.4 percent for cancer of the prostate and from 61.5 percent to 72.0 percent for Hodgkin's disease. Gains for other common cancers were much smaller. Overall, the authors of this report concluded that little if any progress was being made toward the control of cancer in the United States.[37] Given the continuing increase in lung and other respiratory and nonrespiratory cancers attributable to tobacco addiction, this is certainly true and will likely remain true until the tobacco epidemic is controlled.

It is not easy to classify the known causative factors. They include physical factors such as ionizing and certain forms of nonionizing radiation; biologic factors such as several viral causes (e.g., hepatitis B virus, the Epstein-Barr virus, the papillomavirus, the virus of herpes type II, human T-cell lymphotropic virus type I, HIV, and a few others); numerous chemicals and industrial products and some drugs are also implicated (Table 7–6).

The prevention of cancer could theoretically be achieved by removing or excluding known and presumed precipitating factors from the human environment, but this hardly seems to be feasible. The contribution of some important risk factors has been calculated, and on this basis it is possible to say that as much as a third of all cancers could be prevented by eliminating tobacco from our society; tobacco is not only by far the greatest single cause of lung and other respiratory system cancer, it is also a powerful risk factor for cancer at many other sites and in many other tissues and organs. Other important risk factors that could be changed include diet; there is good evidence that high-fat, low-fiber diets increase cancer risks, and that diets high in vitamin A appear to have some protective effect.

Cancer epidemiology and prevention is such a large and complex subject that further detail here would make this book needlessly prolix. Readers seeking more information should consult the excellent review of cancer etiology, epidemiology, and prevention listed in the references at the end of this chapter.[38]

Respiratory Disease

COPD is an important cause of premature death and prolonged disability (Tables 7–1, 7–2). Cigarette smoking is heavily implicated; COPD is far less common among nonsmokers, even if they have other risk factors such as a history of repeated respiratory infection and work in occupations where they are exposed to irritant dusts or fumes. Occupational causes of COPD are second in importance to cigarette smoking as risk factors, and much can be done to eliminate or control this preventable disease by improving workplace safety (see Chap. 4). Other important forms of chronic respiratory disease and their prevention are summarized in Table 7–7.

TABLE 7–6.   Human Carcinogenic Agents and Circumstances

Agent or Circumstance	Occupational	Medical	Social	Site of Cancer
Aflatoxin			+	Liver
Alcoholic drinks			+	Mouth, pharynx, larynx, esophagus, liver
Alkylating agents:				
Cyclophosphamide		+		Bladder
Melphalan		+		Marrow
Aromatic amines:				
4-Aminodiphenyl	+			Bladder
Benzidine	+			Bladder
2-Naphthylamine	+			Bladder
Arsenic	+	+		Skin, lung
Asbestos	+			Lung, pleura, peritoneum
Benzene	+			Marrow
Bis(chloromethyl)ether	+			Lung
Busulphan		+		Marrow
Chewing (betel, tobacco, lime)			+	Mouth
Chinese salted fish			+	Nasopharyngeal
Chromium	+			Lung
Chlornaphazine		+		Bladder
Furniture manufacture (hardwood)	+			Nasal sinuses
Immunosuppressive drugs		+		Reticuloendothelial system
Ionizing radiations	+	+		Marrow and probably all other sites
Isopropyl alcohol manufacture	+			Nasal sinuses
Leather goods manufacture	+			Nasal sinuses
Mustard gas	+			Larynx, lung
Nickel	+			Nasal sinuses, lung
Estrogens:				
Unopposed		+		Endometrium
Transplacental (DES)		+		Vagina
Overnutrition (causing obesity)			+	Endometrium, gallbladder
Phenacetin		+		Kidney (pelvis)
Phenoxyacid/chlorophenal herbicides	+			Non-Hodgkins' lymphoma
Polycyclic hydrocarbons	+	+		Skin, scrotum, lung
Reproductive history:				
Late age at 1st pregnancy			+	Breast
Zero or low parity			+	Ovary

(continued)

TABLE 7–6.   *(continued)*

Agent or Circumstance	Occupational	Medical	Social	Site of Cancer
		Exposure		
Parasites:				
Schistosoma haematobium			+	Bladder
Clonorchis sinensis			+	Liver (cholangioma)
Sexual promiscuity (Herpes virus, papillomavirus)			+	Cervix uteri
Steroids:				
Anabolic (oxymetholone)		+		Liver
Tobacco smoking			+	Mouth, pharynx, larynx, lung, esophagus, bladder
UV light	+		+	Skin, lip
Vinyl chloride	+			Liver (angiosarcoma)
Virus (hepatitis B)			+	Liver (hepatoma)
HTLV-I			+	Leukemia and lymphoma
HIV			+	Kaposi's sarcoma, Various other sites
Epstein-Barr virus			+	Lymphoma

DES = diethylstilbestrol; HIV = human immunodeficiency virus; HTLV = T-cell lymphotropic virus.
(Adapted from Doll and Peto,[8] and Schottenfeld and Fraumeni.[38])

Injury

Injury, the leading cause of death at all ages from 1 to 40 years, occurs in three main settings: traffic, the workplace, and the home; a fourth setting is recreational, which is less common but still important. We must also consider whether the injury occurred as a result of unintentional or intentional actions. The word commonly used to describe unintentional injury is "acci-

TABLE 7–7.   **Chronic Obstructive Pulmonary Disease**

Cause	Percentage Contribution to COPD	Prevention Potential
Smoking	90	Entirely preventable
Chronic respiratory infection	5	Mostly preventable
Occupational or environmental	4	Many cases preventable
Asthma, congenital heart or lung disease (cystic fibrosis, etc.)	1	May not be preventable

dent," but this word suggests circumstances beyond our control; some epidemiologists dislike calling "accidental" the situations where injury occurs as a consequence of factors that are often predictable and therefore preventable (Box 7–5).

The epidemiology of **traffic injury** has been extensively studied; we can classify the contributions to the risk of death or injury among drivers and pedestrians as factors affecting the host, the agent, and the environment (Table 7–8).

Of the preventable factors, those relating to the host—the driver or operator of the vehicle—are the most obvious and generally the most remediable. Alcohol-impaired driving can be reduced, as has been shown in many studies.[39] Alcohol use is a form of risk-taking behavior for some drivers, and driving at excessive speed is another. Both are common among youths. Both prescribed and nonprescribed drugs can impair consciousness or judgment and so act as enabling factors in traffic crashes. Antihistamines, especially if their sedative effect is potentiated by alcohol, can cloud consciousness enough to be dangerous. Diabetics and persons with heart-block, epilepsy, and other conditions that may lead to transient or unpredictable attacks of loss or impairment of consciousness are at higher risk of traffic crashes (and injury from moving machinery) than the rest of the population. Impaired vision,

---

BOX 7–5.   Injury Control—Predictable and Preventable Risks

Host Factors
Risk-taking behavior
Alcohol or other substance abuse
Medical conditions; some medications
Age: Infancy, childhood, old age

Agent Factors
Automobile safety standards
Industrial safety equipment
Firearm control regulations
Recreational equipment standards
Domestic product safety

Environment Factors
Well-designed, controlled-access roads
"Good housekeeping" in the workplace
Home safety standards

TABLE 7–8. Traffic Injury Risk Factors

Exposed Group	Risk Factors
Host	
Pedestrians	Toddlers and young children lack road safety sense
	Adolescents are risk-takers
	Elderly have impaired sight, hearing, mobility
	Anyone may have alcohol-impaired judgment
	All pedestrians are unprotected by "armor"
Cyclists	No adequate protection
	Often defy traffic rules, take risks
Motorcyclists	Inadequate protection
	Excessive speed
	Poor visibility
Car drivers	Excessive speed
	Alcohol-impaired judgment
	Medical conditions
	Risk-taking behavior (seatbelt not used)
Passengers	Risk-taking behavior (seatbelt not used)
Agent	
Unsafe vehicle	Brakes, steering, windshield, etc.
	Overpowered, underpowered
Environmental	
Road conditions	Weather, visibility
	Unguarded intersections
	Poorly graded; tight, narrow curves
	Inadequate control of access roads

hearing, and mobility of the vehicle driver also increase the risk of traffic crashes. Physicians have a legal duty in many jurisdictions to certify elderly persons' (often age 75 and over) and persons suffering from certain medical conditions medical fitness to drive. By fulfilling this duty conscientiously, physicians can help to reduce the incidence of injury and death resulting from traffic crashes. Driver education, nowadays often part of high school education, has produced a generation of drivers who are better trained and more proficient at handling automobiles than their parents and grandparents were.

Vehicle safety is the next remediable aspect of traffic injury; improved vehicle design has helped reduce the toll of serious injury, but the trend toward smaller cars, in which occupants are more exposed to trauma than in larger cars, has partly offset this reduction. The use of safety belts has had significant benefit, reducing the toll of death and serious injury notably in several jurisdictions where careful before and after comparisons have been made.[40] Airbags that inflate on impact are popular in the United States where many people object to laws that compel them to use seatbelts; randomized trials to compare their efficacy to seatbelts are not feasible, but several reports of fatal injury to children when airbags have inflated with explosive force, perhaps exceeding the crash impact, suggest that seatbelts are probably superior because they do not present that hazard to users. In comparisons of similar settings with and without seatbelt legislation, the rates of seatbelt use are much higher where laws require car occupants to buckle up—but the traffic death rates are not necessarily different. Before and after comparisons could be confounded by other variables. Some evidence from studies by transport authorities suggests that high speeds and impaired driving—and failure to use seatbelts even when their use is mandatory—may be responsible for failure to demonstrate an improvement in traffic death rates when seatbelt use is mandatory.

Similar arguments apply to the use of crash helmets by motorcyclists. Serious and lethal head injury is greatly reduced by the use of crash helmets; but in the United States some motorcyclists say that helmets are unsafe because they restrict vision. There is no evidence to support this, but laws mandating use of crash helmets have been repealed in about half the states in the United States where they were introduced, with the predictable result of rising rates of death and permanent brain damage resulting from head injuries sustained in motorcycle crashes.

Domestic injury is commonest as a cause of death at the extremes of age, among toddlers and young children and among the elderly. Among toddlers and young children, this reflects the behavior of this age group, an age of exploration and experiment, in which lack of knowledge of the dangers contributes to high incidence and mortality rates (Box 7–6). Among the elderly, it may not be the injury itself that causes death, but rather the consequences: Old women who fracture their femurs are confined to bed and die of pneumonia or venous thrombosis. But coding rules for death certification attribute the death to the fracture, i.e., to the fall that caused the fractured femur.

BOX 7–6. Why Children Are at High Risk of Injury

Curiosity and ignorance of hazards
Fragile bodies
Pharmacologic sensitivity
Careless parents

Recreational injury is a complex subject, dealt with in textbooks and journals of sports medicine and well discussed in monographs on injury epidemiology.[41] Some forms of recreational injury continue to occur despite extensive publicity about their causes and prevention. Many young people every year continue to suffer the tragedy of paraplegia or quadriplegia as a result of diving into water so shallow that they fracture their cervical spines and transsect their spinal cords. Activities in which the participants deliberately attempt to injure each other, notably boxing, do not deserve to be called either sports or recreations; the evidence that even minimal torsion injury of the brain causes permanent brain damage has led medical associations in several countries to campaign for the abolition of boxing.

Industrial injury is discussed in Chapter 4.

Intentional Injury

Under this heading we can include two varieties: injury directed against others and self-injury, which is often suicidal.

Homicide and Interpersonal Violence

Although long a leading cause of death among young black males, homicide has only recently been recognized as a public health problem in the United States. While violence against others is relatively common among young adult males in most countries, its prominence as a cause of death in the United States is unusual, to say the least, among civilized countries. The great majority of these deaths are caused by handguns, and all agree that easy access to handguns is the prime determinant of this preventable cause of death.[42] It is unfortunate that the United States, in many respects among the most civilized of nations, contains the powerful interest group, the National Rifle Association, that often successfully lobbies against legislation designed to make lethal firearms less readily accessible to youthful and irresponsible purchasers and users of handguns that kill about 20,000 Americans, mostly young adult males, every year. Virtually no research funds have been devoted to this problem in the United States, and the National Rifle Association has even lobbied with some success to prohibit the Centers for Disease Control and Prevention (CDC) from gathering statistics on death and injury resulting from guns—not exactly shooting, perhaps, but trying to bind and gag the messenger. Only in the United States is such a state of affairs tolerated.

Data are patchy and incomplete on domestic violence, spouse abuse, child abuse, sexual assaults against children (nearly always perpetrated by someone known to the child, commonly a family member). Until recently there were almost no data on these classes of injury, which were not recognized as public health problems. Are they increasing in incidence? Their recognition as a public health problem has led to greater consciousness of their existence and to the collection of information for the first time only within the past few years. Larger numbers are being reported each year in many places where facts are now being gathered, but this could reflect expansion of reporting systems rather than a real increase in incidence.

A survey in 1982 in Canada revealed that the frequency of sexual abuse against children is higher than previously had been suspected. By the time they are 16, as many as 40 percent of girls have been the victims of some unwanted sexual act, most often committed by a family member or other person close to the family.[43]

Other forms of domestic violence have been documented in a collaborative study between law-enforcement agencies and the CDC.[44] It is estimated that each year in the United States, between 3 and 4 million women are assaulted by their male partner (spouse, lover, boyfriend). The public health approach consists of recognition and secondary prevention where possible, tertiary prevention most of the time. Secondary prevention consists of identifying high-risk persons and families and counseling with the aim of eradicating the behavioral problems that lead parents to abuse their children, men to abuse their partners, some adults to abuse their elderly and infirm parents or other relatives. Identifying potentially violent individuals is rarely possible before an episode of violence has brought the problem to the attention of the police, emergency room physicians, pediatricians, or others; hence tertiary prevention is often all that can be accomplished. With growing recognition of the determinants of domestic violence, this should improve. The determinants include a family history of violence, alcohol abuse, unemployment, and overcrowded housing conditions; alert social workers can sometimes predict from such a profile that violent episodes will occur in certain families.

Suicide and Attempted Suicide

There are striking international variations in the frequency of suicide as a certified cause of death (Table 7–9); and there has been a considerable increase in the frequency of suicide as a certified cause of death, especially among young people, in some countries, including Canada[45] and the United States, in recent years. The reasons are not clear. Suicide is always commonest at times of social and economic distress but decreases in countries at war. It is particularly common among groups whose culture is disintegrating, for example Native Americans, and citizens of Hungary after the Russian occupation of 1956. There is a relationship to alcohol use (also a signal of self-destructive impulses, perhaps?). Many suicides are found to have high blood alcohol levels. Other forms of self-destructive behavior, notably drug abuse, are common among those who kill themselves.

Epidemiologically and psychologically there are notable differences between completed and attempted suicide. Completed suicide is commoner among males than females, while attempted suicide is commonest among young women. Investigation often shows that these young women merely seek to escape briefly from the problems that oppress them, not to end their lives. Nevertheless, anyone who has attempted suicide should be considered

TABLE 7–9. Suicide Rates per 100,000 for Selected Countries (1991–1993)

Country	Men	Women
Hungary	55.0	18.3
Finland	44.9	11.2
Denmark	29.3	15.6
Austria	32.1	11.2
Switzerland	29.8	11.4
France	30.2	10.9
Japan	22.3	11.1
Canada	20.7	5.5
United States	20.1	4.7
Norway	21.2	7.8
Australia	20.5	5.3
England and Wales	11.1	3.8
Italy	11.5	4.2
Israel	10.6	3.9
Ireland	16.8	3.3
Spain	11.2	3.9
Russian Federation	66.2	12.9
China (selected rural regions)	23.2	30.6
China (urban regions)	7.7	9.3

(Source: World Health Statistics Annual, 1994.)

at risk of repeat attempts, and whether by mistake or intent, the outcome may be fatal after the initial unsuccessful attempt.

Mental Disorders

Suicide is generally regarded as an outcome of severe depression, so the rising incidence of suicide presumably reflects a rising incidence of severe depression. Community studies of the prevalence of mental disorders show a rising trend in depression, anxiety, and neurosis. The occurrence rates (often a mixture of incidence rates and prevalence) of severe psychotic disease, i.e., schizophrenia, manic-depressive psychosis, and paranoid psychosis, appear to remain much the same over time, although changes in patterns of psychiatric care have led to a decline in the numbers of long-stay patients in institutions. The incidence of dementia that requires institutional care may be rising, perhaps at about the same rate as the rising proportion of older persons in the population, i.e., it is probably senile dementia that is increasing, rather than dementia of the Alzheimer's type. Among persons in the age group 75 to 85, new cases of dementia occur at an annual rate of 2.4 per 100, more frequently than strokes, but these are mostly senile dementia.[46] It is not clear whether the incidence rate of Alzheimer's disease is rising, although as Fig. 1–1 (see Chap. 1) shows, it is increasingly often the certified cause of death.

Another form of severe mental disorder that often requires institutional care is the group of disorders called mental retardation; epidemiologic studies have revealed much about this miscellaneous group of conditions. Down's syndrome is commoner among offspring of mothers (perhaps fathers too) at the upper end of the reproductive age range (Fig. 7–4). Because of improved prenatal diagnosis and the availability of abortion, the incidence of Down's syndrome is declining; but improved care of children with this disorder leads to longer life span, so the prevalence is probably still rising. The incidence of most other forms of mental retardation is stable or declining. The prevention of measles and rubella by community-wide immunization programs has led to the virtual elimination of subacute sclerosing panencephalitis and congenital rubella syndrome, thus removing two previously important causes of mental retardation.[47] Recognition of the fetal alcohol syndrome and effective campaigns against consumption of alcohol by pregnant women could greatly reduce this variety of mental retardation.[48] Unhappily, the epidemic of crack-cocaine use has led to the birth of infants affected by cocaine addiction, so although fetal alcohol syndrome may have declined, this has been counterbalanced by rising incidence of crack-cocaine-addicted infants.[49]

Chronic low-level lead intoxication causes intellectual impairment, but this is seldom severe enough to be regarded as mental retardation. Studies in several parts of the world have shown prolonged adverse effects on intellectual development of children exposed to long-term low-level environmental lead contamination.[50]

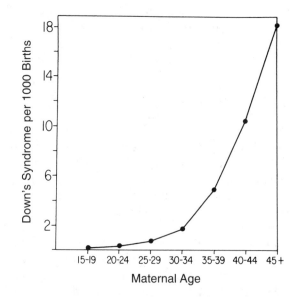

Figure 7–4. The frequency of Down's syndrome relative to maternal age. *(From Porter IH:* Genetic Aspects of Preventive Medicine. *In Last JM (ed):* Maxcy-Rosenau Public Health and Preventive Medicine. *12th ed. E. Norwalk, CT: Appleton-Century-Crofts, 1986, p. 1439.)*

Improved community support systems make it possible to avoid lifelong institutional care for many of the mentally retarded, but there has been overzealousness in "deinstitutionalizing" persons with severe mental disorders, both those who are mentally retarded and those with chronic diseases such as schizophrenia. Unless adequate community support systems are in place, many such persons become derelicts on city streets, the homeless mentally ill[51] (known as "bag people" because they carry all they possess in shopping bags).

Sensory Impairments

A good deal is known about the incidence and prevalence of visual impairment, because the legally blind are entitled to benefits. Table 7–10 summarizes recent data from the United States.[52] Several forms of blindness, especially in developing countries where xerophthalmia and trachoma are common, are preventable. Visual impairment as a result of cataract can be prevented if it is occupationally related and can be treated with increased chance of success by modern methods. Cataract is likely to become more common and to occur at younger ages as stratospheric ozone attenuation leads in future years to increased ultraviolet radiation flux at the Earth's surface (see Chap. 11). Glaucoma can be detected early and treated to prevent deterioration or loss of sight. Diabetes is the commonest cause of blindness in many industrial nations, but this is not preventable at present.

Severe deafness is less well documented. Its causes include several that are preventable, e.g., recurrent middle-ear infection, congenital rubella syndrome, and occupational exposures (Table 7–11).

Impaired Mobility

The various forms of arthritis are the most common cause of impaired mobility, and collectively, disorders of the musculoskeletal system are by far the commonest cause of activity limitation[53] (Fig. 7–5). Osteoarthritis is the commonest serious musculoskeletal system disorder. It is age related, often associated with osteoporosis; it is a degenerative disease, related also to repeated exposure to trauma, often of the "wear-and-tear" variety that is occupational in origin. Osteoarthritis affects the spine, large joints such as hips and knees, and small joints in hands and feet. We may conveniently consider in this category the painful feet that cripple many old people, women especially, as a consequence of a lifetime of walking in poorly fitting shoes. This is the commonest reason why old people become less mobile, spending more time sitting and less standing and walking; one of the commonest complaints of the elderly is "painful feet."

Arthritis of the joints of the feet is just one of several disabling foot disorders of old people; poor circulation can cause a change in the shape and tex-

TABLE 7–10. Blindness in the United States

Potentially Avoidable Blindness

Cause of Blindness	Percent of Total Blindness [a]	Proportion Potentially Avoidable [b]	Percent Total Blindness Avoidable
Retinal degeneration	22	0.16	3.5
Other retinal	18	0.47	8.4
Multiple affections	14	0.10	1.4
Cataract	14	0.75	10.5
Glaucoma not congenital	13	0.50	7.5
Optic nerve atrophy	8	0.18	1.4
Uveitis	4		
Myopia	3		
Other corneal or scleral	2	0.18	2.0
Retrolental fibroplasia	1		
Keratitis	1		
Total	100		34.7

Rate of Annual Additions to Blindness Registers by Cause and by Race (Rate per 100,000)

Cause of Blindness	Nonwhite	White	Total
Retinal disease	4.4	4.2	4.2
Cataract	3.4	1.8	2.1
Glaucoma	5.1	0.8	1.5
Multiple affections	2.1	1.2	1.3
Unknown	2.5	1.6	1.8
Other	6.5	2.7	3.3

[a] Excludes "unknown" and "other," 4.8 and 9.4 percent respectively of total in original tables.
[b] Based on an appraisal of maximal, feasible impact of new technology and research findings since 1970.
(From Kahn HA, Moorhead HB: Statistics on Blindness in the Model Reporting Area, 1969–1970. DHEW Pub. No. (NIH) 73–427. Washington, DC: U.S. Government Printing Office, 1973.[52])

ture of the toenails, leading to horny excrescences that are difficult and painful to trim; and calluses may become acutely sensitive to pressure, another cause of severe pain when walking. Poor circulation, especially among diabetics, also contributes to severe, sometimes dangerous infections, which can become gangrenous. Less severe disorders can be disabling enough to restrict activity and lead old people to become chair-bound, then ultimately bed-bound.

TABLE 7–11. Causes and Prevention of Deafness

Cause	Prevalence	Prevention Potential
Infection		
Congenital rubella	Formerly high	+++
Upper respiratory with middle-ear infection ("glue ear," etc.)	High, especially when health care is inadequate	++
Trauma		
Birth injury	Uncommon	+
Noise-induced hearing loss	Very common	+++
Meatus disease		
Inflammation	Uncommon	+
Wax (cerumen)	Very common	– (but easily treated)
Toxic		
Certain drugs, e.g., streptomycin	Uncommon	+
Neurologic		
Tinnitus	Uncommon	?
"Nerve deafness," senile deafness	Common among elderly	–

▶ DISABLING DISORDERS IN AGING POPULATIONS

All these age-related disabling disorders will become more prevalent as the population ages. In the industrial nations in the 1990s, the proportion of persons aged 65 and over ranges from 7 to 15 percent; it will rise over the next 35 to 40 years as the "baby boom" generation grows older, reaching a peak of over 20 percent, perhaps as high as 25 percent in some countries, about the year 2031, when the students who read this book will be at the summit of their professional careers.

The proportion of the "oldest old," i.e., 85 years of age and over, is also rising and will continue to do so. Many people in this age group need institutional care; they have impairments that make it impossible for them to care for themselves, and often they have no close family members who can help them.[54]

Indeed, increasing proportions of all older people have little or no family or social support system. Data from the National Health Interview Survey in January–June 1984 showed very high proportions, especially of women, living alone[55] (Table 7–12); nearly 20 percent were not in close contact with relatives or friends, either in person or even by telephone. Given the trends in family formation and dissolution, the proportions who are completely isolated from family will rise over the next 35 to 40 years. The trends carry a clear message that many more community resources will be required in the future to meet the needs of the aging population.[56]

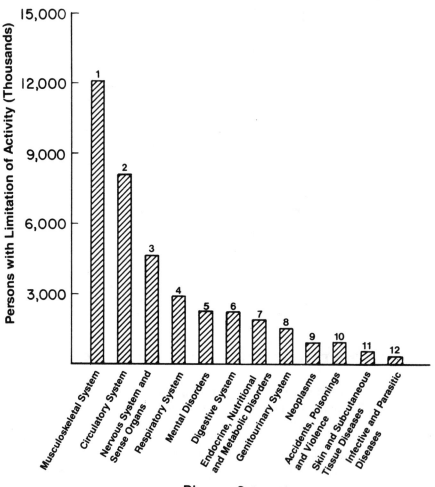

Figure 7–5. Estimated number of persons in the United States in 1984 with limitation of activity attributable to specific disease categories. *(From Holbrook TL, et al:* The Frequency of Occurrence, Impact, and Cost of Musculoskeletal Conditions in the United States. *Chicago: American Academy of Orthopedic Surgeons, 1984.)*

The rising proportion of older people as the "baby boom" generation grows older will make this segment of the population a political force to be reckoned with, if they should be mobilized as a pressure group. This could happen if existing social security provisions are weakened or diluted (Box 7–7).

TABLE 7–12. Domestic Arrangements and Support Systems of Older Americans, 1984

Percent Distribution of People Age 65 Years and Over by Age, Sex, and Marital Status,
According to Whether They Lived Alone or with Others: United States, January–June 1984

Age, Sex, and Marital Status	Total	Living Alone	Living with Others
		Number in thousands	
Estimated population	26,290	8,018	18,272
		Percent distribution	
Total	100.0	100.0	100.0
Age			
65–74 years	61.7	50.2	66.8
75–84 years	30.7	38.6	27.2
85 years and over	7.6	11.2	6.0
Sex			
Male	40.8	20.2	49.9
Female	59.2	79.8	50.1
Marital status			
Married	54.7	0.0	78.6
Widowed	34.1	77.1	15.2
Divorced	6.3	14.1	2.9
Never married	4.4	8.1	2.8

Percent of People Age 65 Years and Over Who Lived Alone by Contacts with Relatives, Friends, and
Neighbors within the Previous 2 Weeks and Whether by Person or Telephone: United States,
January–June 1984

Immediate Family	Relatives		Friends or Neighbors	
	In Person	*Telephone*	*In Person*	*Telephone*
		Percent with Contact		
Total	72.8	84.0	69.5	81.4
No child or sibling	26.8	37.8	50.5	56.6
Sibling(s) only	66.6	80.7	71.0	83.4
Child(ren) only	72.8	85.8	69.2	81.5
Both	84.0	93.5	39.4	85.6

(From the National Center for Health Statistics.[55])

▶ THE HANDICAPPED IN MODERN INDUSTRIAL SOCIETY

Although rather low-key, the changes that have taken place in providing for handicapped persons in recent years have been impressive and effective. There is room for more improvement, but among the advances in recognizing previously unmet needs we can identify the provision of ramps and other means of access to public places, toilet facilities, public transport, etc., for

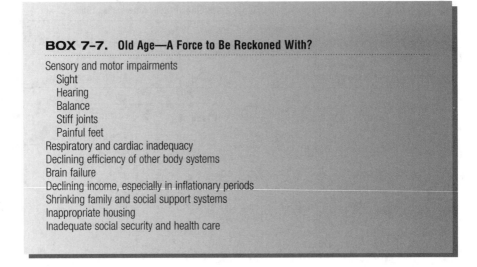

BOX 7-7.   Old Age—A Force to Be Reckoned With?

Sensory and motor impairments
  Sight
  Hearing
  Balance
  Stiff joints
  Painful feet
Respiratory and cardiac inadequacy
Declining efficiency of other body systems
Brain failure
Declining income, especially in inflationary periods
Shrinking family and social support systems
Inappropriate housing
Inadequate social security and health care

persons in wheelchairs; closed-caption television programs and inset sign-language interpreters for the deaf; serious and determined efforts to integrate handicapped persons of all kinds, including those with mild mental impairments, into regular and meaningful forms of employment. The International Year of Disabled Persons, the WHO theme for 1981, did much to raise public consciousness of the needs of the disabled, and many effective public policy decisions were taken then and have been maintained since.

► CONCLUSION

This chapter has outlined some common forms of disabling disorders in modern society. I have alluded to preventive measures that are available for some of these conditions. How widely used are these measures? The NCHS included questions on health promotion and disease prevention in the National Health Interview Survey in 1985; this survey covered a large sample and used a wide range of questions. Answers to some of these questions are summarized in Table 7–13. The picture that emerges is of a nation in which health-promoting behavior is, like the curate's egg, good in parts. There is room for much improvement, especially in self-motivated behaviors such as seatbelt use, exercising, and maintaining a healthful diet. The data suggest that many people rely on medical sources for preventive care and that although knowledge of positive health-promoting behaviors is adequate, it often is not applied. These results are a challenge to health educators and to experts in health promotion. They also offer a prognostic guide: The health problems of the future will arise from the health-related behaviors of the present.

TABLE 7–13. **Health Promotion and Disease Prevention—Behavior of Americans as Revealed in the National Health Interview Survey, January–June 1985 (Percentages)**

	Male	Female
Consider self overweight		
Very	3	12
Somewhat	13	21
A little	20	22
Trying to lose weight	27	46
Sleep 7–8 hr/night	66	65
Sleep < 7 hr/night	23	22
Sleep > 8 hr/night	11	13
Females: Pap smear within last year		45
Within last 1–2 years		27
5 or more years ago		12
Never had Pap smear		7
Females: Breast exam by doctor in last year		50
5 or more years ago		8
Never		7
Wear seatbelts when driving or riding in car		
Always	31	33
Never	37	34
Regular exercise in last 2 weeks		
Walking	39	47
Jogging or running	15	9
General exercise	25	25
Biking	11	11
Swimming	10	8
Exercise or play sport regularly	44	39
Cigarette smoking		
Never	35	54
Former smoker	31	18
Current (all)	33	28
Less than 15/day	9	10
15–24/day	13	12
25+/day	10	6
Alcohol use		
None	23	42
Light (0.01–0.21 oz. absolute alcohol)	13	15
Moderate (0.22–0.99 oz. absolute alcohol)	27	15
Heavy (1.0 oz. or more absolute alcohol)	13	3
Work exposure to toxics	44	23

(From NCHS, Advance Data No. 119, May 14, 1986.)

► **REFERENCES**

1. National Center for Health Statistics: Current Estimates. Washington, DC: U.S. Government Printing Office.
2. Susser MW: *Causal Thinking in the Health Sciences.* New York: Oxford University Press, 1973, pp. 4–5.
3. Last PM: First experiences with ICIDH in Australia's largest nursing home. *Int Rehabil Med* 7:63–66, 1985.
4. Katz S, Ford AB, Moskowitz RW, et al.: Studies of illness in the aged. The Index of ADL, a standardized measure of biological function. *JAMA* 185:914–919, 1963.
5. *Population Projections, 1990–2020.* New York: United Nations Statistical Office, 1992.
6. World Health Organization, Regional Office for Europe: Health Projections in Europe. Copenhagen: WHO, 1986.
7. Hetzel BS, McMichael T: *The LS Factor.* Harmondsworth, England: Penguin Books, 1987.
8. Doll R, Peto R: The causes of cancer. *J Natl Cancer Inst* 66:1191–1308, 1981.
9. Report of the Surgeon General: *The Health Consequences of Smoking. Cardiovascular Disease.* A Report of the Surgeon General. Washington, DC: U.S. Public Health Service, DHHS, 1983.
10. Report of the Surgeon General: *The Health Consequences of Smoking: Chronic Obstructive Lung Disease.* Washington, DC: U.S. Public Health Service, DHHS, 1984.
11. Vessey MP, Doll R: Investigation of relation between use of oral contraceptives and thromboembolic disease. *Br Med J* 2:199–205, 1968.
12. 1993 National Health Interview Survey: CD-ROM Series 10, No. 7, March 1996, SETS Version 1.22.
13. Kolata G: Obese children; A growing problem. *Science* 232:20–21, 1986.
14. Graham S, Marshall J, Haughey B, et al.: Dietary epidemiology of cancer of the colon in western New York. *Am J Epidemiol* 128:490–503, 1988.
15. Goodwin PJ, Boyd WF: Critical appraisal of the evidence that dietary fat intake is related to breast cancer risk in humans. *J Natl Cancer Inst* 79:473–485, 1987.
16. Ardrey R: *The Territorial Instinct.* New York: Harper, 1969.
17. Calhoun JB: Death squared. *Proc Roy Soc Med* 66:80–84, 1973.
18. Woolf SH, Jonas S, Lawrence RS (eds): *Health Promotion and Disease Prevention in Clinical Practice.* Baltimore: Williams & Wilkins, 1996.
19. Feinlieb M, Havlik RJ, Thom NJ: The changing patterns of ischemic heart disease. *J Cardiovasc Med* 7:139–148, 1982.
20. Blackburn H, Luepker R: Heart disease. In Last JM, Wallace RB (eds): *Maxcy-Rosenau-Last Public Health and Preventive Medicine.* 13th ed. E. Norwalk, CT: Appleton & Lange, 1992, pp. 827–848.
21. Thom NJ, Epstein FH, Feldman JS, et al.: Trends in total mortality and mortality from heart disease in 26 countries from 1950 to 1978. *Int J Epidemiol* 14:510–520, 1986.
22. Paffenbarger RS Jr, Hyde RT, Wing AL, et al.: Physical activity, all-cause mortality and longevity of college alumni. *N Engl J Med* 314:605–613, 1986.
23. Review panel on coronary-prone behavior and coronary heart disease: A critical review. *Circulation* 63:1199–1215, 1981.
24. Coates BE, Rawstron EM: *Cardiovascular Diseases: Regional Variations in Britain.* London: H1450, 1971.

25. Comstock GW: Water hardness and cardiovascular diseases. *Am J Epidemiol* 110:375–400, 1979.

26. Dawber TR: *The Framingham Study; The Epidemiology of Atherosclerotic Disease.* Cambridge, MA: Harvard University Press, 1980.

27. Puska P, Salonen JT, Nissenen A, et al.: Change in risk factors for coronary heart disease during 10 years of a community intervention programme (North Karelia project). *Br Med J* 286:1840–1846, 1983.

28. Farquhar JW, Wood PD, Breitrose H, et al.: Community education for cardiovascular health. *Lancet* 1:1192–1195, 1977.

29. Multiple Risk Factor Intervention Trial Group (MRFIT): Multiple risk factor research trial: Risk factor changes and mortality results. *JAMA* 248:1465–1477, 1982.

30. Ferrie JE, Shipley MJ, Marmot MG, Stansfield S, Davey-Smith G: Health effects of anticipated job change and non-employment. Longitudinal data from the Whitehall II Study. *Br Med J* 311:1264–1268, 1995.

31. Proceedings of Eleventh Annual Scientific Meeting, American College of Epidemiology, co-sponsored by NIH Office of Disease Prevention and Office of Research on Women's Health. *Ann Epidemiol* 4:81–175, 1994.

32. Wilson TW: History of salt supplies in West Africa and blood pressure today. *Lancet* 1:784–785, 1986.

33. Prior IAM, Evans JG, Harvey HPB, et al.: Sodium intake and blood pressure in two Polynesian populations. *N Engl J Med* 279:515–522, 1968.

34. Hypertension detection and follow-up program cooperative group: Reduction in stroke incidence among persons with high blood pressure. *JAMA* 247:633–638, 1982.

35. Tomatis L, Aitio A, Day NE, et al. (eds): *Cancer: Causes, Occurrence and Control.* Lyon, France: IARC Scientific Publications (WHO and IARC), 1990.

36. Li FP: Familial aggregation. In Schottenfeld D, Fraumeni JF (eds): *Cancer Epidemiology and Prevention.* 2nd ed. New York: Oxford University Press, 1997, pp 546–558.

37. Bailar JC III, Smith EM: Progress against cancer? *N Engl J Med* 314:1226–1232, 1986.

38. Schottenfeld D, Fraumeni J (eds): *Cancer Epidemiology and Prevention.* 2nd ed. New York: Oxford University Press, 1997.

39. Zador PL, Lund AK, Fields M, et al.: Fatal crash involvement and laws against alcohol-impaired driving. *J Public Health Policy* 10:467–492, 1989.

40. Baker SP, O'Neill B, Karpf RS: *Injury Fact Book.* Lexington MA: Lexington, 1984.

41. Robertson LS: *Injury Epidemiology.* New York: Oxford University Press, 1992.

42. Cook PJ (ed): The effect of gun availability on violent crime patterns: Gun control. *Ann Amer Acad Polit Soc Sci* Vol. 455, 1981.

43. Report of the Committee on Sexual Offences Against Children: *Sexual Offences Against Children.* Ottawa: Supply and Services Canada, 1984.

44. Rosenberg ML, Mercy JA: Assaultative violence. In Last JM, Wallace RB (eds): *Maxcy-Rosenau-Last Public Health and Preventive Medicine.* 13th ed. E. Norwalk, CT: Appleton & Lange, 1992, pp. 1035–1039.

45. Reid J, Camus J, Last JM: Suicide in Canada. Birth cohort analysis. *Can J Public Health* 76:43–47, 1985.

46. Katzman R: Alzheimer's disease. *N Engl J Med* 314:964–973, 1986.

47. Gruenberg EM (ed): *Vaccinating Against Brain Syndromes; The Campaign Against Measles and Rubella.* New York: Oxford University Press, 1985.

48. Stein ZA, Susser MW: Mental Retardation. In Last JM, Wallace RB (eds): *Maxcy-Rosenau-Last Public Health and Preventive Medicine.* 13th ed. E. Norwalk, CT: Appleton & Lange, 1992.

49. Zuckerman B, Frank DA, Hingson R et al.: Effects of maternal marijuana and cocaine use on fetal growth. *N Engl J Med* 320:762–768, 1989.

50. Tong S, Baghurst P, McMichael A, Sawyer M, Mudge J: Lifetime exposure to environmental lead and children's intelligence at 11–13 years: The Port Pirie cohort study. *Br Med J* 312:1569–1575, 1996.

51. The Homeless Mentally Ill. Washington, DC: American Psychiatric Association, 1984.

52. Kahn HA, Moorhead HB: *Statistics on Blindness in the Model Reporting Area, 1969–1970.* DHEW Pub. No. (NIH) 73–427. Washington, DC: U.S. Government Printing Office, 1973.

53. Kelsey JL: Epidemiology of musculoskeletal disorders. New York: Oxford University Press, 1982.

54. Suzman R, Riley MW (eds): *The Oldest Old. Milbank Mem Fund Q* 63:177–451, 1985.

55. National Center for Health Statistics: *Aging in the Eighties; Preliminary Data from the Supplement on Aging to the National Health Interview Survey, United States January–June 1984.* U.S. DHHS, May 1986.

56. Vaupel JW, Gowan AE: Passage to Methuselah. Some demographic consequences of continuing progress against mortality. *Am J Public Health* 76:430–433, 1986.

8

Public Health Services

In most industrial nations, public health services are organized and administered at several levels, as are other important activities. Nations are usually divided into self-contained jurisdictions—states, provinces, cantons—and within each there are further jurisdictional subdivisions, such as metropolitan areas and rural counties. The organization into several levels may apply to all aspects of health services, i.e., personal health care, institutionally based health care, and public health services, but in many nations, including the United States, it applies mainly to public health services.

There are several excellent descriptive and critical accounts of the way the public and personal health care system is organized in the United States. Instead of repeating or summarizing these, I provide the outline of organization in tables, and use the text to generalize about the structural and functional integration of public health services: The details differ from one nation to another, but the broad principles are nearly universal among the industrial nations. Readers can relate these generalizations to particular details of other countries as well as to the United States.

The historical and cultural context of nations influences the evolution and structure of their health services. In the United States, the separation of powers between the administrative, legislative, and judicial branches of government and the sharing of sovereignty between the states and the federal government have been important determinants of the way health services are organized and how they function. The states, which possess what is termed the "police power," rather than the federal government, have the responsibility for laws to protect the people's health; so historically the principal determinant of action to promote the public health has been state power and responsibility. Federal agencies have arisen more recently than those in the states and act by virtue of their power over interstate commerce and the general welfare powers. The U.S. Public Health Service (USPHS) acquired its first public health function, quarantine enforcement, as recently as 1878. The Department of Health and Human Services (DHHS) originated as the

Department of Health, Education and Welfare (DHEW) in 1953 (it was preceded by the Federal Security Administration in the mid-1930s).

Personal health services for care of the sick vary greatly in organization and method of financing. The variations are determined by historical traditions, the relationship between the political system and the medical and other health professional associations, and sometimes by the influence of leaders of the medical profession and of political parties. Hospital and other institutional services are similar in all industrial nations, although there are differences in the extent to which hospitals are established and maintained by public (governmental) authorities, religious and charitable interests or other voluntary nonprofit groups, and private, proprietary (profit-making) corporations. There are also differences in the extent to which hospitals offer ambulatory and outreach services and tertiary care. In some countries, tertiary care is concentrated in a few metropolitan hospitals; in others, including the United States, it is provided in many hospitals, often in competition with one another.

All affluent industrial nations make some tax-supported or subsidized contribution to personal care of the sick. This often involves governmental participation in at least some aspects of personal health services, but the medical profession remains largely independent of government control over patient care in most countries. In the United States, the prevailing political philosophy—the free enterprise ethic—is the rationale for the dissociation of practicing personal physicians from governmental control. Even so, increasing proportions of personal physicians in the United States derive all or some of their income from salary, rather than from fees collected for each item of service rendered to their patients. Moreover, the introduction of the Medicare and Medicaid programs brought about a situation whereby public revenue is used to pay privately practicing physicians for the personal care of certain classes of patients. The details of payment mechanisms for personal health care are so complex and diverse that no brief general account is either possible or useful. Since the mid-1980s, and with gathering momentum in the 1990s, profit-making health maintenance organizations (HMOs) have proliferated in the United States. Some of these do not offer adequate preventive or health maintenance services to their clients or patients—the term HMO is a misnomer for these. However, independent primary care physicians and many HMOs do offer a widening range of preventive services: screening for early evidence of disease and counseling for patients and clients on a widening range of health-promoting and health-protecting actions. Similar ranges of health-promoting and disease-preventing programs are offered by primary care physicians in other countries, for instance, several nations of the European Union. This helps to close gaps left in services provided by local health departments when budget-cutting administrations reduce staff in local health departments, further discussed later in this chapter.

Several critical reviews and many descriptive accounts are available, and some are listed in the references at the end of the chapter. I will discuss services directly concerned with public health, mentioning other components such as personal health services only in the context of their contribution to preventive medicine.

► **ESSENTIAL PUBLIC HEALTH FUNCTIONS**

In 1995–1996, a World Health Organization (WHO)-based Internet discussion group has delineated public health functions. Those that by common consensus are regarded as essential address one or more of the following needs:

1. Prevent epidemics and the spread of disease (within a country or internationally)
2. Protect the population against environmental hazards
3. Prevent injuries
4. Encourage healthy behavior
5. Respond to disasters
6. Assure the quality and accessibility of health services
7. Support the management, planning, development, and evaluation of health-care systems
8. Support and manage the development of health resources including finance, human resources, and technology

These needs are addressed in a manner that, to the extent possible:

1. Addresses priority and emerging health problems
2. Is responsive to the needs of all people, the need for caring and human concern, and the need to be culturally acceptable
3. Is cost-effective, affordable, and of acceptable quality
4. Applies the principles of equity, gender sensitivity, social justice, and sustainability
5. Seeks innovative approaches to service delivery and technology use
6. Addresses the full spectrum of the most important determinants of health
7. Stresses the importance of intersectoral collaboration
8. Includes surveillance of the health situation and monitoring of health outcomes
9. Influences at the global level the manner in which the WHO and its global partners undertake international action, thereby creating a world health conscience via advocacy and resource mobilization and providing global health foresight by anticipating threats and influencing global and national agendas

There are several categories of essential public health functions:

1. Health information management
2. Protection of the environment

3. Health promotion and education
4. Prevention, surveillance, and control of communicable diseases
5. Health legislation and regulations
6. Health research
7. Developing and implementing health policies, programs, and services
8. Developing human resources for health
9. Assessment and standardization of health technology
10. Occupational health
11. Delivering selected health services to selected populations

As you read the following accounts of national, regional, and local public health services, consider the extent to which all the previously mentioned points are satisfactorily covered.

► NATIONALLY ORGANIZED PUBLIC HEALTH SERVICES

The primary concern of public health services at the national level is with practices and policies that affect the nation's health; included in this are some areas of interaction with other nations and with the international health-related agencies, especially WHO (see Chap. 9). An important responsibility of national public health services and the initial reason for their establishment in many countries is to protect the people against imported diseases. This is accomplished by quarantine regulations, including plant and animal quarantine. Until the early 1970s, there were six quarantinable diseases—smallpox, plague, yellow fever, cholera, epidemic typhus, and louseborne relapsing fever. Since the eradication of smallpox and advances in control and treatment of several other diseases, only yellow fever, cholera, and plague are designated quarantinable. Epidemic influenza A, paralytic poliomyelitis, and acquired immunodeficiency syndrome (AIDS), and from time to time other diseases, are subject to international surveillance and reporting by national public health authorities to WHO.

By international agreement, national public health services are also responsible for health surveillance and some aspects of medical care of persons whose work requires their movement between nations, e.g., sailors on ships.

Another function often performed by national public health services is the provision of health care for special groups, such as persons living in isolated or remote regions where private or independent medical practice is nonexistent, indigenous peoples, persons in certain kinds of institutions, members of the armed forces, and certain other groups that vary from country to country (Box 8–1).

BOX 8-1. National Public Health Services

Protect the nation's health
   Quarantine
   Communicable disease surveillance
   Other diseases of importance
      Cancer
      Birth defects
      Heart disease
      Injury control, etc.
Health promotion
   National food policies
   Fitness policies
   Health education
Environmental protection
   Workers' health and safety
   Food safety
Health care of special groups
   Armed services
   Government employees
   Native people
   Remote communities
   Aged, indigent, etc.
Medical research
Health statistics
Standard setting, licensure, etc.

In most nations, public health services have assumed other responsibilities, either as a matter of national policy or by default. These responsibilities usually include formal financial support for basic and applied medical research. In the United States, the two most prominent research institutions in the nation, the National Institutes of Health (NIH), which conduct and financially support research in every aspect of the biomedical sciences, and the Centers for Disease Control and Prevention (CDC), which are responsible primarily for surveillance but also do much research, are both financed from the federal budget.

For historical and political reasons, many other federal government departments have authority and responsibility for important activities affecting the public health. There is similar diversity in most other nations.

Table 8–1 lists the range of health-related services and responsibilities exercised at federal level and the government departments in charge of each in the United States. Most, but not quite all, of the activities discussed in the following paragraphs are listed in this table; those that are missing may be undertaken in some instances by voluntary bodies in a piecemeal fashion

TABLE 8-1.   Health-Related Roles, U.S. Federal Government

Branches of government

Legislative branch	Enacts federal health laws
Judicial branch	Adjudicates disputes
	Safeguards rights
Executive branch	Provides, finances services
	(No "Ministry of Health")

Federal departments, agencies involved in health matters

1. Department of Health and Human Services (DHHS)

   Health Care Financing Administration (HCFA)

   U.S. Public Health Service (USPHS)
      Quarantine
      International health
      Communicable disease control
      Health promotion/protection (Office of Disease Prevention and Health Promotion)
      Health resources and services
      Biomedical research (National Institutes of Health [NIH])
      Health surveillance (Centers for Disease Control and Prevention [CDC])
      Substance control (alcohol, drug abuse)
      Smoking and health
      Mental health
      Population affairs (National Center for Health Statistics [NCHS])
      President's Council on Fitness and Sport
      Health services research

2. U.S. Congress, Office of Technology Assessment (OTA)
   Health technology assessment

3. U.S. Department of Agriculture (USDA)
   Food, meat, etc.

4. U.S. Department of Labor
   Workplace safety and health

5. Department of Defense (DOD)
   Total health care of armed forces

6. Environmental Protection Agency (EPA)

(e.g., promotion of physical fitness) or partly by governmental bodies (e.g., recommended dietary allowances, in lieu of a national food policy).

The medical services administered by the Department of Defense (DOD) and its equivalent in many other nations deserve special mention: These are the only comprehensive health services in the true sense of the word, as they provide a full range of preventive, therapeutic, and rehabilitative services for armed services personnel.

The provision of national health-related data, their collection, storage, processing, retrieval, analysis, and publication in periodic reports on the state of the nation's health, is an important activity in most nations. This may be solely the responsibility of the national public health service, or there may be some sharing with other national governmental agencies such as those devoted to census taking and economic statistics. In the United States, the agency responsible for compiling and analyzing health statistics is the National Center for Health Statistics (NCHS), but related statistics are produced by several other agencies, for instance the Bureau of the Census. The initial collection of many vital and health statistics is at local level, where registrations of vital events (births, deaths, and marriages) and notifications of reportable diseases are transmitted to state registrars; from the offices of state registrars, either the whole statistical data file or summary statistics may be transmitted to the NCHS, where national reports are compiled. Similar procedures exist in other countries. The collection and compiling of hospital statistics is in some respects a joint public and private enterprise initiative; many useful data originate in the computerized records of the Commission on Professional and Hospital Activities (CPHA), which is responsible for the widely used Professional Activity Study (PAS), i.e., summary statistics of all separations from participating hospitals. Other data are collected by the American Hospital Association and summarized in the annual publication, *Hospital Statistics*. Federal government agencies such as the NCHS collaborate closely with these private enterprise and voluntary bodies.

Public health activities related to occupational health may be the responsibility of the national ministry or department of labor, rather than the health department as such, as happens in the United States. Similarly, setting and monitoring national standards for environmental quality of air and water is a responsibility of the Environmental Protection Agency (EPA) in the United States. Both occupational health and environmental health are further supervised and controlled by state authorities.

The protection of standards of purity and wholesomeness of food is a national responsibility in most nations. In the United States, this is the responsibility of the U.S. Department of Agriculture (USDA) and the Food and Drug Administration (FDA), which, as the title indicates, also watches over drug safety and efficacy. Food quality must also be assured at local level, and the monitoring of food preparation, storage, distribution, etc., is among the important functions of health inspectors in local health departments.

In most countries, national public health authorities are responsible for the overall direction of health care for conditions that might threaten the national health or well-being. These conditions include human immunodeficiency virus (HIV) disease, tuberculosis, and sexually transmitted diseases (STDs), and in many countries, severe forms of mental disorder that require institutional care. The day-to-day administration and management of such services is usually delegated to regional and local authorities; the salaries of workers in these services and the operating funds may come from local, regional, or national budgets, or partly from each. As part of the work related to this, there may be a national laboratory service for investigation of specimens collected from patients with specified diseases and perhaps related research activities. In the United States, this is an important function of the CDC. Frequently such laboratory services are coordinated with regional and local services, but the latter are usually service oriented with little research component.

National food policies exist in many countries, especially those that have strong social programs and a socialist form of government and those that have had to institute food rationing in times of war or scarcity. These policies usually include explicit guidelines on dietary requirements of essential ingredients such as vitamins, minerals, protein; and they may be implemented by ministries of health or of food and agriculture. In the United Kingdom, the introduction of national food policies is credited with having achieved spectacular improvements in child health and physical development during the years of scarcity in and just after World War II.

In the United States, there is no national food policy as such, but several national agencies, both governmental and quasi-governmental, notably the Food and Nutrition Board of the National Academy of Sciences, the Senate Committee on Nutrition and Human Needs, and the White House Conference on Food, Nutrition, and Health, all in the late 1960s and early 1970s, helped both to reinforce existing standards and set new ones in important matters such as recommended dietary allowances (see Chap. 5).

National fitness policies are pursued by some nations; these may be directed from the ministry of health or, if there is one, a ministry of sport. In some nations, great value is accorded to prowess in sport and to national achievements in international sporting contests, and there is much emphasis on attaining and maintaining high degrees of physical fitness. In the United States, although there is no national fitness policy as such, fitness and achievement in sport is highly valued in many high schools and colleges; success in competitive sports may be more highly valued in some colleges than scholastic achievements.

Whether or not there are fitness policies, most national governments conduct some form of health education, frequently directed toward reduction of tobacco smoking, improved diets, highway safety, and the like. The health education programs are normally a responsibility of national ministries or departments of health, sometimes of national ministries of education, sometimes the two in collaboration. In the United States, the Office of Disease Prevention and Health Promotion coordinates and conducts a wide-ranging program aimed at improving the health of the American people. Much of the activity of this office centers on health education or other and more sophisticated health-promoting activities (see Chap. 1).

The regulation of standards, licensure of health professionals, accreditation of institutions that care for the sick and train health workers, regulation of drugs, appliances, etc., is usually implemented nationally, but frequently with some regionalization; for example, physicians are licensed to practice at the state or provincial level in the United States and Canada. Specialty certification for health professionals is regulated by the professions themselves; this is a largely voluntary activity in which each specialty within the profession determines its own standards and disciplines its own members when they depart from accepted standards. However, the law is invoked when the need arises: Criminal sanctions may be applied to prohibit practice by persons who do not meet basic educational requirements or who are found guilty of gross professional misconduct. The legal responsibility of licensing bodies may be explicitly set out in laws enacted by the elected government, so the so-called voluntary professional licensing body may be in effect a de facto agency of the government. The regulation of pharmaceuticals and medical appliances is in the hands of the government, although there may be advisory groups whose members include representatives from the industries concerned as well as practicing health professionals and government employees. This description, like much else in this chapter, is an attempt to generalize from the particular details that apply in any given nation such as the United States or the United Kingdom. In fact, although the details differ, the overall pattern is remarkably similar in many nations. This pattern is set at least partly as a consequence of recognition that regulation of activities related to health protection and disease prevention requires the coordinated and collaborative efforts of many interest groups, and collaboration is best achieved by a combination of government and volunteer groups.

Almost all industrial nations have made provision for the costs of health care for certain groups to be borne wholly or partly by public revenue. These groups include old age, invalid pensioners, and the medically indigent. There is considerable variation among nations in the extent to which medical services are provided for such people and in who provides the service—privately practicing physicians or government-salaried doctors. The national ministry or department of health has a supervisory role in the provision of this care. Of all aspects of the work of national health ministries, this is the one most responsive to political ideologies, and consequently it is the most variable, not only among nations but also within the same nation when the balance of power shifts from one political ideology to another. It is possible to make some generalizations, however. In particular, since the late-19th century, there has been a progressive trend toward more active commitment of national resources to the care of the sick and the disabled and the provision of some form of social security. This began in Germany in the 1870s with Bismarck's recognition of the value of adopting such measures, both to promote improved health and to assuage social discontents—and so prevent revolutions.

In summary, national public health authorities are primarily concerned with protecting the public health against diseases that threaten all the people, with national policies, and with regulatory activities, some of which are conducted in collaboration with voluntary professional organizations. There is relatively little or no direct involvement with health promotion or disease prevention activities at the personal level.

► REGIONAL PUBLIC HEALTH SERVICES

In most industrial nations, many of the services and activities just described are organized and administered—and often at least partly financed—at a secondary level within each administrative jurisdiction of the nation, i.e., each separate state or province. Exceptions to this generalization are the countries with a unitary form of government, where there is no devolution of power to regions; Finland and the Netherlands are examples. Regional devolution is often done for convenience, as part of the devolution of power and authority to regionally elected and appointed officials, and in recognition of the fact that many national standards and circumstances have to be modified within regions to meet regional requirements. In the United States, the reason for this arrangement is the historical origin of the federal government as an instrument of the states. The same is true, of course, of other services such as those relating to education. As already noted, collection, and often analysis, of health-related statistics is conducted regionally, and the compiled statistics are sent to a national agency, which condenses them into published form. Notification of communicable diseases, a local responsibility, yields information that usually goes first to state or provincial authorities because responses to outbreaks of communicable disease are usually more efficient if mobilized regionally rather than nationally.

In many countries, regional (state, provincial) regulatory, standard-setting, and supervisory bodies are responsible for environmental air and water quality, food and milk hygiene, etc., and for such activities as health education. This also reflects devolution of power and recognition of regional differences that justify variations of what otherwise would be uniform national standards. At times, this variation can be detrimental if it leads to relaxed standards that ought to be maintained in the public interest. If food, for example, is produced and prepared for consumption in one jurisdiction and consumed in another that has stricter standards, the residents of this second jurisdiction could justifiably criticize the authorities in the less strict jurisdiction for putting their health in jeopardy. For this reason it is best to have overriding national standards, as most nations do. Sometimes, particularly in the United States, landmark decisions in the courts have been invoked to establish standards.

Many state (provincial) government departments other than health have direct involvement in some aspect of public health. Generalization is difficult; as an example, the departments that are involved in New York State are set out in Table 8–2.

TABLE 8–2.   Services Commonly Provided and/or Administered by State (Provincial, Regional) Health Departments

Maternal and child health, including prenatal and postnatal services, family planning, immunization, and well-baby care

Public and personal health education

Communicable disease control, including immunization, tuberculosis and venereal disease control, epidemiology, and laboratory services

Dental health, emphasizing preventive services

Handicapped children's services

Chronic disease screening

Mental health, mental retardation, and alcohol and drug abuse services

Environmental health, including consumer protection and sanitation, air and water quality, waste management, occupational health and safety, and radiation control

Health professions licensure

Health resources management, including the planning, development, and regulation of health services, facilities, manpower, and health statistics activities

Laboratory, including analytic services and laboratory improvement to assist in efforts to prevent, detect, and treat disease

Other Agencies with Public Health Responsibility (New York State)
Department of Education

　Supervises health teaching in schools

　School sanitation

　Licenses physicians and medically related professionals

　Vocational rehabilitation

Department of Labor

　Responsible for health and safety of workers

　In-plant air pollution control

　In-plant protection from radiation

Department of Environmental Conservation

　Protects shellfish

　Controls pesticides

　Rabies control in wildlife

　Air pollution

　Sewage treatment

　Solid wastes

Department of Motor Vehicles

　Promotes highway safety via research and engineering

Department of Mental Hygiene

　Operates mental institutions

　Directs community mental health services

　Tuberculosis case finding among inmates

Department of Correction

　Operates hospitals and institutions for the criminally insane, for defective delinquents

　Conducts tuberculosis case finding among inmates

(continued)

TABLE 8-2.   *(continued)*

Department of Agriculture and Markets
    Licenses milk dealers
    Licenses slaughterhouses
    Inspects restaurants
    Regulates food additives
    Inspects ice cream

Department of Social Services
    Provides medical assistance for the needy

Office of Aging
    Promotes health services for the aging

State University of New York
    Operates health sciences schools and programs and university hospitals
    Operates student health services

Office of Alcoholism and Substance Abuse Services
    Directs community alcoholism and drug abuse treatment services
    Carries on research
    Promotes public understanding of alcoholism and drug abuse

(Modified from Jonas S: Provision of public health services. In Last JM (ed): Maxcy-Rosenau Public Health and Preventive Medicine, 12th ed. E. Norwalk, CT: Appleton-Century-Crofts, 1986, p. 1629.)

▶ THE LOCAL HEALTH DEPARTMENT

The local health department has day-to-day responsibility for health protection at the level of individual communities. The local health department, moreover, is the setting for direct interaction of public health workers and the people whose health they are employed to preserve and protect. The local health department is much more interactive with other health workers in the community than are the national or regional health departments.

There is considerable similarity around the world in the structure and functions of local health departments, although the administrative arrangements (who reports to whom) may vary. Figure 8–1 is an organization chart of a "typical" local health department, and Table 8–3 is a list of the professional groups typically represented in a local health department.

The primary function of a local health department is, of course, to protect the health of the people in the community. But there are always other responsibilities that relate directly to health protection and frequently others again that have been added because they are needed and not otherwise provided in the community. There are activities concerned with health planning and evaluation related directly to health protection often much concerned with resource allocation and budgeting. Less closely connected with the health protection activities, sometimes with no perceptible connection, is the

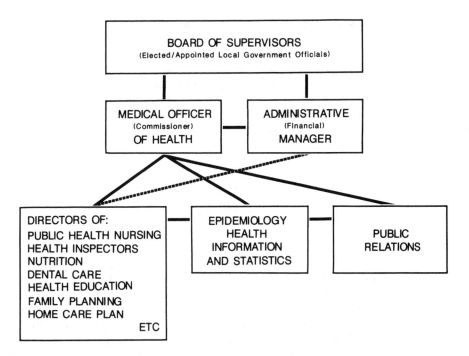

Figure 8–1. Organization chart of a typical local health department.

provision of services of several kinds to particular groups, notably high-risk infants and the frail elderly who remain outside of institutions.

Usually, but not always, the chief executive officer of the local health department is a physician with special training in public health, usually called medical officer of health (MOH) or commissioner of health. This physician is highly specialized and has diverse and important responsibilities, summarized in Table 8–4.

The MOH has the support of a multidisciplinary team, the principal members of which are health inspectors and public health nurses. Others usually include specialists in dental public health, social work, and epidemiology.

TABLE 8–3. **Professional Groups in a Local Health Department**

Physicians	Epidemiologists
Nurses	Hygienists
Dentists	Nutritionists
Health administrators	Health educators
Health inspectors	Social workers
Environmental scientists	Secretarial and other support staff

TABLE 8–4. **Responsibilities and Required Skills of the Medical Officer of Health**

Health promotion, disease prevention
Organization and management of complex staff
Epidemiologic skills—health information-gathering and needs assessment
Public relations and political savvy
Communication skills
Knowledge of public health law, history, philosophy; knowledge of medical, social, and behavioral
   sciences; ability to react calmly in crises and to consider all angles of complex situations

The diverse activities that go on in a local health department all deserve discussion (Box 8–2).

Control of Communicable Diseases

Effective control requires surveillance, case finding, investigation of outbreaks, treatment of infectious cases and of contacts if these can transmit infection, elimination of environmental health hazards that can be foci of infection, and immunization of the susceptible population, which may be done either by health department staff or, in collaboration, by family physicians, etc. This complex array of functions clearly involves specialists in several professions and cooperation between staff in the local health department and many other health professionals, such as family physicians, pediatricians, and hospital-based and laboratory specialists.

Moreover, the nature of the tasks required to control communicable diseases differs and depends upon the type of communicable disease. An outbreak of food poisoning requires one sort of management, cases of STD another, a solitary case of an exotic infection such as a quarantinable disease something else again. The first task in all instances is to verify the diagnosis, which may require laboratory investigations, careful assessment by specialized consultants, observation, etc. Often a presumptive diagnosis suffices for action to be initiated. The public health nurses usually are responsible for assessing the situation in which cases occur to determine what measures are required to contain the outbreak. In control of STDs, the public health nurse's role is the difficult and demanding task of contact tracing; this calls for persistence, tact, and skill in eliciting answers to questions, often from people who are reluctant to disclose details of their casual sexual encounters. The laboratory investigations that confirm the nature of the responsible infectious microorganism are usually done by staff in a laboratory that may be a formal administrative component of the local health department or an independent entity (see also Chap. 2).

Immunization against communicable diseases may be conducted by health department staff or by pediatricians or family physicians. Most local health departments hold regular clinics for immunization (and other aspects

BOX 8-2. Activities of the Local Health Department

Health Needs Assessment—Using All Available Health Information Systems
Control of Communicable Disease
    Immunizations
    Special clinics (STDs, tuberculosis, etc.)
    Environmental sanitation
    Pest control
    Surveillance of cases, contacts
Environmental health
    Waste disposal
    Noise abatement
    Nuisance control
    Water, air pollution monitoring
    Hazardous waste disposal
Food hygiene
    Inspection of food producing, processing
    Restaurant inspection
Health education
    School health
    Public campaigns
Special health-related clinic services
    Family planning
    Dental health
    Maternal and child health
    Geriatric care
    STDs
Preventive screening programs
    Hypertension
    Pap smears
    Chest x-ray surveys for tuberculosis
Home care plans
    Visiting service for invalids, pensioners
Disaster planning
    Coordinated with other services (Police, fire department, hospitals, etc.)
Coordination of voluntary service agencies
    Meals on Wheels
    Aid to dependent, handicapped, etc.

of child and maternal health). As a rule, immunizations and other essential health-protecting services for infants and children are provided at public health clinics without charge; privately practicing physicians, on the other hand, normally charge a fee for the same service. In many communities there is a well-established routine procedure of home visits to all mothers of newborn infants by public health nurses, who advise about ways to protect the health of the newborn infant, specifically about the necessary immunizations, as well as about infant feeding, etc. The advantage of having these health-protecting services provided by the local health department is that comprehensive coverage of the high-risk population groups is more likely to be assured than when the same services are provided perhaps in rather haphazard hit-or-miss fashion by family physicians. The fact that the latter's fees for this essential preventive service may be a deterrent to some who need it is another disadvantage in countries with a fee-for-service system of personal health care.

Environmental Health

Many hazards to health and nuisances are dealt with by local health authorities. These include hazardous waste disposal, noxious trades, and noise abatement. Local control of water and air pollution is another important task of the local health department. These activities are primarily the responsibility of the health or sanitary inspectors.

Food Hygiene

This too is a responsibility of the health inspectors. In most jurisdictions, all establishments that produce, process, distribute, sell, or serve food have to be periodically inspected to ensure that adequate safeguards are in place to protect against food-borne disease.

Health Education

Most local health departments have a line item in their budget to cover the cost of disseminating important health-related facts, such as advice about infectious diseases. This may be a prominent part of some health department's work, for instance including regular health teaching in schools by public health nurses. This may or may not include education on aspects of human sexuality, but it usually includes teaching on nutrition, dental hygiene, reasons why exercise is good for people, why smoking is bad, and so on.

Family Planning

This is a routinely operated clinic in many local health departments, usually staffed by gynecologists as well as by public health nurses and health educators. The need for family planning clinics is clear from the statistics on unwanted and unplanned pregnancies, especially among girls and women who for various reasons do not attend a family physician for advice and treatment of fertility. Family planning clinics are especially valuable for women in low-income groups. Unfortunately their roles and responsibilities have been hampered in some U.S. communities by "right to life" politicization; some family planning clinics have been targeted by terrorists linked to "right to life" extremists.

Dental Clinics

Many local health departments operate dental clinics specifically for low-income families; these provide restorative as well as preventive dental care and are staffed by dentists; preventive dental care, such as fluoride mouth rinses, may be offered to all children, often as part of a school health service that is operated by the local health department. In some countries, school health services are separately administered at a higher level than the local health department, often by the department or ministry of education.

Preventive Screening

Recognition that some remediable conditions are best dealt with if detected very early has led to many initiatives in preventive screening, e.g., of neonates for congenitally dislocated hip, phenylketonuria, hypothyroidism; of women for preinvasive cancer of the cervix; and of men and women for high blood pressure. Some local health departments have initiated screening clinics for these and other conditions, often in collaboration with specialists in the pertinent fields, e.g., pediatricians, gynecologists, and internists. Screening services, however, are more often provided by privately practicing physicians or by prepaid health plans, e.g., HMOs.

Home Care Plans

Persons with disabling disorders who can be kept in their own homes if provided with housekeeping services may be able to rely on homemakers employed by the home care plan in their community; this home care plan may be administered by a voluntary body, as also may related activities such as Meals on Wheels, or it may be a formally constituted part of the work of the local health department. In most communities there is a means-test–based charge for this service.

Disaster Planning

This is not a specific function unique to local health departments, but it is an essential activity in which all local health departments should participate with other pertinent authorities, who usually include law enforcement agencies, fire departments, ambulance transport authorities, senior management and clinical staff of local hospitals, local communications networks, voluntary agencies such as Red Cross, and others, often coordinated by a duly constituted statutory body with a title, e.g., Emergency Services Organization. Both natural and manmade disasters frequently have public health implications. Floods and earthquakes disrupt sanitary services, forest or urban fires can render many people homeless, chemical explosions or large-scale leakages of toxic or radioactive material can cause large numbers of deaths and injuries and make it necessary to evacuate a whole area at very short notice. In recent years, large-scale disasters involving the need to move many people rapidly away from their normal dwelling places have frequently captured the headlines—Seveso, Three Mile Island, Bhopal, and Chernobyl are just a few among many such episodes (Table 8–5; see also Chap. 4). As Table 8–5 shows, very large numbers of people may be killed and injured in some disasters, especially in developing countries; but even when there are no deaths, the need to evacuate large numbers at short notice; to provide emergency accommodation, food supplies, communications, social support to reunite families; and to deal with disaster-related and unrelated medical emergencies, requires well-prepared plans in which local health department staff must participate.

Other Activities

Clearly, local health departments have many roles and responsibilities. A good way to get the flavor and range of these is to study the annual report of the local health department in any community with a population of half a million or more. But this description may not sufficiently emphasize the important role of the health department in helping to coordinate and sometimes orchestrate the work of numerous voluntary organizations. Some of the tasks undertaken by voluntary organizations may occasionally be carried out by local health departments if there is a gap in local coverage of this particular service and the need for it is perceived. The range of these tasks and the organizations that perform them is so extensive that no brief description can do them justice. Table 8–6 displays the more important, but many others

TABLE 8–5.   **Some Recent Natural and Manmade Disasters**

Year	Type of Disaster	Place	Impact
1976	Earthquake	Guatemala	23,000 deaths; 77,000 injured
1976	Explosion in chemical factory	Seveso, Italy	17,000 evacuated; many pregnancies terminated
1978	Hurricane	Sri Lanka	900 deaths; 100,000 homeless
1978	Chemical spill	Mississauga, Canada	Over 100,000 evacuated
1979	Flood	Jamaica	40 deaths; 40,000 homeless
1981	Earthquake	Iran	1000 deaths; 40,000 homeless
1984	Chemical leak	Bhopal, India	2000 deaths; ?70,000 evacuated
1985	Earthquake	Mexico	100,000 homeless
1986	Nuclear reactor meltdown	Chernobyl, Ukraine	30 immediate deaths; 100,000 + evacuated; 500–600 cancer deaths as of 1995
1991	Cyclone, floods	Bangladesh	140,000 deaths
1992	Hurricane Andrew	Florida	74 deaths; $30 billion damage
1993	Flood	Mississippi river basin	41 deaths; $12 billion damage

TABLE 8-6. **Some Agencies Relating to Local Health Departments**

Child health services	Pediatric departments, specialists
	Child protection agencies
Reproductive health	Planned Parenthood, etc.
	Women's groups
Occupational health	Labor unions
Environmental health	Environmental groups
Geriatric services	Senior citizens' councils
	Drop-in centers for seniors
Emotionally disturbed	Distress center
	Samaritan service
	Homeless, e.g., Salvation Army
Handicapped, impaired	Home help services
	Red Cross
	Meals on Wheels
	Other volunteer agencies

exist. Most large communities maintain a directory of all the statutory and volunteer agencies in the health and social service fields, and physicians setting up practice are well advised to obtain the directory for their community and familiarize themselves with the important information it contains.

▶ EVALUATION OF PUBLIC HEALTH SERVICES

The "Disarray" of Public Health

Concerned about the state of public health services in the United States in the late 1980s, the Institute of Medicine (IOM) of the National Academy of Sciences struck a committee for the study of the future of public health. Around that time, similar studies of public health services were conducted in several other nations. *The Future of Public Health,* the report of the IOM's committee, and the report of a study of public health services in the United Kingdom were both published in 1988. Both studies identified serious defects.

In the United States, the problems, characterized as "disarray," included high staff turnover, especially at senior levels; inadequate and uncertain financial support; poor communication between public health departments and schools of public health and other higher learning centers responsible for training and for conducting relevant research on aspects of public health; and gratuitous interference by elected officials when political fortunes changed. Often the consequences included inadequate or even nonexistent responses to new public health problems for which obsolete local public health statutes and regulations provided no solutions. The public health problems to which responses were inadequate included, e.g., the AIDS epidemic, environmental pollution from toxic waste sites, and the rising incidence of dementia. The IOM committee made sweeping recommendations for improvements, including updating public health statutes, development of relevant disease control measures for contemporary health problems, special linkages to environmental agencies, mental health and social services, and services for care of the indigent, etc. Other recommendations dealt with strategies for capacity building of preventive health services, development of political linkages, managerial skills, secure funding, and improved programs of public health education and research.

Similar conclusions and recommendations emerged from the inquiries conducted in the United Kingdom and other countries. Unfortunately, these reports and their recommendations appeared at a time when political and fiscal situations were changing, and the reaction of elected officials in the United States and other countries has been, at best, muted.

Budget Cutting and "Downsizing"

As the demographic transformation of the "baby boom" works its way through the population of the industrial nations, rising proportions of elderly and often infirm people require expensive forms of medical care. Budget-conscious elected officials and health policy analysts have become increasingly concerned about these rising costs. The demographic and epidemiologic changes have coincided with political swings toward fiscal conservatism in many of these nations. In the United States, Canada, the United Kingdom, France, New Zealand, and Australia, conservative governments have reshaped health policies at national, regional, and local levels. Tax revolts and local options in many jurisdictions have made matters worse for those seeking a fair share of tax funds for public health services. The combined effects of national, regional, and local budget cuts and "downsizing" of essential public health services have reduced human and material resources in some public health services to a potentially, perhaps actually, dangerous level. Experienced staff have been laid off and replaced with lower-salaried and less well-trained technical support staff; fully trained public health specialists have been replaced by poorly trained or even untrained workers.

This is a dangerous trend, threatening the health of the public in many ways. In 1995, major outbreaks of food poisoning in several Midwestern states in the United States might have been made worse by less than adequate reactions in some public health departments. Protection of health is so important that allowing public health services to decay in the interests of reducing taxes is irresponsible.

All professional staff members of public health services have a duty to defend the establishments that employ them. It helps to point out that protection of the public's health is as essential as the nation's defense forces are in protecting the citizenry from foreign invaders, and as essential as the police forces are in protecting the citizens from criminals.

Accountability

Public health services use public funds in their operations, and therefore they are publicly accountable. Taxpayers and their elected representatives are interested in knowing whether they are getting value for money. Evaluation of public health services is therefore an important activity. Evaluation of other aspects of health care is equally important; much of the following discussion applies with only slight modification to the evaluation of hospital-based and personal health care services. Evaluation of health services is an important use of epidemiology. Descriptive and analytic (hypothesis-testing) methods and epidemiologic experiments (randomized trials) all play a part in evaluation of health services.

The performance of public health services is routinely monitored in several ways, mostly by simple inspection of health and vital statistics, or even more simply, by surveillance of reports as they come in. This is hardly even worthy of being called descriptive epidemiology, but it is often valuable. The work of the public health department is evaluated by making random spot checks on public water supplies for fecal contaminants, milk for pathogens, routine review of statistics on the numbers and proportions of schoolchildren immunized against communicable disease, and other routine reviews. The notification of a single case of certain communicable diseases, such as typhoid or diphtheria, is an instant warning that public health measures against that disease have not been working.

Another common procedure is to define specific objectives and use the statistics to determine the extent to which these objectives are met. For example, the objectives of the school health service might include provision of specified health education to all students in specified grades and the detection and correction of defects such as impaired vision and hearing. The annual report of the school health service may contain statistical tables that display the number of curriculum hours of health education, the number of detected cases of refractive error, impaired hearing, uncorrected hernia, poor posture, etc. Evidence of uncleanliness, such as presence of head lice, and information on the numbers and proportion of schoolchildren in specified grades who are smokers may also be collected in this way. Information on smoking can be related to the health education classes aimed at reducing smoking.

The previous account is intended to convey the flavor of the way evaluation is often conducted. There are better and more orderly ways to evaluate public health services.

Donabedian categorized evaluation strategies under the headings of structure, process, and outcome. Each can be evaluated and their relationships also can be rigorously assessed (Box 8–3).

BOX 8-3.   Evaluation of (Public) Health Services

Structure	—Physical plant
	—Technical resources
	—Human resources
	—Lines of communication
	—Budget allocations
Process	—Appointment systems
	—Services provided
	Diagnostic tests
	Preventive procedures
	Educational classes
	Etc.
	—Referrals to other agencies
Outcome	—Death (rates)
	Infant, perinatal mortality rates
	Communicable diseases
	Suicides
	Cancer
	Etc.
	—Disease (rates, cases)
	Notifiable diseases
	—Disabilities
	Handicapped, impaired, disabled (and reasons)
	—Disruptions
	Family disruption
	Occupational disruption
	—Discomfort
	Use of substances to relieve distress
	—Dissatisfaction
	Broken appointments
	Requests for change to another service

Structure means physical plant, equipment, staffing, funds for operation, maintenance. *Process* covers all the operating procedures, many of which can be summarized in statistical tables. Included are such indicators as those mentioned previously that relate to the performance of the school health service. Process measures are important because they reveal how much is being done by each aspect of the health service—how many laboratory tests, how many home visits by public health nurses, how many referrals are being received by the home care plan, and so forth. The statistical tables in the annual report of many local health departments contain numerous process measures. *Outcome* measures are the most valuable, and least often adequately recorded. While it is useful to have information on such matters as the number of hours of instruction that public health nurses provide to schoolchildren on the harmful effects of cigarette smoking, a "process" measure, it is much more useful if this process measure can be related to an outcome measure, e.g., reduction in the number and proportion of children who smoke. It would be even better to have objective outcome measures of health improvement consequent on not smoking; this, however, would be technically difficult and subject to confounding variables that would make interpretation virtually impossible.

Evaluation based on outcome measures is necessary for objective appraisal of many aspects of the work of health services. Health outcomes that can be operationally applied and readily measured should have clearly defined qualities. Death, disease, and disability have such qualities, and statistics on these are usually accessible. Other measurable outcomes are discomfort, dissatisfaction, and disruption (from work or family). "Positive" outcomes, for example, reduced teenage pregnancy rates, can be recorded, as well as "negative" ones.

Mortality statistics are very useful. Traditionally we have regarded infant mortality rates as a measure of the efficacy of public health services, but other mortality rates that relate to reproductive outcomes are better. Infant mortality rates are made up of deaths in the immediate postnatal period and throughout the rest of the first year of life; they indicate a mixture of environmental, social, and health-care–related influences on infant health. On the other hand, the perinatal mortality rate, i.e., stillbirths and early infant deaths, is sensitive mainly to the quality of antenatal, natal, and immediate postnatal care; therefore the perinatal mortality rate is a useful outcome measure of the quality of care during pregnancy, labor, and the immediate postpartum period.

If infant mortality rates are used to assess public health or health care services, they must be dissected into early and late infant deaths; those in the first month of life are mainly associated with events relating to childbirth, such as immaturity, birth injury, and birth defects. In the second half of the first year of life, infections predominate among causes of infant death and reflect social and environmental conditions, the status of immunizations against childhood infectious diseases, etc. The second-year death rate is also a useful indicator of the efficacy of public health measures.

Disease incidence rates are another valuable outcome measurement; obviously the success of mass immunization and other disease control programs can be assessed by studying the subsequent incidence rates of the communicable diseases concerned. Similarly, the occurrence and duration of certain disabilities can be accurately recorded. This is possible mainly in occupational health services where there are procedures to routinely record absence from work and the reasons for it. Another setting in which the extent of disability is valuable as an outcome measure is in rehabilitation services, where systematic chart entries are made on the degree of mobility, activity, etc., of patients with chronic impairments; the entries can be abstracted and tabulated to show progress under treatment (see Chap. 7).

Another useful outcome measure is an indicator of satisfaction with the service provided. If clients or patients are dissatisfied, they may not come back. The extent of dissatisfaction can be measured by recording the rate or proportion of broken appointments; validation by asking randomly selected clients why they broke their appointments may reveal that a common reason is dissatisfaction with the service offered to them on earlier occasions. If providers are compassionate and friendly, as well as competent, clients or patients are more often satisfied and come back for return visits when requested to do so. If they do not come back when asked to, the service is a failure and corrective measures are required. Therefore this is a useful performance indicator.

Can evaluation of health services make greater use of random allocation? This is frequently unattainable. Evaluation of the ongoing work of a public health service can seldom make use of anything but descriptive methods; an experiment involving random allocation of clients or patients would have to comply with ethical requirements. On the first occasion when an innovative method, procedure, or practice is used, random allocation of clients or patients and rigorous measurement of outcomes is ethical and desirable. Indeed, failure to evaluate by means of a randomized trial may result in the adoption of a new idea without adequate evidence that it works. For many years we did not know whether cervical cytologic examination to detect and treat preinvasive cancer of the cervix did any good, because the procedure was widely adopted without ever having been evaluated by a randomized trial. After many years and much uncertainty, we are now reasonably sure that this is a worthwhile procedure, but it would have been better to have known many years ago, which would have been possible if a randomized trial had been done.

Randomized trials have been extensively used to evaluate many preventive regimens, notably vaccines for poliomyelitis, measles, rubella, and mumps. Some forms of health promotion and health education, like campaigns to reduce cigarette smoking, have also been tested by randomized trials.

Another form of evaluation is a "natural experiment." This term derives from John Snow's observational epidemiologic studies of cholera among householders whose water was supplied by different companies (see Chap. 2). The different rates of quitting smoking among British doctors and the rest of the British male population after Doll and Hill began their cohort study in 1951 have provided us with a natural experiment in which the influence of quitting smoking at various ages and durations of smoking can be assessed. Similar natural experiments occasionally are possible if a polluting industry is established in a community and safeguards against the effects of the pollution are not in place.

Evaluations should distinguish between efficacy, effectiveness, and efficiency. Efficacy is concerned with the question whether an intervention, procedure, or regimen does more good than harm when used under ideal conditions, or does more good than some previously used alternative. Effectiveness means that the intervention, procedure, or regimen works under normal circumstances; thus, a vaccine may be efficacious but not effective if the cold chain necessary to preserve it in the field is disrupted by exposure to high environmental temperatures. The term efficiency addresses the question of whether the resources are best used in a particular way; for instance, is it more efficient to train primary health care workers to provide an immunization service at village level in a developing country, or to use the same financial resources to build and equip hospitals in regional centers to treat patients with communicable diseases? The answer to this rhetorical question is obvious—though not always so to health planners and political leaders.

A useful way to evaluate national progress toward improved health is to use vital and health statistics to dissect causes of premature death and disability that are amenable to correction at the present state of medical science from those that are not so amenable. Application of this method in Finland, where it was first developed, shows the impressive beneficial effect of applying modern medical knowledge to preventive services; replication of the method in other countries has shown that this is a valuable addition to methods of health service evaluation.

► BIBLIOGRAPHY

This chapter is based in part on material and ideas from Scutchfield FD, Williams SJ: The American Health Care System (pp 1065–1078) and Buttery CMG: Provision of public health services. In Last JM, Wallace RB (eds): *Maxcy-Rosenau-Last Public Health and Preventive Medicine.* 13th ed. Norwalk, CT: Appleton & Lange, 1992, pp 1113–1128.

Other Sources Included

Institute of Medicine, National Academy of Sciences, Committee for the Study of the Future of Public Health: *The Future of Public Health.* Washington, DC: National Academy Press, 1988.

Roemer MI: *An Introduction to the U.S. Health Care System.* 2nd ed. New York: Springer, 1986.

Scutchfield FD, Keck CW (eds): *Principles of Public Health Practice.* Albany: Delmar, 1997.

Two series of occasional articles in the *New England Journal of Medicine,* which appeared in 1996 under the generic titles of "Health Policy Report" and "Quality of Health Care," are useful sources of further information. See especially among the articles in the "Health Policy Report" series, Inglehart JK: Politics and Public Health. *N Engl J Med* 334:203–207, 1996; and in the series on "Quality of Health Care" see Brook RH, McGlynn EA, Cleary PD: Measuring Quality of Care. *N Engl J Med* 335:966–969, 1996; and Blumenthal D, Epstein AM: Quality of Health Care. *N Engl J Med* 335:1328–1331, 1996.

9

World Health

The term "global interdependence" describes the connections that this chapter is about. We are all interdependent—all of us are affected by the actions of others and our actions affect others, including other creatures that share our planet. When we speak of "international health," we recognize that disease has no national boundaries: An outbreak of influenza A or polio in Bangladesh concerns people who live in Belgium or in the Bronx; a toxic spill into the Mississippi River can affect people who eat fish caught off the coast of Africa as well as those downstream; acid emissions from factory chimneys in England kill forests and fish in lakes in Scandinavia, and this ultimately harms human health. Destruction of tropical and boreal forests is changing the climate, disrupting global ecosystems, and threatening human health (see Chap. 11). Dangers to health anywhere on earth are dangers to health everywhere. International health, therefore, means more than just the health problems peculiar to developing countries. I have called this chapter World Health to avoid misunderstanding about its message.

It has long been realized that epidemic infectious disease is not stopped by national frontiers. International conferences aimed at standardizing quarantine regulations and procedures have been held at intervals since 1851; these led in 1907 to the establishment of the Office International d'Hygiene Publique (OIHP), which was the precursor of the Health Office of the League of Nations. In 1948 the functions of the Health Office were assumed by the World Health Organization (WHO), which soon was recognized as the most important international health agency.[1]

There are several good reasons why we should be concerned about world health. The most obvious is self-interest: Some of the world's health problems endanger us all. Those of us who live in affluent industrial nations can easily become complacent or indifferent to the poverty and malnutrition, the preventable disease and premature death of children and women in their reproductive years that occur in many developing nations. Of course, similar problems exist in parts of many rich nations. These deplorable conditions influence the health and well-being of us all, wherever we live. They are at the

roots of much of the political unrest that threatens the world with new outbreaks of violence. Many infectious diseases can be exported to, other nations and obviously threaten people from affluent nations when they travel
to, or work in, the developing world. Political unrest and warfare in many
parts of the third world disrupt public health services, adding to the risk that
dangerous epidemics will occur and spread. Other reasons for international
health programs include the scientific challenge of unsolved health problems and the altruistic impulse that leads some people to devote their lives to
improving the lot of others less fortunate than themselves. This has been an
important motive for medical missionaries; hospitals and clinics run by religious orders provide the only health care available in some communities in
developing countries.

▶ **CLASSIFICATIONS OF NATIONS**

The terms "developing" and "developed" country are loosely used in relation
to gross national product (GNP). The World Bank classifies nations into low-
income economies (including the two most populous nations on earth, India
and China) with per capita GNPs of about $350 in 1991 U.S. dollars; lower-
middle-income nations with per capita GNPs up to $2500; upper-middle-
income nations with per capita GNPs up to $3500; and high-income nations,
most of them members of the Organization for Economic Cooperation and
Development (OECD), with per capita GNPs on average of $21,500.[2] A fur-
ther classification is into severely indebted nations and oil-exporting nations,
recognition of the dependence of all nations on oil-derived energy (Table
9–1). About 3.1 billion people, well over half the world's population, live in
countries in the poorest group. A further 1.4 billion live in the lower-middle-
income nations and 630 million in the upper-middle-income nations. About
820 million people live in the high-income nations, which are rich at least in
part because of their ability to exploit the resources, such as oil, minerals,
and food, of the poorer nations. Putting it another way, over 80 percent of
the world's people live in nations that collectively have less than 20 percent
of the world's wealth and productive capacity. An even more striking fact is
that the poorest 40 percent of the world's people collectively have less wealth
than the world's richest 400 people. Moreover, the gap between rich and
poor nations (and people) is getting wider (see Chap. 6).

Another collective term sometimes used to describe the developing nations is the "third world"; this term originated in French (*tiers monde*) and
evokes memories of the time soon after the end of World War II when our
planet became divided along geopolitical lines into the so-called "free
world," the communist and socialist nations that were politically aligned with
the Soviet Union, and the rest, the "third world," sometimes also called non-
aligned nations. The Brandt Commission[3] gave us another concept, a division of the world into the "North," the industrially developed nations, nearly

TABLE 9–1. Population and Socioeconomic Indicators, 1991–1993

	Pop. 1991 (Millions)	GNP 1991 $U.S.	Life Expectancy 1991	Growth 1991–2000 %	Urban 1991 %
Low-income economies					
China, India	2016	350	66	1.5	46
32 others	1111	350	55	2.4	28
Low-middle income economies	773	1590	67	1.8	54
Upper-middle income economies	627	3530	69	1.1	73
Severely indebted economies	486	2350	67	1.8	68
Fuel-exporting economies	262	14,820	66	3.0	52
High-income economies	822	21,050	77	0.5	77

(Source: World Bank World Development Report, 1993.[2])

all in the northern hemisphere, and the "South," comprising almost all of Africa, Latin America, South, Southeast, and Southwest Asia, which are industrially and economically less developed or undeveloped. The United Nations' Children's Fund (UNICEF) simply ranks the nations in order of their infant and early child mortality rates—which correlate closely with per capita GNP.[4] Clearly, all descriptive terms for the nations of the world have limitations.

Economic and social development and health improvement are hard to achieve among the poorest nations. In the mid-1990s, many nations in Africa (south of the Sahara) and in parts of the former Soviet Union are deteriorating; some are suffering because of inadequate natural resources that have to be shared among too many people, some because of poor planning and misuse of available resources, and some because of corruption or political or military turmoil.[5] The prospects for improvement in the short term are not bright for many of the poorest nations, which often are poor because they lack the natural resources that ultimately produce wealth.

▶ AGENCIES INVOLVED IN INTERNATIONAL HEALTH

International and national agencies under the control of governments, nongovernmental organizations (NGOs), and private voluntary organizations are all active in international health.[6] The government-sponsored international agencies include several United Nations (UN) organizations, the best-known of which is WHO. Other UN agencies with well-defined and very important health-related roles are UNICEF, the United Nations Development Programme (UNDP), the Food and Agriculture Organization (FAO), the United Nations Fund for Population Activities (UNFPA), the Office of the UN High Commissioner for Refugees (UNHCR), the UN Fund for Drug Abuse Control (UNFDAC), and the International Bank for Reconstruction and Development, better known as the World Bank. The most important international NGO is probably the International Commission of the Red Cross/Red Crescent (ICRC). Several high-income nations have their own agencies that provide direct financial and logistic support for health-related activities in the developing world. These bilateral agencies include the U.S. Agency for International Development (USAID), the Swedish International Development Authority (SIDA), the Canadian International Development Agency (CIDA), and similar agencies based in Switzerland, Japan, Saudi Arabia, Australia, and a few other nations. Many agencies, both governmental and NGOs, are affiliated with WHO; examples include the U.S. Centers for Disease Control and Prevention, the Public Health Laboratory Service in the United Kingdom, the Canadian Addiction Research Foundation, and some national professional health-related associations.

The NGOs and private voluntary organizations provide funds and human and technical resources for international health work of many kinds, mainly supported by voluntary subscriptions and donations. Many churches and missionary groups also play a prominent role; their activities include general and specific programs, such as hospital and community-based therapeutic and preventive services, aid for persons with specific diseases such as leprosy, trachoma, cataract, and aid for destitute children. Several foundations, notably the Rockefeller, Wellcome, and Ford Foundations, have a long record of contributions to the advance of medical research and education in developing countries.

WHO is supported by all nations and is concerned with all aspects of human health. Its achievements since 1948 have been impressive. WHO has made at least one contribution of lasting historical importance, the eradication of smallpox[7]; this was accomplished in 1979 after an international collaborative effort that was supervised, coordinated, and directed by WHO. If WHO had done nothing else, the total and permanent eradication of this disease, one of the great scourges of mankind since prehistoric times, would have justified its existence. Given enough money, material, and manpower, WHO could eradicate other diseases and improve the human condition in many other ways. WHO aspires to eradicate poliomyelitis and dracunculosis and to eliminate leprosy and several other diseases by 2000.[8]

Communicable disease control is much emphasized among the activities of WHO; there are programs aimed at controlling all the principal communicable diseases of developing and tropical countries: malaria, schistosomiasis, onchocerciasis, leprosy, leishmaniasis, trypanosomiasis, yaws, tuberculosis, yellow fever, parasitic diseases, sexually transmitted diseases, viral hemorrhagic fevers, zoonoses, and emerging infections including, of course, human immunodeficiency virus (HIV) disease.[9] WHO's Global Programme on

AIDS (acquired immunodeficiency syndrome) became a direct UN agency in 1993. There are programs on maternal and child health, on nutritional disorders, on occupational and environmental health problems, mental disorders, etc. Other programs deal with education and training of health workers, with information and technology transfer, and quality control of biologic products and pharmaceutical preparations. A section is concerned with epidemiologic surveillance, health status analysis and trend assessment, health statistics, disease classification systems, etc.[10] An activity often done in collaboration with organizations such as ICRC and UNHCR is emergency and disaster relief. Natural or man-made disasters often displace large numbers of people, rendering them homeless and depriving them of means to subsist and survive. In the mid-1990s there are an estimated 20 million refugees and another 50 million displaced persons, i.e., displaced from their normal place of residence but still within the borders of their own country. These include people affected by natural as well as man-made disasters, mostly living in refugee communities in various parts of the world.[11] It is difficult to find any aspect of health affairs that is not dealt with somewhere within the scope of work of WHO. You can explore for yourself by visiting WHO's home page on the World Wide Web **(http://www.who.ch).**

The work of WHO is conducted at the headquarters in Geneva, in the six regional offices (Fig. 9–1), at country offices, and in the field. All offices have permanent staff, reinforced by temporary advisers, short-term consultants, and technical experts. The six regions are defined by geographic and political criteria, and within each there is considerable economic and cultural diversity; this can both help and hinder the collaborative efforts of countries within a region. The rich nations can help the poor, but cultural and ideologic differences sometimes impede understanding and cooperation.

The activities of WHO took a new direction after a resolution approved by the World Health Assembly in 1977 and an international conference in Alma-Ata, U.S.S.R., in 1978.[12] At this conference, it was agreed that a realistic target to aim for would be the provision of primary health care for all the world's people by 2000 (see Chap. 1). This goal is summarized in the slogan "Health for all by the year 2000," and induced much effort and thought about ways to achieve better health for people everywhere. Internationally recognized experts on every aspect of health and disease considered how to achieve "health for all." Many strategies and tactics were formulated at national, regional, and international levels, and action began on them. Within the regions of WHO, specific objectives were set, relating to the existing health problems and health resources; the objectives of the mainly rich and developed European region differed from those of the mainly developing African and Southeast Asian Regions.

Unfortunately the work of WHO has been severely compromised by defaulting donor nations that collectively owe more than $2 billion to this and other UN agencies.[13] The United States is by far the largest defaulter, with out-

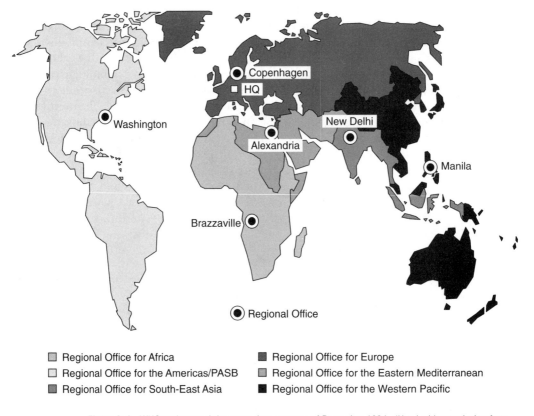

Copenhagen
HQ
Washington
New Delhi
Alexandria
Manila
Brazzaville
Regional Office

☐ Regional Office for Africa   ■ Regional Office for Europe
☐ Regional Office for the Americas/PASB   ■ Regional Office for the Eastern Mediterranean
■ Regional Office for South-East Asia   ■ Regional Office for the Western Pacific

Figure 9–1. WHO regions and the areas they serve as of December 1994. *(Used with permission from World Health Report 1995.)*

standing debts to UN agencies of about $1.4 billion in 1996. (Most of the U.S. arrears to WHO, but not other UN agencies, were paid early in 1997.) One reason for failure to pay is perception of excessive waste and bureaucracy that have often been the topic of adverse criticism. The combination of severe budget cuts and widespread criticism contributes to low morale of WHO staff, which of course makes matters worse.[14] Many people believe a change in leadership is needed, but this is opposed on grounds of national pride and politics.

► THE STATE OF THE WORLD IN THE MID-1990s

Spectacular improvements in health have occurred since the beginning of the 20th century; many are attributable to advances of medical science and application of public health measures such as sanitation, vaccination, and clean water. Some formidable obstacles to good health and well-being, however, still persist. Wars and political instability are at the heart of some of the most intractable problems. Some resurgent infections are due to organisms (or their vectors) that are resistant to antibiotics (or pesticides). Other problems are due to uncontrolled excesses in exploiting the environment, destroying what was naturally present and poisoning vegetation, wildlife, even human communities. Some emergent infectious diseases may have arisen because of ecosystem disruption. We cannot consider the health problems of the developing world in isolation from those of the industrial nations—all are interconnected.

Population Growth

Throughout history and probably since long before recorded history, the growth rate of human numbers was linear, save for occasional disruptions such as the epidemics of plague in the 14th century, which killed about a third of the population of Europe. At varying times from the late 18th century onward, the rate of growth became exponential and since about 1950 it has become hyperexponential[15] (Fig. 9–2). These trends have been observed all over the world, beginning in the late 18th century in western Europe, the early 19th century in eastern Europe, and the early 20th century in Africa, South

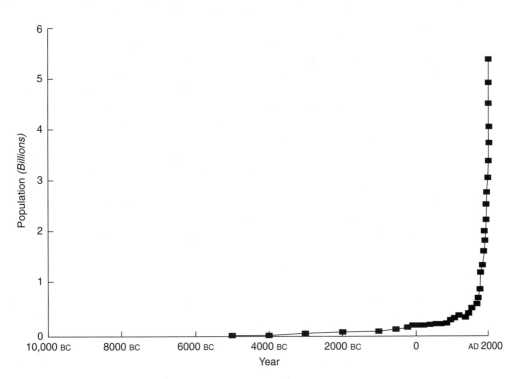

Figure 9–2. Estimated human population from the last ice age to present. *(Used with permission from Cohen JE: How Many People Can the Earth Support? New York: Norton, 1996.)*

and Southeast Asia, and Latin America.[16] In North America the pattern has been distorted by migrations. Birth rates began to greatly exceed death rates early in the 19th century in the United States. The causes of this surge in numbers are debated by demographers. Some believe that improved nutrition, related to favorable climatic conditions and opening up to agriculture of vast areas in the Americas and Australasia, was the primary determinant; others think the reasons are more complex, including reduced risks of infant death from infections related to ecologic changes. The transition to an exponential growth rate preceded most of the modern advances of medical science.[17] It therefore was not due initially to control of infectious disease by antibiotics and immunization programs, although these helped to accelerate the trends, first in the industrialized countries and then in much of the developing world (see Fig. 3–2). The hyperexponential growth in the second half of the 20th century may be due to a combination of optimism about the future after World War II (giving rise to the "baby boom"), earlier age at childbearing, and effects of vaccines, antibiotics, and in developing countries, child-survival strategies such as oral rehydration therapy for infant diarrhea.

This cannot continue indefinitely. Other living creatures fluctuate in numbers according to the supply of needed nutriment and pressure from predators. Humans are subject to the same biologic laws and, like bacterial colonies, flour beetles, fieldmice, shoals of herring, and roving herds of caribou, we must strike a balance between reproductive rates and the supply of food and other essentials. The difference between humans and the other life forms whose reproductive performance has been studied, is that humans have greater capacity to adapt to a wide range of environmental conditions. This has made it possible for humans to settle all over the planet on a scale unmatched by any other species; but it has also meant that almost no part of the earth's surface has remained untouched (and unspoiled) by human occupation. Humans have transformed the planetary ecology as a result. The ultimate consequences of this cannot be determined, but it is prudent to prepare for adverse effects, some of which I discuss in Chapter 11. Human health cannot be sustained at its present level unless environments required for survival are sustainable too.[18] There is a growing consensus that there will be serious adverse ecologic effects of the recent population explosion, probably soon. We may have to pay a heavy price for our reproductive success.

Migrations

Several times in human history there have been massive movements of large numbers of people about the earth, great redistributions, probably related to an imbalance between numbers and the supply of needed resources of food, fuel, raw materials, or valued commodities.[19] Evidence from archeology and folklore suggests considerable migration from Asia to Southeastern Europe about 2000 B.C.; another migration probably played a role in the fall of the Roman Empire (A.D. 200 to 600) when an invasion of people from Asiatic

Russia to Europe took place. In the first 300 years of European colonization of the Americas, there was an involuntary migration of an estimated 10 to 12 million slaves from Africa to South, Central, and North America. The most recent mass migrations have accompanied the unprecedented population growth of the past 200 years. These began with the initial European colonization of the Americas, gathered momentum toward the end of the 19th century with large-scale migration from Europe to the Americas and Australasia, and continue until the present, interrupted only by the two world wars. This movement has been turbulent, at times chaotic. It includes not only the massive flow of people from and among many European nations to other parts of the world, but also at least as much movement, perhaps more, between certain Asian nations, from Asian nations to Europe and the Americas, from Latin America into the United States, and within Africa. Much of the migration is not documented in detail, though the approximate numbers and their origins and destinations are known. It is beyond my capacity to produce a table to show in full the main features of this migration: Table 9–2 deals only

TABLE 9–2. **World Migrations—A Summary**

Period	Place	Numbers (thousands, approx.)
3000–2000 B.C.	Asia Minor → Greece	Unknown
c. A.D. 300–900	Asia → China and Europe	Unknown
1450–1800	Europe → Americas	?100–150
1800–1850	Europe → Americas, Australia	?200
1550–1850	Africa→ Americas (slaves)	10–12 million

European Emigrations, 1851–1980

Period	Numbers (thousands)
1851–1860	2171
1861–1870	2805
1871–1880	3239
1881–1890	7785
1891–1900	6770
1901–1910	11,371
1911–1920	7791
1921–1930	6785
1931–1940	1226
1941–1950	2275
1951–1960	4922
1961–1970	2521
1971–1980	5949

Since the mid-1960s, migration of "guest workers" into Europe from North Africa, the Middle East, the Caribbean, etc., has equaled or exceeded emigration, making the figures difficult to interpret.
(Source: UN Demographic Yearbooks.)

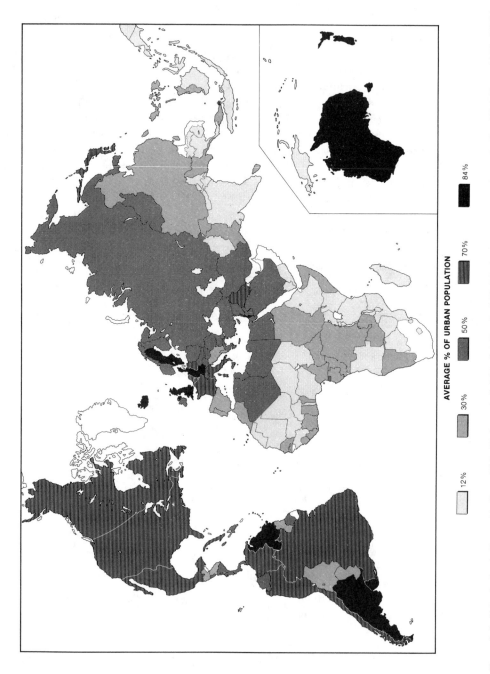

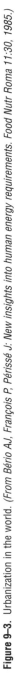

Figure 9-3. Urbanization in the world. *(From Bério AJ, François P, Périssé J: New insights into human energy requirements. Food Nutr Roma 11:30, 1985.)*

with earlier times. This is a poorly understood sociodemographic phenomenon that has had, and continues to have, profound effects on the well-being and health of huge numbers of people in many countries. In the late 20th century, population pressure, acute shortages of land, food, water, and natural resources, and political unrest and many wars are forcing large numbers to move, but many have no obvious place to go. This imbalance could have explosive consequences. Environmental stress, when too many people attempt to extract a living from a fragile ecosystem, causes many conflicts[20]; the 1995 genocide in Rwanda may have been an extreme example or a premonitory indication of a growing trend in our overcrowded world.

Rural-to-Urban Migrations

Within many developing and developed nations there has also been a massive redistribution from rural to urban areas. In the early 20th century, over 90 percent of the population in most countries, especially in the developing world, lived in rural areas. By 2000, the proportion of people living in urban areas will exceed the proportion in rural areas.[21] By the mid-1980s about 45 percent of the world population was already urbanized (Fig. 9–3). Some of this rural-urban movement has been due to drought or other natural disasters that have led people to flee from the land in search of work in cities. In the Indian subcontinent, Southeast Asia, much of Latin America, and many African nations, it has been due in part to economic and political disturbances, sometimes with warfare or rural banditry. Many millions of dispossessed subsistence farmers and displaced or unwanted rural agricultural laborers have moved to squalid shanty towns on the outskirts of third-world cities, swelling the urban populations and overloading already inadequate water supplies and sanitary services. Whenever they can, people living under such conditions as these seek to escape by migrating—legally or illegally—to industrially developed nations in Europe or North America.

The growth of cities, especially in the developing nations, is an oppressive problem. The population living in cities of 1 million and over in 1950 to 2015 is shown in Table 9–3; In developing nations, water and food supplies, sanitary services, fuel, and shelter are often inadequate to cope with such

TABLE 9–3. Number of Cities with More than One Million Residents, by Region, 1950–2015

	1950	1970	1990	2015
Africa	3	16	59	225
Latin America	17	57	118	225
Asia	58	168	359	903
Europe	73	116	141	156
North America	40	78	105	148

(Source: UN Statistical Office [Population Division], 1995.)

numbers. These megacities are excellent breeding grounds for infectious diseases, drug abuse, and social unrest. Moreover, the rural areas of many of the developing nations in which these cities are located are experiencing equal or greater rates of population growth and cannot relieve the pressure.

Health Problems of Developing Nations

A useful way to arrange and classify the nations of the world, suggested by the late UNICEF Director-General James Grant,[4] is according to their prevailing infant mortality rates. Infant mortality rates correlate closely with levels of economic development, literacy, housing conditions, access to pure water supplies, and several other variables dependent on economic development; the availability of health care is not directly related to infant mortality rates, although it is often related to the level of economic development.

Table 9–4, which arranges selected nations in order of under-5 child mortality, also shows their growth rates, per capita GNP, literacy levels, access to clean water, and the supply of doctors. The World Bank's recognition of the relationship between economic development and health[3] is an important contribution if it leads to greater investment in material and human resources to improve health. Many developing nations are caught in a vicious circle of unrelieved poverty that causes or contributes to most of the ill health, which aggravates the poverty. Development assistance that relieves the poverty may be the first step toward improvement of health. The low status of women,[22] leading to female illiteracy and poor understanding of ways to protect their infants' health, must also be dealt with.

Interaction of Infection, Malnutrition, and Population Growth

Many health problems of the developing world arise from the interaction of three forces: infectious diseases, especially of infants and young children; malnutrition; and uncontrolled population growth (Box 9–1).

Infectious diseases take a terrible toll. There are about one billion cases each year of the common infectious diseases: diarrhea, respiratory infections, malaria, schistosomiasis, tuberculosis, and intestinal parasites. In Africa, more than one million deaths occur each year from malaria alone. About three million children die each year from diarrhea, four million die from respiratory infections, and another three million from a combination of malnutrition and vaccine-preventable diseases, especially measles.[23] About 150,000 deaths are due to neonatal tetanus. There are also about half a million maternal deaths each year in the developing world, and many of these, leaving infants motherless, are followed by the death of these infants.

Malnutrition is widespread in some of the poorest nations, notably those affected by droughts and famine in Africa, where matters have been made worse by civil unrest and warfare. All forms of malnutrition occur—protein-calorie shortage, marasmus, and vitamin-deficiency diseases (see Chap. 5). Malnutrition enhances susceptibility to infection, and infection enhances

TABLE 9–4.   Basic Indicators, Selected Countries, in Descending Order of Mortality Rates for Children Under Five

Country	Mortality Rate (under 5)		Infant Mortality Rate (under 1)		Total Population (millions) 1994	GNP per capita (U.S. $) 1993	Life Expectancy at Birth (years) 1994
	1960	1994	1960	1994			
Angola	345	292	208	170	10.7	700	46
Sierra Leone	385	284	219	164	4.4	150	39
Nigeria	204	191	122	114	108.5	300	50
Zaire	286	186	167	120	42.6	220	52
Uganda	218	185	129	111	20.6	180	45
Pakistan	221	137	137	95	136.7	430	61
Ghana	213	131	126	76	16.9	430	56
India	236	119	144	79	918.6	300	60
Nepal	290	118	190	84	21.4	190	53
Bangladesh	247	117	151	91	117.8	220	55
Indonesia	216	111	127	71	194.6	740	62
Kenya	202	90	120	61	27.3	270	56
Brazil	181	61	118	51	159.1	2930	66
Egypt	258	52	169	41	61.6	660	63
Iran, Islamic Republic of	233	51	145	40	65.8	2200	67
Viet Nam	219	46	147	35	72.9	170	65
China	209	43	140	35	1208.8	490	68
Thailand	146	32	101	27	58.2	2110	69
Mexico	148	32	103	27	91.9	3610	71
Russian Federation	n.a.	31	n.a.	28	147.4	2340	68
Sri Lanka	130	19	90	15	18.1	600	72
Hungary	57	14	51	13	10.2	3350	69
Cuba	50	10	39	9	11.0	1170	75
United States	30	10	26	8	260.6	24740	76
Spain	57	9	46	8	39.6	13590	78
France	34	9	29	7	57.8	22490	77
Israel	39	9	32	7	5.5	13920	76
Australia	24	8	20	7	17.9	17500	77
Italy	50	8	44	7	57.2	19840	77
Netherlands	22	8	18	6	15.4	20950	77
Norway	23	8	19	6	4.3	25970	77
Canada	33	8	28	6	29.1	19970	77
United Kingdom	27	7	23	6	58.1	18060	76
Switzerland	27	7	22	6	7.1	35760	78
Germany	40	7	34	6	81.3	23560	76
Denmark	25	7	22	6	5.2	26730	75
Japan	40	6	31	4	124.8	31490	79
Finland	28	5	22	4	5.1	19300	76
Sweden	20	5	16	4	8.7	24740	78

(Source: UNICEF, 1996.)

BOX 9–1. The Vicious Circles of Population Pressure, Malnutrition, and Infection

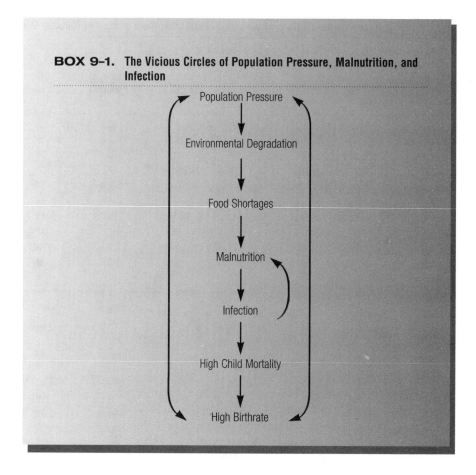

metabolic demand for protein and calorie intake, so there is a vicious circle in the infection-malnutrition complex that causes many child deaths, mainly in the under-5 age-group, in developing countries.

Children continue to die of measles and diarrhea, despite the fact that there are inexpensive ways to prevent and treat these diseases. As part of the "Health for All" strategy, the WHO Expanded Programme on Immunization set targets to be achieved in immunization coverage of infants and children. Considerable progress has been made in many countries, but this must be a continuing effort, for new generations of susceptible infants are added each year. Some countries lag far behind in immunization coverage but in others it gets high priority. In El Salvador, the civil war stopped briefly each year for child immunizations, but there has been no respite from conflict in other wars.

Oral rehydration therapy, a simple and inexpensive supplement that replaces fluid and electrolytes lost during bouts of diarrhea, has saved many lives; this technique is easily taught even to illiterate village women. International health agencies have justifiably invested much effort in teaching women about oral rehydration therapy, and the benefits are apparent in many rural communities. The program has the virtue of being easily applied by minimally trained health workers.

The fact that so many children now live where previously they died helps to persuade parents that fewer children have to be conceived to provide the workforce needed to maintain farms or paddy fields. Protecting and preserving the lives of infants and children is the first step toward dealing with the most urgent problem of all, uncontrolled human reproduction.

The rate of population growth is influenced by complex cultural factors, religious beliefs, levels of education and literacy, especially female literacy, which depends on the status of women. Once they are able to read, women are better able to understand the basic principles of contraception; they are also better able to understand that disease and premature death are not inevitable facts of life. The education that is needed to change traditional values is another urgent priority. Television can play a valuable role by contributing to the education and value changes needed to improve the status of women (Box 9–2).

Special efforts are needed in some nations to improve the status of women. In many rural agrarian societies, women's lives are determined for them by the elders of the family or tribe; most are destined to spend their lives in a combination of childbearing and heavy manual labor, working crops, carrying fuel wood and water long distances, crouched over smoky cooking fires in ill-ventilated village huts, inhaling toxic fumes in greater amount than if they smoked 40 cigarettes a day.[24] They may be denied access

---

BOX 9–2. **Factors Influencing Women's Health in Developing Countries**

Culture, Tradition
   Religion (Religious fundamentalism)
   Low status of women
   Illiteracy
   Menial tasks
   Heavy manual labor
Marriage Customs
   Childbearing begins at puberty
Environmental Problems
   Water polluted
   Smoke from cooking fires
   Gathering fuel
   Collecting water
Violence

to education, so have no way to learn how much they are missing by reading about the better situation of women and their families in other countries. In African countries where AIDS has taken a heavy toll, many able-bodied men have already died or are dying, leaving women on their own (often infected with HIV) to till the land, harvest the crops, and raise the children.[25] The ultimate legacy of the AIDS epidemic in many developing countries will be a generation of orphans (see Chap. 3).

High population density favors the spread of communicable diseases, so population pressure not only drains food resources and leads to widespread malnutrition but also sets the stage for epidemics. These three problems, population pressure, malnutrition, and infection thus constantly reinforce one another. Economic development and education of women may best help to break these vicious circles by concentrating on the control of infections, but the control of infections cannot achieve much without opportunities for employment—which requires improved education and higher levels of literacy. The solution is as challenging as the problem is complex (Box 9–3).

New Problems

The combination of population pressure, malnutrition, and infection has sapped the vitality of the developing nations for generations. Now there are

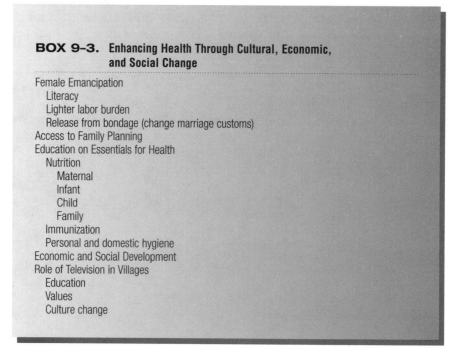

BOX 9–3. Enhancing Health Through Cultural, Economic, and Social Change

Female Emancipation
   Literacy
   Lighter labor burden
   Release from bondage (change marriage customs)
Access to Family Planning
Education on Essentials for Health
   Nutrition
     Maternal
     Infant
     Child
     Family
   Immunization
   Personal and domestic hygiene
Economic and Social Development
Role of Television in Villages
   Education
   Values
   Culture change

new problems. Industrial development, often without the restraining laws and regulations of the rich industrial nations, is causing serious environmental damage and occupational diseases. And some of the worst health-harming habits of the industrial nations, notably cigarette smoking and traffic injury, are increasingly common[26] (Box 9–4).

Industrial development is needed, but unfortunately many multinational corporations want to set up petrochemical plants, textile mills, and factories, not because they aim to assist these nations toward economic development, but because they are assured of a supply of cheap labor and can avoid regulations and laws that have been enacted in the industrial nations to protect the health of workers and to preserve environmental quality. Factories in the developing nations frequently employ children and women for low wages, have no workers' compensation, and have few if any occupational health and safety standards. Workers who are injured on the job are dismissed without compensation and their places filled by others from the virtually limitless pool of unemployed workers among the rural and new urban poor. Environmental quality is often damaged by unrestrained discharge of toxic waste products.

The habits and customs we recognize as harmful to health are eagerly embraced by people in developing nations, who often perceive them as outward signs of their own emergence into better times. Women are persuaded that artificial formula is better than breastfeeding; for over 30 years, transnational infant formula manufacturers have engaged in a persuasive advertising campaign to promote infant formulas, even though it is well known that mothers in rural villages lack the means to purchase, sterilize, or store formula under safe and hygienic conditions.[27] Despite campaigns by UNICEF and national public health and child care agencies, some manufacturers of

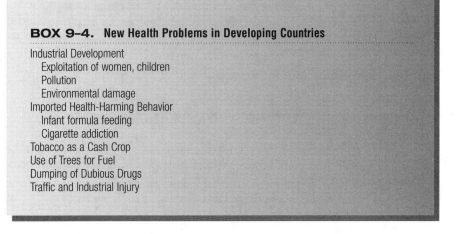

BOX 9–4. New Health Problems in Developing Countries

Industrial Development
    Exploitation of women, children
    Pollution
    Environmental damage
Imported Health-Harming Behavior
    Infant formula feeding
    Cigarette addiction
Tobacco as a Cash Crop
Use of Trees for Fuel
Dumping of Dubious Drugs
Traffic and Industrial Injury

breast-milk substitutes continue to promote the use of infant formula rather than breast milk. There is no excuse for this practice, which reveals starkly the moral bankruptcy of those who set the marketing policies for these manufacturers.

Addiction to cigarette smoking is probably the worst of the unhealthy practices of industrially developed nations to be exported. The tobacco companies are able to promote their deadly product without restraint in most developing nations; advertising is directed specifically at children, and the use of cigarettes is equated with social and economic success—with the result that in some developing nations over half the child population of both sexes is already addicted to cigarettes.[28] Tobacco is securely established as a lucrative cash crop, displacing badly needed subsistence agriculture, and trees are depleted to provide fuel for flue-curing tobacco to make cigarettes.

Another problem caused by immoral and unethical conduct by some transnational corporations is the export to developing countries of pharmaceutical preparations that have been denied a licence in the country where they were manufactured, usually because of doubts about their safety or efficacy.[29] In cities in Latin America and Southeast Asia, these drugs are often sold in open stalls in marketplaces. Apart from the harm they may do, some of these drugs are broad-spectrum antibiotic combinations that help to produce resistant strains of pathogenic microorganisms that may then be exported back to the industrial nations whence came the harmful antibiotics in the first place—fitting retribution were it not for the resulting harm to health.

There has always been a heavy toll of accidental death and injury in developing countries, e.g., from burns and scalds that occur when cooking is done over open fires inside village huts. With the influx of automobiles, often on roads never built to carry them and with drivers who have never been properly taught to drive, the toll of traffic injury and premature death is also rising. City traffic density is very high in many developing countries and will doubtless continue to rise, but adequate roads will probably not be constructed for many years, and it is unlikely that cars will be separated from pedestrians, cyclists, and carts drawn by animals. Industrial accidents also occur with increasing frequency because untrained workers and unsafe machinery are a dangerous combination. For all these reasons, the burden of accidental death and injury is rapidly increasing.

► FAILURES OF PLANNING AND ORGANIZATION

The solution to many health problems in developing nations is elusive, at least in part because of poor planning, inadequate organization, and misplaced values. These human factors contribute to several problems, of which the following are the most obvious, although this is not an all-inclusive list (Box 9–5).

BOX 9–5. **Man-Made Problems ("Human Factors")**

Unequal Access to Care
Treatment Preferred to Prevention
Maldistribution in Health Professions
    Rural vs. urban
    Specialized vs. primary care
Investment in Inappropriate Technology
Inappropriate Training Programs
Lack of Health Information
Administrative Inadequacies
Communication Breakdowns
Wrong Priorities
    Military vs. social expenditure

Inequitable Access to Health Care

The poor, especially the rural poor, frequently have great difficulty gaining access to any form of health care other than traditional village healers. Health care services of all kinds are mainly concentrated in the cities, and frequently those who use them must pay a fee. While the few wealthy people have abundant health care of good quality, the rest of the population may lack even elementary health services.

Treatment Gets Higher Priority Than Prevention

Of course this is not unique to developing countries. In developing countries, however, expensively equipped modern hospitals to treat complex and difficult medical and surgical cases can do harm because they attract not only an unfair share of the small budget available for health services, but also a disproportionate share of the skilled and well-trained health care workers. Moreover, they contribute to the "brain drain": To acquire the necessary skills to work in specialized health care settings, medical graduates have to be trained abroad, and many never return to their homeland. Training for primary care and public health workers may be underfunded or nonexistent.

Maldistribution Among the Health Professions

In many countries, there is serious maldistribution among the branches of health care practice.[30] There may be a surplus of physicians and a shortage of nurses, as well as greater numbers of specialists than generalist physicians. This problem is particularly acute in nations where low status of women leads to high female illiteracy rates, low rates of recruitment into the nursing profession, and thus to a situation in which there may be several practicing doctors to each nurse, rather than the other way around. Nursing is viewed as a low-status occupation, akin to domestic service; midwifery, on the other hand, may have high status, even when practiced by traditional village midwives who lack proper professional training. There may also be serious shortages of technicians, e.g., medical laboratory assistants.

Inappropriate Investment in High Technology

Political decisions may lead to investment in expensive technical devices such as electron microscopes and diagnostic imaging equipment, which is not only expensive and requires expensively trained technical staff, but is even more expensive to maintain. There may be no funds for maintenance or persons qualified to do repairs, so the investment is wasted.

Inappropriate Training Programs

Although international planners sponsored by WHO and other agencies have recommended emphasis on training primary health care workers, national pride, tradition, and reluctance to change established educational systems may lead to continuation of training programs in a pattern along the lines of the United States or Western Europe. The graduates of such training programs are attracted to nations where they can practice the kind of medicine or nursing that they have been taught and are reluctant to work in the rural areas of their own countries where there is more need for their services. This can be a particularly difficult problem for health planners and policy makers, because there is an understandable reluctance to train indigenous health workers to supposedly lower standards than those prevailing in rich nations. This situation requires a value change, recognition that training programs for primary health care workers are not of a lower, but a different standard and have different aims, i.e., to promote, protect, and preserve health, rather than to diagnose and treat disease.

Lack of Health Information

Sometimes the population and its distribution are not accurately known, let alone its diseases and causes of death. A high priority is to establish and maintain comprehensive health information systems, or if this is not feasible, at least to set up registration areas in which the numbers of persons, diseases, premature deaths, and disabilities can be accurately and continuously ascertained. When this is done, health planners can argue for an adequate allocation from the national budget that will enable them to begin dealing with prevailing health problems.

Administrative Deficiencies

Sometimes there is no trained cadre of administrators. Some former colonies of European nations were left with no civil service when the colonists departed. Many of these nations have been plagued by political and military unrest, and health and other essential services are led by untrained office staff or members of the armed forces, among whom a common view is that "anyone can be an administrator." Sometimes the administration is corrupt, further aggravating the situation. India is an exception; one legacy of the British colonial period was a well-trained civil service; but excessive bureaucratization has impaired its efficiency.

Breakdown of Communication

All forms of communication may be faulty: road and rail communication from the center to the periphery, the posts, telephone service, even contact between professionals in different sections of the service. Thus it can happen that someone who encounters a problem is unaware that another professional person elsewhere in the same country, even the same city, or the same building, possesses the solution (or it may be in the library, or to which there is no easy access).

Wrong Priorities

National budgets may be meager, and often funds are misallocated. There is an obscene imbalance between expenditures on social and health services and on military weapons in many developing countries (as there is in the world as a whole). Since the 1960s, the scale of expenditure on armed services and imports of sophisticated armaments from the industrial nations to the developing nations has sharply increased.[31] Many wars now in progress are in developing countries, some of them being surrogate conflicts in which the geopolitical designs of the great powers are being played out with the lives and over the land of people in some of the poorest and most backward nations on earth.

Chronic so-called low-intensity warfare is another pervasive problem. On average, more than 400,000 people have died in wars every year since the end of World War II, almost all of them in developing countries. Increasing proportions are noncombatant women and children, and in several combat zones in Africa, Central America, and Southeast Asia, children not yet even in their teens, often kidnapped or captured when their parents have been killed or their villages overrun, have been pressed into military service.[32] Another consequence of these conflicts is the terrible toll in death and maimed limbs caused by land mines that continue to kill indiscriminately long after hostilities have ceased and "peace" is restored.[33]

Problems of Industrial Nations

The previous accounts earlier could be misleading unless balanced by a brief summary of problems afflicting industrial nations that, like those described earlier, are mainly man-made. Our complex society shows many signs of disintegration, of processes resembling the sequence that Durkheim called *anomie*. We do not know or care about our neighbors, even our blood relations, who sometimes are abandoned when they most need help. Young people numb their minds with addictive drugs and alcohol, children are reared increasingly often in homes with but a single parent. Life in the high-rise tenements of our densely packed city slums offers the pablum of television—situation comedies and sexy dramas, advertisements for headache pills, hemorrhoid ointments, and nostrums that relieve bad breath, and escape to the unreal worlds of fantasy but no constructive suggestions about ways to improve the human situation. Health and social problems are sometimes attributed to dissatisfaction with modern urban living; we blame substance abuse, vandalism, and mindless violence of urban society on this without being able to specify what we mean.

We consign elderly dependent members of what would have been extended families in earlier generations to impersonal homes for the aged, and our elected leaders, with our connivance, seek ways to cut the costs of caring for these survivors of the generation that nurtured and defended us. Our elected leaders, also with our connivance, expend our revenue on weapons of mass destruction that have collectively enough power to kill everyone on earth many times over. These, too, are world health problems of massive proportions, as challenging and as difficult to deal with as any of the health problems of the third world. It is an indictment of our lifestyle that we do not recognize these as health problems.

Problem Solving in the Developing World

Probably because the problems are tangible rather than a reflection of prevailing values, progress toward solutions is sometimes more impressive in developing than in industrial nations. There is much to inspire confidence and hope (Box 9–6).

"Health for All" gave a focus to what were previously rather aimless efforts. The Expanded Programme on Immunization and oral rehydration therapy have achieved measureable results already; the tropical disease research program, chasing elusive goals such as vaccines against malaria and schistosomiasis, has achieved more than optimists could have hoped for a few

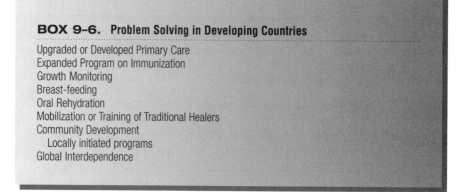

BOX 9–6. Problem Solving in Developing Countries

Upgraded or Developed Primary Care
Expanded Program on Immunization
Growth Monitoring
Breast-feeding
Oral Rehydration
Mobilization or Training of Traditional Healers
Community Development
    Locally initiated programs
Global Interdependence

years ago. Less glamorous but as important, the infrastructure of primary care services and health information systems in developing countries is beginning to work. Instrumental in this is collaboration among WHO, other official agencies, and NGOs, which have responded to the challenge of meeting specific goals with finite deadlines. A significant achievement has been the shift of emphasis of leadership from the international agencies to local communities, giving control over their own health affairs back to the people who will directly benefit, in contrast to preserving the traditional approach in which expatriate advisers, with varying degrees of paternalism, made all the decisions and implemented all the plans. A central feature of this reorientation of aims and methods has been the development of primary health care—a direct and explicit reaction to the "Health for All" initiatives. A few years ago, many developing countries had virtually no primary health care workers other than traditional healers; now increasingly there are battalions of rural health workers, often modeled on the Chinese barefoot doctor pattern. Trained for a few months in first aid, health education, and elementary principles of personal preventive medicine, these health workers are concerned mainly with promoting better health, and only secondarily with the treatment of the various incidental illnesses and injuries that afflict the people in the villages where they work. An important part of this approach is to upgrade the skills of traditional healers. One of the most valuable forms of development assistance that industrial nations can offer to the third world is to help with these training programs for primary health care workers.

Another priority is to promote the concept of global interdependence, recognizing that actions of groups, communities, and nations in one part of the world affect those who live at a distance, perhaps ultimately impact us all wherever we may live. All agree that despoiling the environment and profligate consumption of nonrenewable resources will ultimately harm us and our descendents, especially if this is accompanied by pollution and destruction of other living creatures with which humans are interdependent. But little can be done about this when people must slash and burn tropical rain forests in order to ensure their immediate need to grow food required for survival, when boreal forests are clear-cut in order to maximize short-term profits and provide jobs, however briefly, and when elected leaders plan with a time horizon no further off than the next election.

Another priority is to focus attention on major problems, rather than attempting to deal superficially with a great many at once, including perhaps some of little consequence. Programs that protect the health of infants and children have the highest priority in developing countries.

▶ CAREERS IN INTERNATIONAL HEALTH

The previous discussion conveys an idea of what it takes to be an effective international health worker. All the knowledge, skills, and attitudes that make a competent public health worker are needed. These include knowledge and skills in infectious disease control, nutrition, population dynamics, environmental health, behavioral sciences (including an understanding of anthropology), and most fundamental of all, a good grounding in methods of surveillance used in epidemiology as it is applied in tropical settings. Some special surveillance methods are needed, for instance, the ability to identify the environments where important diseases can flourish, e.g., the existence of anopheline breeding sites as a risk for malaria. Along with this, the ability to examine thick blood films for malaria parasites is also required. Other kinds of surveillance have been added. For example, the use of a simple tape measure to record upper arm circumference in growth monitoring programs is a clue to nutritional status. This is a skill that can easily be taught to village health workers, so that enthusiastic assistants at the periphery reinforce the ranks of professionally trained experts.

Managerial skills are equally important, for without good organization, the service cannot be efficient. The international health worker's training includes management and administration, and evaluation methods are an integral part of this. It is useless to have plans, however good they may be, unless there is provision for evaluating their success.

International health attracts a special kind of health worker, with unusual commitment and dedication to hard work, uncomfortable, even dangerous working conditions, and uncertain long-term career prospects. Health workers from industrially developed nations may be able to work for an international agency such as WHO or UNICEF, through the aid programs sponsored by their own national government or through one of any number of NGOs, church missionary societies, and the like.

Although international health work may not include active clinical involvement, the young health professional who undertakes work in a developing country without possessing good clinical skills is handicapped. It is important to be able to demonstrate the qualities that accompany good clinical skills, high among which is a capacity for making swift—and correct—decisions. Emergencies may require wide-ranging ability, but it is more likely that there will be occasions calling for the use of dental forceps, a spatula to remove foreign bodies from the eye, the ability to recognize exanthemata, and the peculiar odor of diphtheria. Outbreaks of disease must be recognized early and controlled effectively. The health worker who cannot cope with these everyday situations has little credibility when attempting to promote health and prevent disease.

► ADVICE FOR INTERNATIONAL TRAVELERS

Among the many useful publications produced by WHO is *Vaccination Certificate Requirements and Health Advice for International Travel.*[35] Many countries require travelers who enter from other parts of the world to produce an International Vaccination Certificate or other proof that they are free of contagious diseases considered to be a threat. It is always advisable in any case for international travelers to take suitable precautions against diseases to which they may be susceptible in developing countries that they plan to visit. Table 9–5 summarizes compulsory and advisable vaccination requirements. The WHO booklet, revised annnually, also contains commonsense advice about travel to countries where standards of hygiene and sanitation may be suspect and where the sun may burn more because it comes through the atmosphere more vertically than in higher latitudes. There are also helpful remarks about the cultural and social differences that can come as a shock to those accustomed only to the luxuries of contemporary western civilization.

TABLE 9–5. International Vaccination Certificate Requirements and Recommended Immunizations for International Travel

Required for Travel	Country or Region
Smallpox vaccination	No longer required anywhere
Yellow fever	Parts of Africa, South and Central America
	Strongly recommended for travel outside urban areas
Cholera	Not required except for travel from highly endemic areas to certain destinations
Strongly recommended vaccines	
Polio	
Tetanus	
Typhoid and paratyphoid	
Recommended vaccines	
Hepatitis B	
Indicated in special circumstances	
Measles, mumps, rubella	
Plague	
Typhus	
Meningococcus	
Bacille Calmette-Guérin (BCG)	
Diphtheria, pertussis	
Influenza	
Rabies	
Japanese B	
Other precautions	
Antimalarial medication	
Mosquito repellant	
Medication for diarrhea, fungus eruptions of skin	

(Source: International Travel and Health; Vaccination Requirements and Health Advice. Geneva: WHO, 1996.)

► **REFERENCES**

1. World Health Organization: *The Work of WHO*. Geneva: WHO, 1995.
2. World Bank: *World Development Report, 1993; Investing in Health*. New York: Oxford University Press, 1993.
3. Brandt Commission Reports: *Common Crisis; North-South Cooperation for World Recovery*. London: Pan Books, 1983.
4. Grant J (ed): *The State of the World's Children, 1983*. New York: UNICEF and Oxford University Press, 1983.
5. Kaplan RD: *The Ends of the Earth. A Journey at the Dawn of the 21st Century*. New York: Random House, 1996.
6. Basch PF: *Textbook of International Health*. New York: Oxford University Press, 1989, pp. 326–354.
7. Henderson DA: The eradication of smallpox. In Last JM (ed): Maxcy-Rosenau Public Health and Preventive Medicine. 11th ed. New York: Appleton-Century-Crofts, 1980, pp. 95–110.
8. World Health Organization: *World Health Report, 1996*. Geneva: WHO, 1996.
9. World Health Organization: *Ninth General Programme of Work*. Geneva: WHO, 1995.
10. World Health Organization: *World Health Situation Analysis and Trend Assessment*. Geneva; WHO, 1995.
11. Office of the United Nations High Commission for Refugees: *Annual Report, 1995*. Geneva: UNHCR, 1995.
12. World Health Organization and UNICEF: *Primary Health Care*. Geneva and New York: WHO/UNICEF, 1978 .
13. Godlee F: *The World Health Organization: WHO in Crisis. Br Med J* 309:1424–1428 1994. [And subsequent articles.]
14. Ermakov V: Reform of the World Health Organization. *Lancet* 347:1536–1537, 1996.
15. Cohen JL: *How Many People Can the Earth Support?* New York: Norton, 1996.
16. McEvedy C, Jones R: *Atlas of World Population History*. London: Allen Lane, Penguin Books, 1977.
17. McKeown T: *The Role of Medicine; Dream, Mirage or Nemesis*. Princeton, NJ: Princeton University Press, 1979.
18. King M: Health is a sustainable state. *Lancet* 336:664–667, 1990.
19. Cavalli-Sforza LL, Cavalli-Sforza F: *The Great Human Diasporas*. Reading, MA: Addison-Wesley, 1995. (See also Ascherson N: The Black Sea: *The Birthplace of Civilization and Barbarism*. New York: Random House, 1995, for a very readable account of the movements of people in a pivotal part of the world.)
20. Homer-Dixon TF: Environmental changes as causes of acute conflict. *International Security* 16:76–116, 1991.
21. UN Statistical Office: *Population Statistics and Projections*. New York: United Nations, 1995.
22. United Nations Development Programme: *Human Development Report, 1995*. New York: Oxford University Press, 1995.
23. Bellamy C (ed): *State of the World's Children 1996*. Annual Report of UNICEF. New York: Oxford University Press, 1996.
24. de Koning HW, Smith KR, Last JM: Biomass fuel combustion and health. *Bull World Health Org 185* 63:1:11–26.

25. Gupta GR, Weiss E, Whelan D: HIV/AIDS among women. In Mann J, Taratola D (eds): *AIDS in the World, II.* New York: Oxford University Press, 1996, pp. 215–228.
26. World Health Organization: *Bridging the Gaps. The World Health Report 1995.* Geneva: WHO, 1995.
27. World Health Organization: *Women, Health and Development. A Report by the Director-General.* Geneva: WHO Offset publication No. 90, 1985.
28. World Health Organization: WHO's Tobacco Control Programme. Geneva: WHO, 1995.
29. Silverman M, Lee PR, Lydecker M: *Prescriptions for Death; The Drugging of the Third World.* Berkeley: University of California Press, 1982.
30. Bankowski Z, Fülop T: *Health Manpower Out of Balance.* (Report of the 20th CIOMS Conference, Acapulco, 1986.) Geneva: CIOMS/WHO, 1986.
31. Sivard RL: *World Military and Social Expenditures.* Washington, DC: World Priorities Inc, 1994.
32. Bellamy C: Children in war. In Bellamy C (ed): *State of the World's Children 1996.* New York: Oxford University Press, 1996, pp. 12–41.
33. Stover E, Cobey JC, Fine J: The Public Health Effects of Landmines; Long-term Consequences for Civilians. In Levy BS, Sidel VW (eds): *War and Public Health.* New York: Oxford, 1997.
34. World Health Organization: *Vaccination Certificate Requirements and Health Advice for International Travel.* Geneva: WHO, 1995.

10

Ethics and Public
Health Policy

Ethics is the set of philosophical beliefs and practices concerned with distinctions between right and wrong; with values, human rights, dignity and freedom; with duties to others and to society. We all distinguish between what we regard as acceptable ("right") and unacceptable ("wrong") conduct, although standards and criteria of right and wrong vary greatly. Almost all human cultures observe a taboo against incest. In many other respects, values, behavior, and policies differ widely over time and from one nation or culture to another: Consider, for instance, infanticide, abortion, cannibalism, public executions, capital punishment, torture, slavery, child labor, permitted and prohibited diets, modes of dress, and the status and roles of women. In our culture, rules about many aspects of acceptable conduct derive from ancient roots such as the Ten Commandments, whence evolved laws to protect society from harm caused by violations.

► VALUES, ETHICS, MORALITY, AND LAW

Values are what we believe in, what we hold dear, what binds us to others of our kind; values are the foundation of morality. The law, which is based on morality, tells us what we are allowed to do. Ethics tells us what we *ought* to do. The distinction between ethics, morality, and law is based on the intellectual and emotional level at which we accept or abhor behavior: Whether we regard conduct as "right" or "wrong" depends on our ethics. Societal values are the basis for many laws, whether enacted by legislation or based on decisions in a lawcourt.

Community standards are also influenced by social values, which vary over time and among groups in society. An example is changing American values regarding alcohol, which led to the constitutional amendment on prohibition, then to its repeal.

In the past 150 years, as discussed in Chapter 1, there have been striking changes in health-related values as a direct result of advances in public health science. In the second half of the 19th century, in a time of improved literacy and plentiful newspapers, the discoveries of epidemiologists and bacteriologists soon became part of general knowledge and popular culture, epitomized in the term "filth diseases."[1] Values changed, and so did public health policy and law. The results were improved standards of personal hygiene and food handling and sanitary disposal of sewage. Since the 1950s, many epidemiologic studies demonstrating the relationship between tobacco and cancer have transformed other values and behavior. Smoking has become socially unacceptable and has been legislated or regulated out of existence in elevators, airplanes, cinemas, and many restaurants across America and in other nations. The transformation of values and behavior regarding human sexuality since the onset of the HIV/AIDS epidemic in the 1980s has been remarkable and is a triumph of effective health education, spearheaded in the United States by former Surgeon General C. Everett Koop.[2]

In Chapter 1, I set out my concept of a necessary sequence (Box 10–1) for the control of any public health problem.[3] It is worth repeating here:

- Awareness that the problem exists
- Understanding what causes the problem
- Capability to deal with the problem
- A sense of values that the problem matters
- Political will to control the problem

Vickers,[4] discussing the progress of public health, described the final two necessary steps as "redefining the unacceptable," a splendid phrase that captures the important role of human values. This also makes explicit the ethical foundations of public health.*

Laws usually uphold the values of society, but some actions that are legal may be unethical. A man holding an elected office in government may legally advise his wife about investments on the basis of privileged information he possesses, unless this is prohibited by rules relating to conflict of interest; but though his conduct may be legal, it is unethical. It is illegal in most jurisdictions for a physician to assist a suicidal act, but it is ethical for a physician to act in a way that avoids prolonging needlessly the distress sometimes associated with the process of dying (this common situation has been the subject of much debate; as the debate leads our values to change, our laws might follow).

---

* Recent conversations with colleagues have revealed that some use the word "values" to describe only the most fundamental and mainly immutable human beliefs, and use the word "attitudes" to describe other more flexible views such as those towards smoking and human sexuality. I use "values" to encompass all gradations that are pertinent to this discussion.

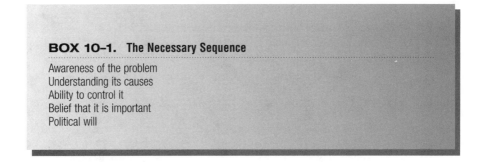

BOX 10–1. **The Necessary Sequence**

Awareness of the problem
Understanding its causes
Ability to control it
Belief that it is important
Political will

► FOUNDATIONS OF BIOMEDICAL ETHICS

Many of our ideas about ethics have descended to us from Aristotle, whose *Ethics*[5] (fourth century b.c.) discussed actions aimed at achieving good or desirable ends. The biblical precepts of the Old Testament and the teachings of Jesus of Nazareth were the source of other fundamental beliefs and values. Hence we sometimes speak of Greco-Judeo-Christian ethics. These concepts were modified by John Stuart Mill and Immanuel Kant, whose names are associated with theories of ethics called utilitarian ("greatest good for the greatest number") or consequential (what the consequences of decisions and actions will be); and deontological (recognizing our duty to behave in certain ways, usually because they conform to religious beliefs or other widely held moral values).

Ethical Theory

Much of modern bioethics is founded on four principles enunciated by Beauchamp and Childress[6]: respect for autonomy, nonmaleficence, beneficence, and justice (Box 10–2).

Respect for autonomy means concern about human dignity and freedom and the rights of individuals to make choices and decisions for themselves, rather than having others decide for them.

Nonmaleficence is the principle of not harming, derived from the ancient medical maxim, *primum non nocere* (first do no harm); this may have had greater force in former times when medical care was often hazardous, but it remains relevant today.

Beneficence is the principle of doing good, which members of the professions related to public health believe to be the purpose of our work (a view shared by those in many other callings).

Justice in the ethical sense means social justice or distributive justice: fairness, equity, and impartiality.

Another approach to biomedical ethics is through the **virtues,** many of which were defined by Aristotle. This approach to health care ethics is based

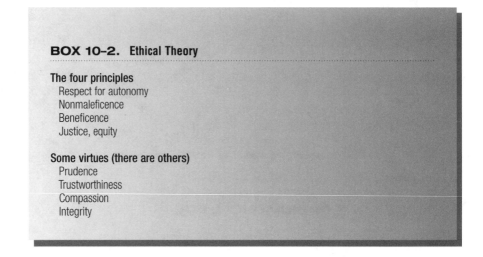

BOX 10–2. Ethical Theory

The four principles
  Respect for autonomy
  Nonmaleficence
  Beneficence
  Justice, equity

Some virtues (there are others)
  Prudence
  Trustworthiness
  Compassion
  Integrity

mainly on four virtues: prudence, compassion, trustworthiness, and integrity. All obviously should be upheld by public health workers.

We adhere to Beauchamp and Childress's four principles as far as we can in many aspects of health care, but the principles sometimes conflict. For example, we invoke the principles of beneficence and justice in control of communicable diseases, but we must sometimes restrict individual freedom by imposing quarantine on persons who have been in contact with contagious disease. In decisions about resource allocation, the principle of justice (equity) ought to prevail, but expensive high-technology care of individual patients is regarded by many clinicians as the highest priority for their patients, whereas public health specialists seek a fair share of health budgets for disease prevention and health promotion for everyone. Entirely new situations have arisen in modern medical practice. Some are a consequence of advancing medical science and technology, e.g., the problems presented by organ and tissue transplants, intensive care life support systems, genetic engineering, and new reproductive technologies. Principle-based biomedical ethics is often found to be inadequate in these situations.

Troubling problems arise from conflicting values. An example with important implications for medical ethics relates to female reproductive behavior and health. Should women have the right to choose whether to become or remain pregnant or have imposed upon them a view they may not share, that it is sinful to interfere with natural reproductive processes, whether to reduce the risk of pregnancy or to terminate an unwanted pregnancy? There is wide variation in the extent to which individuals and groups regard interference with pregnancy as tolerable, sinful, or criminal; the variation is related to conflict between two values, "right to life" and "freedom of choice." These alternatives seem to be irreconcilable in the United States, where ad-

vocates for the two extremes have polarized opinions and the issues have become politicized to a greater extent than in nations where tolerance of the
views and behavior of others is more highly valued.

Some of the ethical problems and ambiguities encountered in public
health practice and research are as difficult to resolve as any encountered in
clinical practice. There may be no "right" or "wrong" answer. In the absence
of an unequivocal answer, it helps to apply logically the principles of biomedical ethics rather than to rely on *ex cathedra* statements of "expert" opinion.
However eminent the experts may be, *ex cathedra* statements are often flawed.

In the account that follows, space limitations preclude lengthy discussion, so I consider mainly rather common ethical problems. These have
arisen and been confronted so many times that heuristic or rule-of-thumb solutions have often been found.

▶ INDIVIDUAL RIGHTS AND THE NEEDS OF OTHERS: COMMUNICABLE DISEASE CONTROL

The concept of contagion has been recognized for centuries. The usual reaction has been to identify "contagious" persons and sometimes to segregate or
isolate them. These customs date from the biblical leper's bell and the medieval lazaretto. In the 14th century, the Venetians added the practice of
quarantine; this restricted the freedom of movement of apparently healthy
people in contact with persons thought to be suffering from certain infectious diseases. In the 18th century, these procedures were codified by Johann
Peter Frank[7] and subsequently reinforced by laws and regulations in nations
around the world.

Identifying persons with communicable diseases means that they are labeled, and this can stigmatize them. Isolation and quarantine restrict freedom. Individuals, families, even entire communities may be identified and
stigmatized, isolated, or quarantined—and shunned by their neighbors. During an outbreak of Ebola virus disease in Kikwit, Zaire, in 1995, some of those
who had been in contact with cases were attacked, even shot at and denied
help by neighbors who feared this deadly infection—a modern echo of the
ancient fear of contagion.

Identifying and isolating cases is an accepted feature of communicable
disease control, held to be necessary to protect the population. Generally
there has been little objection to these measures. The need to protect society
has been recognized as a higher imperative than the rights of an individual
case or contact. When smallpox, cholera, polio, typhoid, diphtheria, and
other contagious diseases were prevalent, few people questioned the actions
of public health authorities who notified and isolated cases, quarantined contacts, often severely infringing the freedom and dignity of entire families. In
polio epidemics in the early 20th century, public health authorities in New

York exercised the "police power" of public health to search private homes and detain family members in contact with cases of polio.[8] In both world wars, prostitutes and "loose" women suspected of transmitting venereal disease to servicemen were arrested and imprisoned.[9] Some diseases, e.g., tuberculosis and scabies, have long carried a social stigma because of a supposed connection to drunkenness, lawlessness, dirtiness, or fecklessness.

▶ ETHICAL RESPONSES TO HUMAN IMMUNODEFICIENCY VIRUS (HIV) DISEASE

Reactions to HIV disease have been different. The first wave of the AIDS epidemic in the United States hit an already stigmatized group, male homosexuals, who had just begun to overcome age-old prejudice against them. Hostile attitudes to persons with AIDS often were aggravated by homophobia and repugnance for anal intercourse, the main mode of transmission among gay men. Eloquent and effective advocacy for gay rights, combined with the rising demand for equity and justice for minority groups, heightened awareness of the need to provide health care for all without discrimination. Widely publicized victimization of people with AIDS—gay men hounded out of their jobs, hemophiliac children rejected by schools, even rejected by communities—aroused public opinion in favor of compassionate and humane approaches. A second wave of the HIV epidemic affected intravenous drug abusers, who attracted less sympathy although their HIV-infected infants have generally been regarded as innocent victims. Even if HIV infection is a consequence of behavior that many public health workers might abhor, we have an ethical duty to apply our professional skills impartially and nonjudgmentally. I discuss the epidemiology of HIV infection in Chapter 3.

Societal reactions to AIDS and HIV infection have provoked much discussion about the ethics of management and control. The diagnosis must not be lightly made, nor HIV tests lightly undertaken. Informed consent to testing is a *sine qua non:* Both voluntary testing and communicating the results of a positive test must be accompanied by careful counseling of all persons concerned and their sexual partners.[10] It is important to protect the privacy of HIV-positive persons and to safeguard the confidentiality of their medical records to minimize the risk of disclosing information that could harm them or members of their families. The diagnosis of HIV infection has grave implications: Even the label "HIV-positive" is harmful to individuals. The diagnosis ought to be an irrevocable edict against promiscuous sexual behavior. Health workers have an ethical duty not to discriminate against persons infected with HIV. The duty to care for them is no less than the duty to care for persons with any other communicable diseases. HIV infection is much less contagious than tuberculosis or streptococcal infection, from which in former times many physicians and nurses died after being infected by patients.

Health workers who argue for the right to know the HIV status of their patients so they can take precautions should be aware that the risk of occupationally acquired HIV infection is about 1000 times smaller than the risk of hepatitis B or C. As of 1993, fewer than 100 cases of AIDS worldwide, out of an estimated 13 to 14 million, had been confirmed as occupationally acquired; the risk of infection following episodes of accidental needlestick is about 3 per 1000 episodes.[11] Furthermore, applying the ethical principle of justice, if health workers have the right to know the HIV status of patients or clients, then clients or patients have the right to know the HIV status of health workers.

For epidemiologic surveillance, public health authorities need data on the prevalence of HIV infection. The World Health Organization (WHO) and many national authorities agree that unlinked anonymous HIV testing is the best way to generate prevalence data.[12] Aliquots of blood taken for other purposes are tested for HIV antibody after stripping personal identifiers. Suitable populations for surveillance include pregnant women and newborn infants. The WHO recommendations regarding anonymous unlinked HIV tests for surveillance purposes have been adopted in most nations. In The Netherlands and briefly in the United Kingdom, it was held that anonymous unlinked testing is unethical, because identifying and counseling cases and their sexual partners was regarded as a more important duty than determining community-wide prevalence trends.

The rules for testing and reporting of HIV infection are a variant on rules and procedures for identifying, notifying, and initiating control measures for other sexually transmitted diseases, or indeed for many other communicable diseases. HIV infection, in contrast to AIDS, is not notifiable in most countries. With the exception of Cuba, where HIV-positive persons have been subject to quarantine (although with weekend leave and marital visiting rights), there have been no serious intrusions on personal liberty. There are, however, other harms: restrictions on medical and life insurance, employment, and freedom to move from one nation to another. Although it makes no epidemiologic sense and violates human rights, most HIV-positive persons are denied entry visas to many countries, including the United States.[13]

The Tragedy of HIV-Contaminated Blood and Tissue

The first cases of AIDS were identified in 1981, although reexamination of pathologic specimens from as far back as the 1960s has shown that a few cases may have occurred as long as 20 years before the epidemic declared itself. Its mode of transmission was implied by results of case-control studies reported in 1983[14] but not confirmed until early in 1985. In the meantime, many people in the United States, Canada, France, Germany, Japan, and other countries received transfusions of HIV-contaminated blood and blood products such as factor 8 for hemophilia; others were infected by semen used in donor artificial insemination, and even by transplanted corneas. The tendency in all the nations listed previously has been to blame administrators and clinical directors of blood transfusion services and the like. In France, some were imprisoned after being found guilty of negligence or malpractice, in trials that had the atmosphere of witch-hunts.[15] Perhaps some clinicians and administrators were negligent, for instance, if they continued to use possibly contaminated blood after early suspicions about this route of transmission were confirmed. Other tragedies have occurred in the offices of dentists and surgeons who carried out procedures with instruments that somehow had been contaminated with HIV by earlier patients.[16] These tragedies remind us of the need for eternal vigilance and, where appropriate, the use of Universal Precautions to eliminate, or at least minimize, the risk of such mishaps in the future. The occurrence in the United Kingdom of several cases of Creutzfeld-Jakob Disease (CJD),[17] putatively linked to bovine spongiform encephalopathy (BSE), reminds us that other dreadful diseases can be transmitted by contaminated human tissues: A confirmed cause of CJD is use of human growth hormone prepared from human pituitary glands before genetically engineered alternatives were available.

The issues in these two situations include violation of the public trust, accountability, honesty, and truth-telling. Elected officials, especially in France, might be regarded as having violated the public's trust in their decision-making powers. They evaded accountability by shifting the blame to hematologists and others—at least one of whom had warned the elected members of the government, had been ignored, then served time in prison when his elected masters blamed him for using HIV-contaminated blood and blood products. Some elected and appointed officials in several countries may not have been fully honest with the public, nor always have been open and truthful, choosing instead to tell part but not all of the truth. In the BSE/CJD fiasco in the United Kingdom, government ministers appear to have withheld from the public at least part of what they knew; subsequently facts came to light that demonstrated their earlier economy with the truth.

▶ INDIVIDUAL RIGHTS AND COMMUNITY NEEDS: ENVIRONMENTAL HEALTH

Most nations have laws or regulations aimed at protecting people against tainted foodstuffs, unsafe working conditions, and unsatisfactory housing, though the strength of such laws and regulations is variable and enforcement is often lax. It may be necessary for aggrieved parties to resort to litigation before an issue can be resolved. Community values and standards have lately shifted toward greater control over environmental hazards to health, reflecting growing concern about our deteriorating environment. In Canada, the Law Reform Commission proposed laws to protect the public from the consequences of "crimes against the environment"[18] but adherence to environmental ethics would be a better solution: Those who pollute the environment harm themselves as well as others; it is in everybody's interest to uphold standards such as those proposed in the European Charter on Environment and Health.[19]

Sometimes health is adversely affected by environmental conditions, but correcting these conditions might have undesirable economic repercussions, such as massive unemployment, and may be opposed by the people whose health is threatened. Public health officials then are in the situation portrayed by Dr. Albert Stockmann in Ibsen's play, *An Enemy of the People*, reviled for actions aimed at protecting health. Control of the public health hazard ought to have highest priority and is clearly the best course of action in such situations, but if this leads to massive economic loss (in itself harmful to health) the principles of beneficent truth telling, justice, and nonmaleficence are helpful: What are the full facts about the situation, who will be helped, which of the competing priorities will harm the fewest people?[20]

► BENEFITS, COSTS, HARMS, AND RISKS

Faced with an outbreak of smallpox in 1947, the public health authorities of the City of New York vaccinated five million people in a period of about six weeks. The human costs were 45 known cases of postvaccinial encephalitis and four deaths[21]—an acceptable risk in view of the enormous benefit, the safety of a city of eight million among whom thousands would have died had the epidemic struck, but a heavy price for the victims of vaccination accidents and their next of kin.

Similar harm:risk:benefit ratios must be calculated for all immunizing agents, indeed for all forms of health care. Consider measles: There may be a risk somewhere between one in one million and one in five million of subacute sclerosing panencephalitis as an adverse effect of measles vaccination.[22] Measles is close to elimination in North America. If we continue to immunize infants against measles after it has been eliminated, there will be occasional harmful consequences, perhaps an episode with fatal cases of septicemia caused by a contaminated batch of vaccine. This fact, and the cost of measles vaccination in face of competing claims for other uses of the same funds, are incentives to stop vaccinating against measles; but the risk of stopping measles vaccination is the return later of epidemic measles, perhaps not until there is a large population of virgin susceptibles. History could repeat itself: Mortality rates of over 40 percent occurred when measles was introduced into the Americas by European colonists. High death rates would be unlikely in the era of antibiotics, but the morbidity and complication rates would be troublesome in an unimmunized population.

The risks of adverse reactions to other immunizing agents are greater than the risks of measles vaccine, but the risks of not immunizing are almost always much greater[23] (Table 10–1).

One duty of all who conduct immunization campaigns is to ensure that everybody is aware of the risks as well as having the benefits clearly explained to them; in short, informed consent is essential. This is very important when children are not admitted to school without evidence of immunization, i.e., when immunization is mandatory rather than voluntary.

TABLE 10-1. **Estimated Rates of Adverse Reactions to Immunizations**

Vaccine	Reaction	Rate per 100,000
BCG	Disseminated infection	< 0.1
	Osteomyelitis	< 0.1–30
	Suppurative adenitis	100–4000
DPT	Convulsions	0.3–90
	Encephalitis	0.1–3
	Brain damage	0.2–0.6
	Death	0.2
Measles	Convulsions	30
	Encephalitis	0.0–0.03

Adverse outcomes of pertussis immunization:

	Cases per million	
	With immunization	Without
Effect (birth–6 months)		
Hospitalization	1060.0	11,098.0
Death	12.5	130.6
Encephalitis	2.4	25.5
Residual defect	0.8	8.5
(6 months–5 years)		
Cases of pertussis	34,048.0	356,566.0
Hospitalizations	6,529.0	38,787.0
Deaths	44.0	457.0
Encephalitis	162.0	87.0
Residual defects	54.0	29.0

BCG = bacille Calmette-Guérin; DPT = diphtheria-pertussis-tetanus.

In some countries, the threat of litigation in the event of mishaps is a deterrent to immunization and a threat to the manufacturers of vaccines. But health care providers can be sued for negligence if they fail to immunize vulnerable persons or groups, as well as for damages if there are adverse reactions—a Hobson's choice. In Britain, France, Switzerland, New Zealand, Australia, and some other countries, the threat of litigation has been removed by no-fault legislation, which provides a standard scale of compensation for mishaps associated with use of immunizing agents. A bill with similar provisions was enacted by the U.S. Congress in 1986, and implementation began in 1990.

Acceptable Risks

We titrate risks against benefits in many other situations, e.g., the use of diagnostic x-rays. Epidemiologic evidence demonstrates that even a single diagnostic dose of x-ray in early pregnancy can harm the developing human fetus.[24] In some medical conditions this small future risk is acceptable because the alternative is a larger immediate risk, such as complications of untreated renal disease. Diagnostic imaging techniques such as ultrasound have removed what was previously a difficult clinical decision when x-rays were the only resort for the obstetrician who suspected fetal malposition or disproportion.

Health administrators and hospital staff who are aware of it accept the small risk of malignant disease among radiographers and other health workers occupationally exposed to x-rays and the risk of fetal loss among operating room staff exposed to waste anesthetic gases—but not all occupationally exposed groups are duly informed of these risks.

Mass Medication

Risk-harm-benefit calculations are required for all forms of mass medication, not only immunizations. The possibility of adverse effects or idiosyncratic reaction always exists. Opposition to fluoridation of drinking water is based in part on the unfounded fear that fluoride can cause cancer or some other dread disease. Epidemiologic analysis shows no association between fluoridation and cancer.[25] Opposition to fluoridation is more a political than a public health issue, in which the catchphrase of the antifluoridation movement, "keep the water pure," is difficult to rebut. Another political argument is that fluoridation is a paternalist measure, imposed on the population whether they like it or not. According to the ethical principle of respect for autonomy, individuals in a free society should have the right to choose for themselves whether they want to drink fluoridated water. Responsible adults can choose, but for infants and small children, fluoridated drinking water makes the difference between healthy and carious teeth. Applying the ethical principle of beneficence, public health officials argue that infants and small children should receive fluoride to ensure that their dental enamel can resist cariogenic bacteria.

Some people conscientiously object to mass medication such as fluoridation of drinking water and immunization of their children against communicable diseases. Opting out can be difficult. Opting out of fluoridation means the trouble and expense of using special supplies of bottled water. To opt out of immunization can mean exclusion of one's children from schools that make entry conditional on producing a certificate testifying to successful immunization. The argument for immunization is strengthened by reports of epidemics of paralytic polio among members of religious sects opposed to immunization.[26] Children, it can be argued, should not be exposed to risks because of their parents' beliefs. Often courts have intervened to save the lives of infants and children requiring blood transfusions that their parents object to for religious reasons; but the circumstances are different when immunizations are offered to healthy children to protect them against diseases that are rare anyway. This is a difficult dilemma when the immunizing agent has adverse effects. The principles of beneficence and nonmaleficence appear to cancel each other out. There remains another argument based on the principle of justice: All infants deserve the protection of vaccines, even though a few may be harmed by adverse effects.

► PRIVACY AND HEALTH STATISTICS

Many people are troubled by the thought that intimate information about them is stored in computers, accessible in theory to anyone who can operate a keyboard and navigate around passwords. Of course the same information has long existed in narrative form in medical charts where it was almost as easily accessible to unauthorized readers as it now allegedly is to unauthorized computer operators. A hundred people or more may be authorized to make entries in the hospital chart of the average patient in an acute, short-stay general hospital bed, and all must read the chart if their entry is to make sense in context. In this respect, the confidentiality of the doctor-patient relationship, the cornerstone of the argument for privacy, is a myth.[27] Proponents of computerized medical record storage and retrieval systems assert that computerized records are more secure than paper records; but if unauthorized access does occur, many people's privacy, not just one person's, can be violated. Moreover, computers can "crash" and a whole library of records may be lost or become inaccessible. Other arguments rest on the premise that personal privacy rights can be violated no matter how the records are stored: People have the right to keep to themselves such facts as the nature of their diseases. This argument, and the powerful emotional reaction against invasions of privacy in formerly totalitarian regimes, set public opinion in the European Union (EU) strongly against maintaining or creating national disease registries. Proposed EU directives would have made it illegal to compile or store medical data for longer than the immediate need in treating sick people and would have prohibited use of medical records for any purpose other than that for which the records were originally collected, without the explicit consent of the persons whose records would be accessed for epidemiologic research, record linkage studies, etc. European societies of epidemiologists and public health specialists successfully argued against this[28]; the 1995 EU Directive[29] supports epidemiologic surveillance and research, whereas earlier versions would have made many forms of it illegal.

Computer storage and retrieval of health-related information greatly enhances the power of analysis to reveal significant associations between exposures and outcomes.[30] Much recently acquired knowledge about many causal relationships has come from routine analyses of health statistics and from epidemiologic studies that have used existing medical records. Examples include the associations between rubella and birth defects, cigarette smoking and cancer, exposure to ionizing radiation and cancer, adverse drug reactions, such as the thromboembolic effects of the oral contraceptive pill, excess child deaths resulting from use of certain antiasthmatic drugs, and increased risk of hypertension in middle age among low birth-weight and premature infants.[31] Community benefit outweighs any harm attributable to invasion of privacy, especially as the harm is theoretical—confidentiality and personal integrity remain intact. In some nations, e.g., Sweden, Australia, and Canada, government-appointed guardians of privacy oversee the uses of medical and other records when these are requested for research purposes.

Resistance to use of routinely collected medical records for epidemiologic analysis has come not only from the grass roots and the guardians of privacy, but also from special-interest groups who would prefer that inconvenient facts should not be disclosed. Industrial corporations have tried to prevent disclosure of adverse effects of occupational or environmental exposures to toxic substances that it has not been in their interest to have widely known. Even governments, which ought to have the public interest as their highest priority, have attempted to suppress information derived from analyses of health statistics when it is politically inconvenient for such information to be publicized. Out-of-court settlements of class action suits, e.g., in tort claims against chemical companies that pollute underground aquifers, have been awarded on condition that the medical records be sealed in perpetuity—a pernicious form of censorship of information that it would be in the public interest to divulge. Public health workers and epidemiologists must be alert to the risk of these forms of censorship and must be prepared to defend access to these sources of health-related information.

Applying the principle of beneficence, it is desirable not only to maintain data files of health-related information but to expand them: Available ideas as well as available information should be used for the common good. Statistical analysis of health-related information has been so convincingly demonstrated to be in the public interest that there is no rational argument against continuing on our present course and expanding further the scope of these activities. This argument applies with particular force to the use of linked medical records, potentially the most powerful method of studying diseases that are rare or have long incubation times, or both.

Health workers have an ethical duty to protect the confidentiality of the records that they use. Irresponsible disclosure of confidential details that can harm individuals is not only unethical but can arouse public opinion against collection and use of such material. Properly used, health statistics and the records from which they are derived do not invade individual privacy. The argument that individual rights are infringed upon in the interests of the community is a "false antithesis"[32]—individual rights are congruent with community needs because, as members of the community, all individuals benefit from analyses based on individual health records.

► CONFIDENTIALITY AND THE LAW

Sometimes the law reinforces this ethical position while respecting autonomy by safeguarding privacy. A U.S. Court of Appeals ruled in favor of preserving the confidentiality of medical records used by the Centers for Disease Control and Prevention in an epidemiologic study of toxic shock syndrome attributed to the use of certain varieties of vaginal tampon. Lawyers for the manufacturer of these tampons had tried to subpoena the records so that they could call the women as witnesses and presumably challenge their testimony. The court ruled that it would not be in the public interest to establish a precedent in which records of epidemiologic importance could be used in an adversarial situation: This would be a deterrent to future epidemiologic studies and to participants in such studies.[33] However, in 1989 a U.S. Circuit Court granted a tobacco company access to clinical records (albeit stripped of personal identifiers) that had been the basis for another epidemiologic study.[34] In 1996, in a product liability suit against manufacturers of silicon breast implants, plaintiffs were denied access to epidemiologic records from the "Nurses' Health Study" on the grounds that this would jeopardize future cycles of this valuable ongoing study.[35] The variation in rulings is confusing. The issue of confidentiality of medical records and their subsequent use for epidemiologic analysis remains open; the threat that courts may allow access by hostile interest groups could be a deterrent to future epidemiologists unless this aspect of law is clarified.

In 1990, the Society for Epidemiologic Research agreed, after much debate, that research data should be shared with outside parties who might wish to reanalyze raw data.[36] Reasons for reanalysis should not influence the right of access.

▶ ETHICAL GUIDELINES FOR EPIDEMIOLOGISTS

These and other problems have preoccupied epidemiologists who have identified ethical issues and formulated appropriate responses. In addition to the Society for Epidemiologic Research, the Industrial Epidemiology Forum,[37] the Swedish Society of Public Health Research Workers, the International Epidemiological Association,[38] among others, have developed guidelines. In 1991, the Council for International Organizations of the Medical Sciences (CIOMS) published *International Guidelines for Ethical Review of Epidemiological Studies*[39] and in 1992 CIOMS revised its *International Guidelines for Ethical Review of Research Involving Human Subjects.*[40] The 1993 revision of the National Institutes of Health's *Institutional Review Board Guidebook*[41] has a section on the special circumstances of epidemiologic and public health studies. Research funding agencies in other countries have been concerned about the same issues. The National Health and Medical Research Council in Australia,[42] the Canadian Medical, Social and Natural Sciences Research Councils,[43] and the European Medical Research Councils have produced codes of conduct, guidelines, or position papers dealing with ethical requirements. The American College of Epidemiology has had a committee on ethics and standards of practice since 1991; this committee has explored the feasibility of developing a formal code of conduct and has conducted a survey of epidemiologists to determine the nature and frequency of ethical problems that they encounter. Similar initiatives have been taken by the American Public Health Association and other national societies.

None so far adequately address the "gray area" between formal (hypothesis-testing) research and routine surveillance. In public health practice and in such settings as cancer registries, it can be difficult to say when routine practice ends and research begins.

All epidemiologic studies, whether for surveillance or for research, involve human subjects and must therefore abide by the Helsinki Declaration[44] and its revisions respecting autonomy and human dignity. Research and surveillance must not harm people,[45] and informed consent is a *sine qua non,* as important in public health practice as in clinical medicine.

Informed Consent

The process and procedures for obtaining informed consent[46] should be clearly understood by all health workers. The process consists of transfer of information and understanding of its significance to subjects of medical interventions, followed by explicit consent of the subjects (or responsible proxies) to take part in the intervention. The task of informing should be conducted by somebody senior and responsible, not delegated to a junior nurse or a medical student. Consent is usually active, i.e., agreement to take part; sometimes it is passive, i.e., people are regarded as research subjects unless they explicitly refuse. Consent need not be written: The act of offering an arm and a vein for withdrawal of a sample of blood implies consent; the essential feature is understanding the purpose for which the blood is taken. Concepts of autonomy vary: In some cultures, patients regard their personal physician as responsible for all decisions about their health, including participation in research. In other cultures a village headman, tribal elder, or religious leader is considered to have responsibility for the group, in which individuals may not perceive themselves as autonomous. Nevertheless, each individual in such a group should be asked to give consent to whatever procedure is being conducted as part of a public health intervention or epidemiologic research project.

Variations From Informed Consent Rules in Epidemiologic Studies

The 1993 CIOMS Guidelines list ten items of information that must be communicated to and understood by potential research subjects before informed consent is regarded as valid. The latest edition of the National Institutes of Health's Institutional Review Board handbook and the Canadian counterpart of this add another five items (Table 10–2).

Epidemiologists must respect these rules and the Helsinki Declaration, but when studying very large populations it is not feasible to obtain the informed consent of every individual whose records contribute to the statistical analysis.[47] Sometimes the records are those of deceased persons. Epidemiologists then abide by the code of conduct of the International Statistical Institute for official statisticians.[48] This is made formal by requiring those who work with official records to take an oath of secrecy, i.e., never to divulge per-

TABLE 10–2. Informed Consent: What Must be Communicated (CIOMS Guidelines)

Aims, methods of research
   Duration of research
   Benefits for subjects and others
   Foreseeable risks, harms
   Possible advantageous alternatives
   Confidentiality details
   Extent of responsibility to provide care
   Treatment for research-related harm
   Compensation for research-related harm
   Freedom to refuse or withdraw

Additional National Institutes of Health Communication details for informed consent
   Circumstances allowing investigator to terminate
   Possible costs to subject
   Consequences of subject's decision to withdraw
   Research findings will be communicated to subject
   Approximate number of subjects in study

sonal information they see in the course of their work. This protection of privacy extends to communities and groups that would be identifiable in the context of routine reporting: Statistical tables are published in a form that precludes identification of small or local jurisdictions.

In the EU, there has been public and political concern about access to and use of official statistics such as death certificates and hospital discharge data. There have even been proposals to respect the privacy of the dead by withholding from death certificates the cause of death when the cause carries a stigma such as syphilis or AIDS.

Although respect for privacy is important in surveillance and research, sometimes privacy must be invaded, e.g., when sexual partners must be traced as part of control measures for sexually transmitted diseases. Epidemiologists attempt to obtain informed consent to these invasions of privacy.

► IMPARTIALITY AND ADVOCACY

Epidemiology, like all science, is objective, so it ought to be impartial. Can it be "value-neutral"? Epidemiologic findings sometimes reveal dangers to health that require active campaigns aimed at changing the status quo, perhaps in opposition to established custom, and social, economic, commercial, industrial, political interests and institutions. The discovery that smoking causes lung cancer is a good example: Public health scientists who identified this massive public health problem sometimes became advocates for better health and opponents of the tobacco industry and of the institutions of society that encouraged the use of tobacco. Advocacy and scientific objectivity are uneasy bedfellows, but most public health research workers believe their duty to protect the public health is a higher imperative than to remain "value-neutral." In many situations since the early days of debate about smoking and lung cancer, epidemiologists have had to wrestle with the problem of reconciling scientific objectivity and impartiality with advocacy of measures to enhance health. I do not believe epidemiology is a "value-free" science.[49]

▶ RESEARCH INTEGRITY

Consider the data in Table 10–3. Such distributions could come from a case-control study or a randomized, controlled trial. The distributions in Table 3A do not quite reach a level of statistical significance at the 5 percent level; those in Table 3B do, but barely. A scientist eager to achieve a "significant" result might yield to the temptation to exclude an observation, perhaps on the grounds that it is an outlier, or find reasons to move an observation from one cell to another in the table. This may seem to be almost a venial sin, but it is not. It is to be hoped that it is rare. It becomes more serious when data are altered after the fact, when some observations in a series are deliberately discarded, and when data are fabricated. Violations of research ethics are com-

TABLE 10–3. How to Achieve "Statistical Significance"

In each of the following distributions, moving one observation achieves a level of "statistical significance" at the 5 percent level.

	A. "Not Significant" Differences		B. "Significant" Differences	
	+	−	+	−
+	20	30	20	31
−	30	20	30	19
Total	50	50	50	50
	$p > 0.05 (= 0.072)$		$p < 0.05 (= 0.045)$	
	+	−	+	−
+	6	14	5	14
−	44	36	45	36
Total	50	50	50	50
	$p > 0.05 (= 0.080)$		$p < 0.05 (= 0.041)$	

ing to light increasingly often; they range from sloppy research design to scientific fraud and misrepresentation. Pressure to get results that will lead to publications required to ensure promotion or tenure encourage some in academia to depart from impeccable scientific standards. There has been enough concern about serious violations to prompt the Institute of Medicine of the National Academy of Sciences[50] to issue guidelines that include a mandatory requirement to faithfully observe preset protocols, maintain and preserve research logbooks, and adhere to other measures aimed at eliminating unethical and dishonest conduct.

▶ CONFLICTS OF INTEREST, CENSORSHIP, AND SECRECY IN PUBLIC HEALTH SCIENCE

Conflicts of interest have worried several professional associations, especially in the United States. Research that had been completed and submitted for publication has been "leaked" to an industrial corporation or pharmaceutical company, which has then hired its own scientists and paid for negative criticism aimed at discrediting the work. Attempts have been made to prevent even casual dissemination (let alone publication) of results that might be damaging to commercial interests. It is impossible to know how often original research results have been suppressed altogether because of intimidation, bribery, or more subtle pressure, because if suppression is completely successful no one outside the immediate circle of those involved will hear about it. This and related problems have preoccupied biomedical science editors.[51] This problem may be more widespread and more serious than crimes like scientific fraud and plagiarism.

▶ OCCUPATIONAL HEALTH

The specialist in occupational health or industrial medicine is responsible for safeguarding the health of workers, usually is employed by management, is answerable also to government regulatory agencies, and is subject to pressure from workers and their unions, public interest groups, and often the media. Remaining impartial among these potential or actual adversarial groups requires a delicate balancing act and considerable political skill. Recognizing this, the American Occupational Medical Association adopted a Code of Conduct[52] in 1976. The International Commission on Occupational Health produced a code of ethics for all occupational health workers[53] in 1992. Both codes of conduct aim to foster exemplary behavior, although neither explicitly recognizes the needs of such vulnerable groups as pregnant women and underage workers; this is a troubling problem, particularly in developing countries.

► POPULATION SCREENING

Screening is the application of diagnostic tests or procedures to apparently healthy people with the aim of sorting them into those who may have a condition that would benefit from early intervention and those who do not. An ideal screening test would sort people into two groups, those who definitely have and those who definitely do not have the condition. In our imperfect world, screening tests sometimes yield false-positive or false-negative results. A false-positive test exposes individuals to the anxiety, costs, and risks of further investigation and perhaps unnecessary treatment, and imposes economic burdens on the health care system that it would be better to avoid. A false-negative screening test could have disastrous consequences if persons suffering from early cancer are wrongly reassured that there is nothing wrong with them. An important use for epidemiology is the calculation of false-positive and false-negative rates and the predictive power of screening tests (see Chap. 2). These calculations must be borne in mind when deciding whether it is ethical to apply a particular test as a population screening procedure. If a disease has a low prevalence (less than 1 in 1000) the screening test is expensive and the predictive power of a positive test is low (say, less than 80 percent), we must question whether screening is ethically as well as economically acceptable. The cost of confirmatory tests as well as the feasibility of treatment must also be considered. Interviews can be used to screen populations for Alzheimer's disease, but confirmatory diagnostic imaging is costly so it is important to know ahead of time who will pay for it.

Screening for evidence of inapparent disease implies the use of interventions that will change the lives of people who had previously thought they were well; they may react in several ways to the knowledge that they have a disease or condition requiring treatment. They may assume a "sick role"—develop symptoms, lose time from work, and become unduly worried about themselves.[54] People who previously considered themselves to be healthy may perceive as gratuitous or paternalist the intervention of the well-meaning specialist who found something wrong—especially when the intervention makes them feel worse, as treatment for hypertension sometimes does. Questions of medical etiquette as well as ethics arise. Screening programs are often conducted by staff in public health rather than personal health care services. Public health workers must communicate results to personal physicians responsible for the care of individuals with positive tests. At the very least, a positive test can arouse anxiety (though it can also allay anxiety); it can be inconvenient, expensive, uncomfortable, distressing, and worrying. A false-positive test can lead to needless anxiety and expense. Counseling must be planned as part of screening programs to minimize anxiety.

More complex questions and ethical ambiguities arise in genetic screening and counseling. It is feasible to screen for Huntington's disease, Tay-Sachs disease, and Duchenne's muscular dystrophy among other conditions. In Huntington's disease, a positive screening test has appalling implications for the person concerned, though early experience with volunteers from high-risk families has suggested that some at least prefer to know than not to know their fate.[55] If Tay-Sachs disease or Duchenne's muscular dystrophy are detected by screening early in pregnancy, the most humane action is termination of the pregnancy.

► HEALTH PROMOTION

Health promotion is the process of enabling people to increase control over and improve their health. Health advocates regard it as a step toward autonomous decision making for people who were formerly passive recipients of public health measures like purifying drinking water, mass vaccination programs, dietary additives, tuberculin tests, and other routine public health interventions. Health promotion ought to be an entirely beneficent activity; but Abelin[56] has identified some possible untoward consequences. The population may not all share the same values as those who offer health promotion programs and may be made to feel alienated. Prolongation of life as an end in itself ignores the quality of that life. Health promotion may be more effective among educated professionals than uneducated working class people so may widen gaps in health status between socioeconomic groups. Advocates for health promotion programs need to be aware of these and other potential drawbacks.

► HEALTH EDUCATION

What could be more beneficent than spreading information about risks to health and actions that can be taken to reduce these risks? Health education encourages all to take greater responsibility for their own health. Often laws or regulations are synergistic with health education about immunizations and admonitions against tobacco addiction. But other issues arise when health educators, with or without the help of laws or regulations, seek to control addiction to tobacco or alcohol use. Some civil libertarians hold that everyone has a right to use alcohol or tobacco. This may be true so long as their use does not harm others, such as the fetus or child of smoking parents or road users who may be killed or maimed by impaired drivers. Economic interests in communities dependent on the alcohol and tobacco industries, it is argued, also must be considered when deciding how to deal with public health problems associated with tobacco and alcohol use and abuse. These are complex economic, political, and ethical questions. No cash crop is as lucrative as tobacco; but in many parts of the developing world as well as in the United States, tobacco has replaced food crops; in Africa, trees are depleted to provide fuel for flue-cured tobacco, contributing to the advance of deserts.[57] These facts, and the worldwide toll of tobacco-related premature deaths, support the argument that the economic well-being of tobacco-producing communities is best ensured by converting to food crops. The ethical principles here are beneficence and justice.

Another concern is that those who fall ill after ignoring health education messages may be blamed for their illnesses or made to feel guilty. It is important for health workers to be nonjudgmental when this possibility exists.

▶ POPULATION POLICIES, FAMILY PLANNING PROGRAMS, REPRODUCTIVE FREEDOM

National population policies range from encouragement of couples to have or refrain from having children (often with related laws on access to and use of contraceptives) to vaguely visualized policies implied by the appearance in newspapers and women's magazines of articles on birth control that contain statements about the efficacy of contraceptive methods. Most Western nations provide funds from taxation or other revenue for support of family planning clinics that are accessible without charge to low-income women—but not always to sexually active unmarried teenage girls in the United States.

There are many variations in constraints on access to such clinics by girls around the age of puberty who are or may soon become sexually active. There are also great variations in the nature and extent of sex education, especially education about contraception, and in access to effective contraception. These variations are associated with corresponding variations in unwanted teenage pregnancy rates, which are up to ten times higher in the United States than in almost all other Organization for Economic Cooperation and Development (OECD) nations.[58]

The arguments for early and honest education about sexuality are compelling. Children become sexually mature in their early teens and at the same age begin to question and rebel against parental authority. The tactics of the religious right wing—pious statements ("just say no") and authoritarian orders forbidding sexual activity and denying access to contraception—are a sure way to increase the risks of early teenage pregnancy and to spread sexually transmitted disease.

Some nations, notably India and China, and one of the most crowded, Singapore, have provided economic incentives or have introduced coercive measures such as enforced sterilization or abortion, aimed at restricting the rate of population growth. Other nations have adopted pronatalist policies, often because of a perceived threat of being overwhelmed by extraneous population groups.

In nations that have government-supported family planning programs, public health workers are responsible for managing and implementing government policies. Even if population policies are implicit rather than explicit, their general direction is usually clear. In a free society, public health workers have an ethical duty to consider each patient or client as an individual with her own unique life situation, problems, and requests, not a "case" to whom the official policies necessarily apply. The aspirations of women and couples to have or refrain from having children are powerful and very personal. Staff members of family planning clinics have an ethical duty to offer advice and treatment and an equally important duty not to enforce their own or official views on individual clients.

Difficult questions arise when we have to balance the mother's rights and those of the fetus. At one extreme are those who would prohibit alcohol and substance use altogether during pregnancy and would indict smoking parents or pregnant women for child or fetal abuse. Law courts have occasionally forced pregnant substance abusers to submit to treatment, which some feminists regard as upholding the view that women exist merely as containers for a fetus. Debates about maternal and fetal rights often reveal irreconcilable differences, and there is no consensus on the "correct" ethical response.

▶ EQUITY AND JUSTICE IN RESOURCE ALLOCATION

Public health is inherently concerned with social justice, with fair and equitable distribution of resources to protect, preserve, and restore health. Public health workers therefore frequently become advocates for health care systems that provide access to needed services without economic or other barriers. Historically, public health workers have often provided the impetus to establish a social security system with unimpeded access to health care for all members of society regardless of income, with access based only on need. In nations that have social security systems, public health workers are prominent among the organizers and administrators. If personal health services are offered to population groups that do not attract fee-for-service practice, these are often run by staff from public health services. When analysis of health statistics reveals regions or districts and population groups that have unmet needs, public health workers often take the initiative to meet these needs.

The principles of equity and justice go further. The allocation of health care budgets is often based on political or emotional grounds and on the ability of eloquent spokesmen for high-technology diagnostic and therapeutic services to promote these interests. Funds sometimes are allocated for expensive equipment and devices, while much needed public health services such as water purification plants in need of renovation or logistic support for immunization programs go without funds. It is an ethical imperative for public health workers to be as aggressive as circumstances require in obtaining an equitable share of resources and funds for public health services.

▶ INTERNATIONAL HEALTH

International health is concerned with the interdependent relationships among all the people and nations on earth (see Chap. 9). For many years the rich nations have provided support for health care, public health, and medical research in the poorer nations. Until recently few questioned this; it was regarded as mutually beneficial. There has been concern about the "brain drain"—the hemorrhage of talent from poor nations that send their best and brightest young people abroad for advanced training and lose many of them permanently to the rich nations. This has been regarded as a necessary price for development assistance. Now other difficulties are perceived. Questions have been raised about the appropriateness of technology transfer from rich to poor countries, about "ethical imperialism,"[59] the use by research workers from rich countries of the large populations and the challenging unsolved health problems of the poor countries, with the aim of addressing priorities as perceived in rich countries but without regard for problems and priorities in the poor.

Other problems are associated with the disparity between rich and poor nations. These include the export from rich to poor nations of problems attributable to affluence and industrial development—tobacco addiction, traffic injury, exploitation of workers (often women and children who work for starvation wages), and environmental pollution.

Other problems arise from differing values and behaviors. The status of women may be quite different from that in Western industrial nations; customs such as female genital mutilation, child marriage, and infanticide may occur. Sometimes developing nations are ruled by a repressive military dictatorship without regard for any kind of impartial justice, including equity in health care. International health workers who encounter such phenomena are in a difficult position. To speak out against these customs or against the actions of repressive rulers is unlikely to help the local people and may expose the health worker to the risk of being deported, or even arrested, tortured, or imprisoned. Yet it is morally repugnant to remain silent.

International health workers should be able to speak out more forcefully against the export of health-harming practices from industrial to developing nations, such as promotion of infant formula in societies that lack facilities to sterilize infant feeds, dumping of drugs that have not been approved for use in industrial nations, and advertising of tobacco.

▶ PATERNALISM AND PUBLIC HEALTH

Beneficence is the dominant ethical principle of public health. We believe in doing good, and historically we have an impressive record—the sanitary revolution, the control of almost all major communicable diseases, the elimination of many such diseases from large areas they formerly dominated, and the worldwide eradication of smallpox. The new challenges presented by the "second epidemiological revolution"[60]—coronary heart disease, many cancers, traffic injury, etc., as the main causes of premature death and chronic disability—have led us to respond by aiming to change human behavior. Many of the behaviors we seek to change are pleasurable to those who practice them, and our efforts to initiate change are often resented. If we wish to promote better health, we should be sure that our advice and recommendations are based on solid evidence of efficacy. There is a long tradition of advocacy by public health workers, but in the past this may have been as often associated with preaching as with teaching. The aim of public health services ought to be to enlighten the people about risks to health and to assist people in gaining greater control over environmental, social, and other conditions that influence their own health. We have an ethical duty to work with people, empowering them, doing whatever may be necessary to promote better health—doing things with, not to, people. This is the main thrust of the Ottawa Charter for Health Promotion.[61]

▶ IS THERE A "RIGHT TO HEALTH?"

Social activists proclaim the concept of health as a human right, but there are problems with this view. If there is a right to health, there must be a duty to provide this right; whose duty is it? The answer may be that it is the duty of the individual whose health is the "right" in question—but this encourages victim-blaming when health is impaired. A further difficulty is defining what we mean by "health." There is confusion between health and quality of life. Nobody would describe the theoretical physicist Stephen Hawking as healthy; he has been afflicted with amyotrophic lateral sclerosis for many years, but they have been very productive years, and judging from his own testimony,[62] they have been happy years. There are innumerable examples of severely disabled people whose lives have been happy and productive—and as many "healthy" people who lead miserable lives. Public health workers might be wise to avoid discussing the "right to health." However, it is beneficent for public health workers to strive for economic, environmental, social, and political conditions that will maximize good health, as by implementing the Ottawa Charter for Health Promotion or the "Targets" document of the European Region of WHO[63] (see Chap. 1).

▶ METHODS IN ETHICS

How should we deal with the ethical problems that arise in public health practice and research? Essentially the answer is the same in public health as in clinical practice. Several books provide guidance,[64] although often there is no easy answer (Box 10–3). Often we must decide what to do while aware

BOX 10-3. How to Deal With Ethical Problems

Identify the nature of the problem
Identify the available options
Whose problem is it?
    Person's?
    Community's?
    Health care worker's?
    Organization's?
    Institution's?
Gather and evaluate all available information
Set priorities
Consider consequences of decision
Choose among the available options, and act
Evaluate the action

that some will be unhappy or even harmed by our decision (for instance the index case, when we must trace contacts of sexually transmitted diseases). Decisions can be very difficult. An orderly and systematic approach is therefore essential.

First, we should clearly identify the problem(s). We should identify the available options and decide whose problem(s) we are dealing with—particular persons, communities, health care workers, organizations, institutions, etc. We must gather all the available information and evaluate it carefully, trying as far as possible to set priorities among the options that have to be considered. We must also consider the consequences of the decisions that have to be taken, relating these to prevailing values, beliefs, community standards, etc. Having done all these things, we must choose among the options, and act. Finally, we must evaluate or review the consequences, often on an ongoing basis—remembering that often there is no "right answer" but a series of alternatives each of which is in some way both satisfactory and unsatisfactory. One of the most difficult aspects of biomedical ethics is that the more securely we may think we grasp the philosophic principles, the harder it may become to arrive at a satisfactory answer to the problem. Ethical problem solving often requires high tolerance of ambiguity.

▶ THE PHILOSOPHICAL BASIS FOR PUBLIC HEALTH

All public health workers should ask themselves "Why am I doing this?" The aims of public health are to promote and preserve good health, to restore health, and to relieve suffering and distress. We often judge our success by reduction of infant mortality rates and increased life expectancy, but we seldom try to measure, record, and analyze data on relief of distress (e.g., associated with chronic unemployment or homelessness). Clinicians responsible for intensive care services and for care of the elderly have been obliged to consider the question of quality of life when life-prolonging measures are used. There is growing concern about the quality of death as well as with the quality of life.[65] In public health, a similar reorienting of focus is to use less tangible outcome measures than life expectancy. A set of health expectancy indicators[66] has been suggested as one useful approach. We must also consider the impact of "improved" human reproductive performance on other living creatures with which we share the earth.[67] Human reproductive success is endangering planetary ecology and therefore our own survival as a species: Health must be sustainable for other species, not merely for humans.[68]

Spectacular gains over infant mortality have been achieved from the expanded program on immunization, oral rehydration therapy, growth monitoring, etc. Innumerable infants and small children who would have died just a few years ago are living. What will become of them? Will they fall victim to the demographic trap[69]—starve, because there are so many more mouths to feed? Will they get an education? Will they have a lifetime of meaningful work? Will they die eventually, rich in years and experience, surrounded by a loving family? The answers to these questions will depend on our response to challenges more subtle than reduction of infant and child mortality rates.

► CONCLUSION

This review hints at the range and complexity of ethical issues in public health practice and research. I do not address the relationship between person-oriented and population-oriented ethics, where there is dissonance in our values and priorities. We spare no effort or expense in striving to prolong lives of infants with incurable liver disease by finding donors for liver transplants; we maintain indefinitely on life-support systems some patients who are in a persistent vegetative state from which they cannot recover.[70] Yet we do little to prevent many diseases that commonly take the lives or destroy the joy of life for much larger numbers of people, such as infants who are the victims of fetal alcohol syndrome and young adults who are permanently brain-damaged by serious injuries in traffic crashes. In many states in the United States, the freedom of individuals to ride motorcycles without wearing crash helmets is considered more important than the right of society to protect its resources by reducing the risk that these individuals, mostly young men, will not become a drain on public resources if they sustain head injuries in traffic crashes that leave them permanently brain-damaged. We spend large amounts and invest much effort in interventions for advanced coronary heart disease but devote little intellectual effort or money to measures that might reduce the magnitude of this public health problem.

This raises philosophic questions about the dissonant aims of medicine and public health, questions that go to the heart of the values, beliefs, and meaning of our culture. Similar questions about dissonant values and aims were raised during the Cold War by thoughtful critics of the arms race who wondered whether our investments in weapons to preserve our freedom were enslaving us in fear and paranoia. Similar questions are raised now by critics of environmental development policies that rely on exploitation rather than on learning to live an interdependent existence with other living creatures on our planet. I take up this topic in the next chapter.

► **REFERENCES**

1. Milton Rosenau credits Murchison (1858) with first use of this term; see Rosenau M: *Preventive Medicine and Hygiene.* New York: Appleton, 1913, p. 684.
2. *Report of the Presidential Commission on the Human Immunodeficiency Virus Epidemic.* Washington, DC: June 1988.
3. Last JM: The future of public health. *Nippon Koshu Eise: Zasshi (Japanese J Public Health)* 38:10(suppl 1):58–95, 1991.
4. Vickers G: What sets the goals of public health? *Lancet* 1:599–604, 1958.
5. Aristotle; Thompson JAK (trans): *Ethics.* Tredennick H (rev). New York: Viking Penguin, 1976.
6. Beauchamp TL, Childress JF: *Principles of Biomedical Ethics.* 4th ed. New York: Oxford University Press, 1994.
7. Frank JP; Lesky E (trans): *A System of Complete Medical Police.* Baltimore: Johns Hopkins University Press, 1976.
8. Paul JR: *A History of Poliomyelitis.* New Haven: Yale University Press, 1971, pp. 148–152.
9. Brandt AM: *No Magic Bullet; A Social History of the Venereal Diseases in the United States Since 1880.* New York: Oxford University Press, 1987.
10. Ontario Ministry of Health: *Testing and Reporting for AIDS and HIV Infection.* Toronto: Ontario Ministry of Health, 1989.
11. Fitch KM, Alvarez LP, Medine RA, et al.: Occupational transmission of HIV in health care workers. A review. *Eur J Public Health* 5:175–186, 1995.
12. World Health Organization, Global Programme on AIDS: *Guidelines for Monitoring HIV Infection in Populations.* Geneva: WHO, 1989.
13. Duckett M, Orkin AJ: AIDS-related migration and travel policies and restrictions. A global survey. *AIDS* 3(suppl):S231–S252, 1989.
14. Jaffe HW, Choi K, Thomas PA, et al.: National case-control study of Kaposi's sarcoma and *Pneumocystis carinii* pneumonia in homosexual men; part 1: Epidemiological results. *Ann Int Med* 99:145–151, 1983.
15. Bader J-M: France: Prison Sentences for Doctors. *Lancet* 360:1087, 1992.
16. Chant K, Lowe D, Rubin G, et al.: Patient-to-patient transmission of HIV in private surgical consulting rooms. *Lancet* 343:1548–1549, 1993.
17. Will RG, Ironside JW, Zeidler M, et al.: A new variant of Creutzfeld-Jakob disease. *Lancet* 347:921–925, 1996.
18. Law Reform Commission of Canada: *Crimes Against the Environment.* LRCC Working Paper #44. Ottawa: 1985.

19. World Health Organization: *European Charter on Environment and Health.* Copenhagen: World Health Organization, Regional Office for Europe, 1989.

20. Last JM, Parkinson MD: Health officials and their responsibilities. In Beauchamp D, (ed): *Encyclopedia of Bioethics.* 2nd ed. New York: Macmillan, 1995, vol. 2, pp. 1113–1116.

21. Greenberg M, Appelbaum E: Postvaccinian encephalitis. A report of 45 cases in New York City. *Am J Med Sci* 216:565–570, 1948.

22. *WHO Weekly Epidemiological Record* 3:13–15, 1984.

23. U.S. Department of Health and Human Services Task Force: Pertussis: CPS, a case study. In *Determining Risks to Health—Federal Policy and Practice.* Dover, MA: Auburn, 1986.

24. Meyer MB, Tonascia J: Long-term effects of prenatal x-ray of human females. *Am J Epidemiol* 114:304–336, 1981.

25. Kinlen L: Cancer incidence in relation to fluoride level in water supplies. *Br Dent J* 138:221–224, 1975.

26. White FMM, Lacey BA, Constance PDA: An outbreak of poliomyelitis infection in Alberta, 1978. *Can J Public Health* 72:239–244, 1981.

27. Siegler M: Confidentiality in medicine. A decrepit concept. *N Engl J Med* 307:1518–1521, 1982.

28. Allebech P: New regulations on databases. *Epidemiol Monitor* November 1993, p. 3.

29. Directive 95/46/EC of the European Parliament and of the Council; *On the Protection of Individuals with Regard to the Processing of Personal Data and on the Free Movement of Such Data.* Luxembourg, 24 October 1995.

30. Newcombe H: *Handbook of Record Linkage.* Oxford: Oxford University Press, 1987.

31. Barker DJP, Martyn CN, Osmond C, et al.: Growth in utero and serum cholesterol concentrations in adult life. *Br Med J* 307:1524–1527, 1993.

32. Black D: *An Anthology of False Antitheses.* London: Nuffield Provincial Hospitals Trust, 1984.

33. Curran WJ: Protecting confidentiality in epidemiologic investigations by the Centers for Disease Control. *New Engl J Med* 314:1027–1028, 1986.

34. U.S. Court of Appeals (2nd Cir 1989): *American Tobacco Company, RJ Reynolds Tobacco Company, and Philip Morris Inc. v. Mount Sinai School of Medicine and the American Cancer Society.*

35. U.S. District Court (ND Ala) CV-92-P-10000-S.

36. *Epidemiol Monitor* May 1990; 11:1–2. See also *Science* 1990.

37. Fayerweather WE, Higginson J, Beauchamp TL (eds): *Ethics in Epidemiology.* New York: Pergamon, 1991; also *J Clin Epidemiol* 44(suppl 1), 1991, pp. 51S–169S.

38. Last JM: Guidelines on ethics for epidemiologists. *Int J Epidemiol* 19:226–229, 1990. See also *APHA Epidemiology Section Newsletter,* Winter 1991.

39. Bankowski Z, Bryant JH, Last JM (eds): *Ethics and Epidemiology; International Guidelines.* Geneva: CIOMS, 1991.

40. *International Guidelines for Ethical Review of Biomedical Research Involving Human Subjects.* Geneva: CIOMS, 1992.

41. National Institutes of Health, Office of Extramural Research, Office for Protection from Research Risks: *Protecting Human Research Subjects; Institutional Review Board Guidebook.* Washington, DC: GPO, 1993.

42. Commonwealth of Australia, National Health and Medical Research Council, Medical Research Ethics Committee: *Report on Ethics in Epidemiological Research.* Canberra: GPO, 1985.

43. Medical Research Council of Canada, Natural Sciences and Engineering Research Council of Canada, Social Sciences and Humanities Research Council of Canada: *Code of Conduct for Research Involving Humans* (draft, March 1996). Ottawa: GPO, 1996.
44. World Medical Association: *Declaration of Helsinki,* adopted by the 18th World Medical Assembly, Helsinki, Finland, June 1964; amended by the 29th World Medical Assembly, Tokyo, Japan, October 1975, the 35th World Medical Assembly, Venice, Italy, October 1983, and the 41st World Medical Assembly, Hong Kong, September 1989.
45. Last JM: Obligations and responsibilities of epidemiologists to research subjects. *J Clin Epidemiol* 44(suppl 1):95S–102S, 1991.
46. Faden RR, Beauchamp TL: *A History and Theory of Informed Consent.* New York: Oxford University Press, 1986.
47. Last JM: Epidemiology and ethics. In Bankowski Z, Bryant JH, Last JM (eds). *Ethics and Epidemiology; International Guidelines.* Geneva: CIOMS & WHO, 1991, pp. 14–28.
48. International Statistical Institute: Declaration on Professional Ethics. *Int Stat Rev* 54:227–242, 1986.
49. Last JM: Ethical challenges for epidemiologists. *Jpn J Epidemiol* 6: (in press), 1996.
50. Institute of Medicine, National Academy of Sciences: *Report of a Study on the Responsible Conduct of Research in the Health Sciences.* Washington, DC: National Academy of Sciences, Institute of Medicine, 1989.
51. Guarding the guardians. Proceedings of First International Congress on Peer Review in Biomedical Publication. JAMA 263:1317–1441, 1990.
52. *Code of Ethical Conduct for Physicians Providing Occupational Medical Services.* Washington, DC: American Occupational Medical Association, 1976.
53. International Commission on Occupational Health: *International Code of Ethics for Occupational Health Professionals.* Singapore: ICOH, 1992.
54. Haynes RB, Sackett DL, Taylor DW et al.: Increased absenteeism from work after detection and labeling of hypertensive patients. *N Engl J Med* 299:741–747, 1978.
55. Turner DR, Willoughby JO: Ethical issues in Huntington disease presymptomatic testing. *Aust N Z J Med* 20:545–547, 1990.
56. Abelin T: Health promotion. In Holland WW, Detels R, Knox G (eds): *Oxford Textbook of Public Health.* 2nd ed. New York: Oxford University Press, 1991, 3, pp. 558–589 .
57. McNamara RS: *The Challenges for Sub-Saharan Africa.* Washington, DC: Consultative Group on International Agricultural Research, 1985.
58. Jones EF, (ed): *Teenage Pregnancy in Industrialized Countries.* New Haven: Yale University Press, 1986.
59. Angell M: Ethical imperialism? Ethics in international collaborative research. *N Engl J Med* 319:1081–1083, 1988.
60. Terris M: The Changing Relationships of Epidemiology and Society. *J Public Health Policy* 6:15–36, 1985.
61. World Health Organization: A Charter for Health Promotion (The Ottawa Charter). *Can J Public Health* 77:425–430, 1986.
62. Hawking S: *A Brief History of Time.* New York: Bantam, 1988.
63. *Targets for Health for All 2000.* Copenhagen: World Health Organization Regional Office for Europe, 1985.

64. See for example Gillon R (ed): *Principles of Health Care Ethics.* Chichester, England: John Wiley, 1995.

65. Saunders C: The dying patient. In Gillon R (ed): *Principles of Health Care Ethics.* Chichester, England: John Wiley, 1995, pp. 775–782.

66. Robine JM, Mathers CD, Bucquet D: Distinguishing health expectancies and health-adjusted life expectancies. *Am J Public Health* 83:797–798, 1993.

67. Last JM, Homo sapiens—a suicidal species? *World Health Forum* 12:2:129–139, 1991.

68. Last JM: Redefining the unacceptable. *Lancet* 346:1642–1643, 1995.

69. King MH: Health is a sustainable state. *Lancet* 336:664–667, 1990; see also King MH, Elliott C: Legitimate double-think. *Lancet* 341:669–672, 1993.

70. Annas GJ, Bioethicists' statement on the U.S. Supreme Court's Cruzan decision. *N Engl J Med* 323:686–687, 1990.

Human Health in a Changing World

Throughout its 4 billion year existence, the earth's atmospheric composition and climate have changed many times. Sometimes air and ocean currents that determine climate and weather have been altered by tectonic plate movements.[1] On a few occasions, sudden climate changes leading to great extinctions have followed the impact of large meteors or massive volcanic activity that filled the air with gases like sulfur dioxide and dust, which blocked sunlight. Variation in solar radiation flux, oscillation of the earth's axis, passing clouds of interstellar dust may induce ice ages and periods of interglacial warming.[2] Minor seasonal and annual fluctuations are associated with many intervening variables that make weather forecasting the most inexact of all sciences.

Recently a consensus has developed among scientists in the relevant disciplines that human activity is adversely affecting the earth's climate.[3] Moreover, there is compelling evidence that human activity is changing the biosphere in other ways besides climate. The changes represent a new scale of human impact on the world quite unlike anything in recorded history.[4] Collectively the changes endanger health and future prospects for many other living creatures. Global warming and stratospheric ozone depletion have attracted the most attention, but the changes go beyond these two processes.

The term **global change** encompasses several interconnected phenomena[5]: global warming ("climate change"); stratospheric ozone attenuation; resource depletion; species extinction and reduced biodiversity; serious forms of widespread environmental pollution; desertification; macro- and microchanges in the ecosystem, including some that have led to emergence or reemergence of dangerous pathogens (Table 11–1 and Box 11–1). These phenomena are mostly associated with industrial processes or are due to the increased pressure of people on fragile ecosystems, or both.[6] All are interconnected and several are synergistic—some processes reinforce others.

TABLE 11–1. **Health-Related Features of Global Change**

Feature	Quality of Evidence	Impact
Global warming Climate change Sea level rise Heat waves, etc.	Fair to good: based on models and empirical observation	Entire world
Ozone depletion UV radiation increase	Good: based on observations	Entire world
Resource depletion Fresh water Food supplies	Fair to good	Hits developing countries hardest
Environmental pollution	Good, but health impacts not always firmly linked to pollutants	Mainly regional, e.g., Eastern Europe, Former Soviet Union, industrializing nations
Demographic changes Population growth Migration Aging	Good, but many details based on estimates	Developing countries, especially Africa
Emerging, reemerging pathogens	Good	Varies; human immunodeficiency virus and some others global, some are regional
Other factors: Rise of transnational corporations, advances in technology, communication, political volatility, religious fundamentalism, regional conflicts	Fair to good	Mainly regional, but some are global

Underlying all forms of global change, indeed part of it, is a population explosion. In little more than the length of an average lifetime, the population has quadrupled, from about 1.6 billion in 1900 to an estimated 6.4 billion by the year 2000.[7] It is not clear whether our numbers have already reached or even exceeded the earth's carrying capacity; but responsible opinion inclines to the view that we have reached the limits for comfortable human existence. The earth might sustain many millions more than the present number, but life for all but a very small minority would be of greatly diminished quality, and long-term sustainablity would be at best a precarious possibility.[8] Not only are numbers increasing at an unprecedented rate, people are moving around in the world on a scale never seen before, and this too is part of global change.

Every health-related component of global change merits discussion; I also mention some of the complex interconnections among them in this

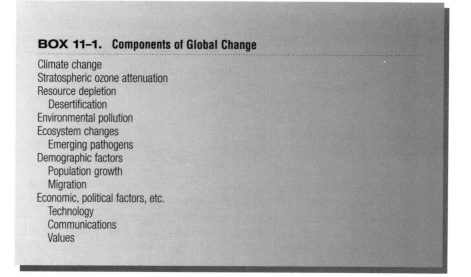

BOX 11–1. Components of Global Change

Climate change
Stratospheric ozone attenuation
Resource depletion
   Desertification
Environmental pollution
Ecosystem changes
   Emerging pathogens
Demographic factors
   Population growth
   Migration
Economic, political factors, etc.
   Technology
   Communications
   Values

brief account. Readers are urged to consult the sources I cite. The demographic, human health, social, economic, and other impacts of global change have been the subject of many important reports.[9,10] There are some obvious actions we should take to enhance readiness to deal with public health aspects of global change, and there are implications for public policy generally.

▶ CLIMATE CHANGE

Some evidence on the causes and consequences of climate change was published by the Intergovernmental Panel on Climate Change (IPCC) in 1990[11,12] and in supplementary reports and other documents. The situation is described and discussed in greater detail in the Second Assessment Report of IPCC, *Climate Change 1995, Impacts, Adaptations and Mitigation of Climate Change; Scientific-Technical Analysis.*[13] Much of the information in this chapter is taken from that report, and from *Climate Change and Human Health,*[14] a more detailed discussion of the health-related aspects of climate change, also published in 1996. There have been many other reports: by national governments,[15] in scientific articles,[16] and in reports, books, and articles produced by nongovernmental organizations such as the Union of Concerned Scientists,[17] Friends of the Earth, the Worldwatch Institute,[18] and the Sierra Club.

In the late 1980s, when concerns about global warming and other aspects of global change began to attract widespread public interest, some contrary views and rebuttals were published,[19,20] sometimes, but not always, sponsored by organizations that opposed actions aimed at mitigating global change. Others have expressed doubts because the current prognostic consensus might turn out to be like past climatic predictions which have often been wrong or misguided.[21] But as the empirical evidence mounted that global climate change is already occurring, these contrary views have become more muted. It is difficult at the end of 1996 to find a prominent scientist who is willing to contest the conclusions about climate change derived from the available evidence.

▶ GLOBAL WARMING

Svante Arrhenius recognized in 1896 that the earth's atmosphere acts like a greenhouse, allowing passage of short-wavelength solar radiation into the biosphere, trapping longer-wavelength infrared radiation. Without the greenhouse effect the earth's surface temperature would swing from over 50°C in strong sunlight to −40°C at dawn. The concentration of greenhouse gases in the troposphere has risen rapidly since the beginning of the industrial era because several of these gases, notably carbon dioxide, are products of fossil fuel combustion and other human activities (Table 11–2). Industrial activity and the combustion of petroleum fuels in automobiles have increased exponentially since the 1950s, accelerated by industrial and commercial development in India, China, South Korea, Taiwan, Indonesia, Thailand, Brazil, Mexico and other countries. Currently about 6 billion metric tons of carbon dioxide, the principal greenhouse gas, are added to the troposphere annually, increasing amounts every year (Fig. 11–1). This is despite promises made by most national leaders at the United Nations (UN) Conference on Environment and Development (UNCED)[22] in Rio de Janeiro in 1992 to stabilize carbon emissions at or below 1990 levels. No nation on earth has deliv-

TABLE 11–2. A Sample of Greenhouse Gases Influenced by Human Activities

	CO_2	CH_4	N_2O	CFC-11	HCFC-22	CF_4
Preindustrial concentration	280 ppmv	700 ppbv	275 ppbv	0	0	0
Concentration in 1994	358 ppmv	1720 ppbv	312[a] ppbv	268[a] pptv	110 pptv	72[a] pptv
Rate of change in concentration[b]	1.5 ppmv/yr 0.4%/yr	10 ppbv/yr 0.6%/yr	0.8 ppbv/yr 0.25%/yr	0 pptv/yr 0%/yr	5 pptv/yr 5%/yr	1.2 pptv/yr 2%/yr
Atmospheric lifetime (yr)	50–200[c]	12[d]	120	50	12	50 000

[a] Estimated from 1992–1993 data.
[b] The growth rates for CO_2, CH_4 and N_2O are averaged over the decade beginning 1984; halocarbon growth rates are based on recent years (1990s).
[c] No single lifetime for CO_2 can be defined because of the different rates of uptake by different sink processes.
[d] This is adjusted to take into account the indirect effect of methane on its own lifetime.
(Source: Intergovernmental Panel on Climate Change, 1996a.)

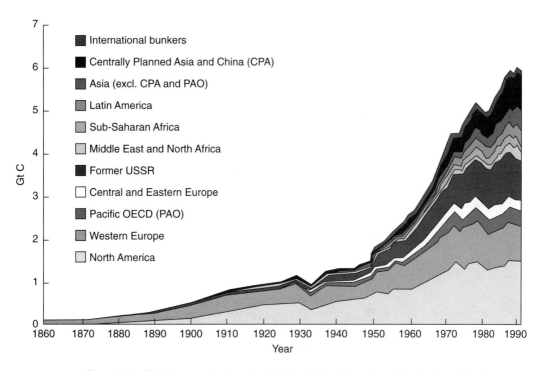

Figure 11–1. Global energy-related carbon dioxide emissions by major world region in gt C/yr. *(Source: IPCC, 1996, with permission.)*

ered on commitments to reduce greenhouse gas emissions to at least 1990 levels by the year 2000. In the United States and Canada, emission rates have continued to rise at a higher rate each year since 1992. Moreover, tropical rain forests, that are among the most important carbon sinks are being rapidly depleted, often by slashing-and-burning, which adds even more carbon gases to the greenhouse. Phytoplankton, another important carbon sink, are damaged by increased ultraviolet radiation (UVR) flux resulting from depletion of stratospheric ozone, an example of reinforcement of one form of global change by another. When they signed the 1995 Framework Convention on Climate Change, most national leaders reiterated their earlier promises, but none has acted yet to do so. The 1995 IPCC reports add a sense of urgency to the need for action.

In 1995, the atmospheric concentration of carbon dioxide reached a higher level than at any time in the last 140,000 years, and the average ambient atmospheric temperature was the highest since record keeping began[23] (Fig. 11–2). It is estimated by global climate models, using a variety of methods, that the average global ambient temperature will rise by about 0.5°C in the first half of the 21st century and may rise 2°C by 2100.[2] These are conservative estimates; and these are *average* global temperatures; the increase, and seasonal and diurnal swing, are expected to be greater, as much as 6 to 8

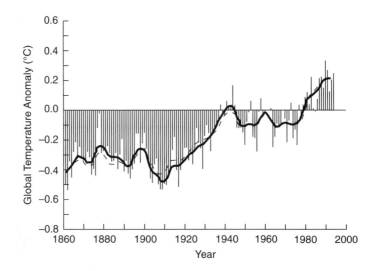

Figure 11–2. Global average temperature trends. *(Source: IPCC, 1996a, with permission.)*

degrees Celsius in temperate zones and perhaps even more near the poles. If arctic permafrost thaws as a result, a great deal of methane would be released, adding to the existing burden of atmospheric greenhouse gases and accelerating the warming process.

Global warming has direct and indirect and predominantly adverse effects on health (Fig. 11–3).

Heat-wave deaths are dramatic and obvious. In 1995, there were severe heat waves in the United States, notably in Chicago where several hundred people died[24]; they were mostly frail elderly people living alone in poor-quality housing and they lacked air conditioning. Larger numbers died in the Punjab and Uttar Pradesh in India, and in several cities in China. The death toll in heat waves is inevitably higher in crowded Asian cities because only small proportions of wealthy people have air conditioning. The total numbers affected, however, are relatively small compared to those affected by other consequences of global warming.

Vector-borne diseases can be expected to threaten scores, even hundreds of millions, of people in a warmer world. Increased average ambient temperate extend the range, distribution, and abundance of insect vectors such as mosquitoes, allow the pathogens they carry to breed more rapidly, and may enhance their virulence. Rainfall patterns are changing, too, so many regions will be not only warmer but wetter and will thus provide optimal breeding conditions for many insect vectors, especially mosquitoes. Because of these changes, malaria is expected to become prevalent in temperate zones and at altitudes in tropical and subtropical regions from which it is now absent, notably large highland cities in East Africa (Nairobi, Lusaka, Harare, Soweto, etc.). There will be tens of millions more at risk of malaria

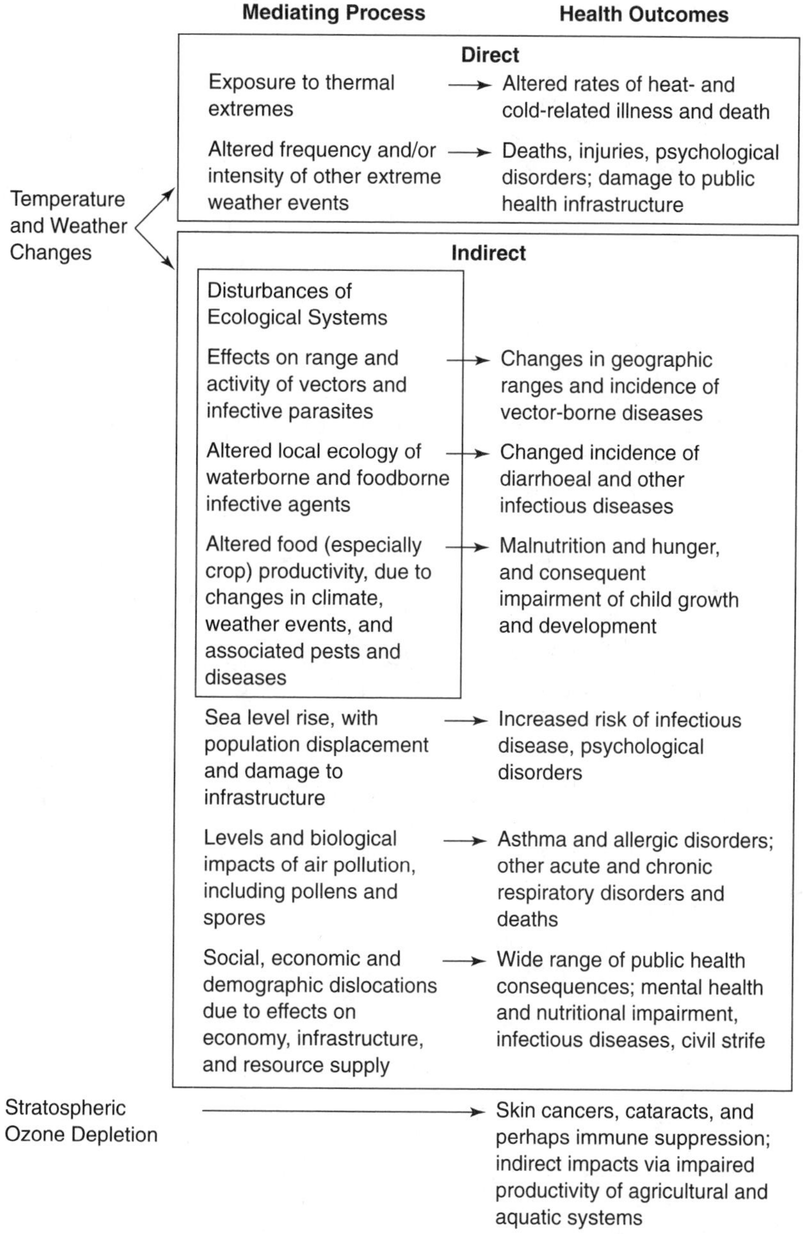

Mediating Process   **Health Outcomes**

Temperature and Weather Changes

Direct

Exposure to thermal extremes → Altered rates of heat- and cold-related illness and death

Altered frequency and/or intensity of other extreme weather events → Deaths, injuries, psychological disorders; damage to public health infrastructure

Indirect

Disturbances of Ecological Systems

Effects on range and activity of vectors and infective parasites → Changes in geographic ranges and incidence of vector-borne diseases

Altered local ecology of waterborne and foodborne infective agents → Changed incidence of diarrhoeal and other infectious diseases

Altered food (especially crop) productivity, due to changes in climate, weather events, and associated pests and diseases → Malnutrition and hunger, and consequent impairment of child growth and development

Sea level rise, with population displacement and damage to infrastructure → Increased risk of infectious disease, psychological disorders

Levels and biological impacts of air pollution, including pollens and spores → Asthma and allergic disorders; other acute and chronic respiratory disorders and deaths

Social, economic and demographic dislocations due to effects on economy, infrastructure, and resource supply → Wide range of public health consequences; mental health and nutritional impairment, infectious diseases, civil strife

Stratospheric Ozone Depletion → Skin cancers, cataracts, and perhaps immune suppression; indirect impacts via impaired productivity of agricultural and aquatic systems

Figure 11–3. Possible major types of climate change and stratospheric ozone depletion on human health. (*Source: McMichael AJ, Haines A, Sloof R, et al.[14]*)

annually in Indonesia and other populous South and Southeast Asian nations. Many other tropical and subtropical vector-borne diseases could increase in incidence, prevalence, and probably in severity and mortality (Table 11–3). In the Americas, the incidence and probably mortality rates of several arbovirus diseases are expected to rise. The threat is worsened by the introduction of new vector species; *Aedes albopictus,* a hardy culicine mosquito, entered the southern United States in the early 1980s in a consignment of used automobile tires imported for retreading; it rapidly proliferated. It is an ideal vector for arbovirus diseases including hemorrhagic dengue and viral encephalitis.

Warmer climates favor agricultural pests, including fungus diseases, weeds, and many insects. Weeds would probably benefit more than cereal crops in a carbon-dioxide–rich environment, and both fungus diseases and insects would be more difficult to control because they reproduce more rapidly in warm environments. This is one of several ways in which global warming threatens food security.[25]

TABLE 11–3. Major Tropical Vector-Borne Diseases and the Likelihood of Change of Their Distribution with Climate Change

Disease	Vector	Population at Risk (million)	Number of People Currently Infected or New Cases per Year	Present Distribution	Likelihood of Altered Distribution with Climate Change
Malaria	Mosquito	2400	300–500 million	Tropics/Subtropics	+++
Schistosomiasis	Water snail	600	200 million	Tropics/Subtropics	++
Lymphatic filariasis	Mosquito	1094	117 million	Tropics/Subtropics	+
African trypanosomiasis (sleeping sickness)	Tsetse fly	55	250,000–300,000 cases per year	Tropical Africa	+
Dracunculiasis (guinea worm disease)	Crustacean (Copepod)	100	100,000 per year	South Asia/ Arabian Peninsula/ Central-West Africa	?
Leishmaniasis	Phlebotomine sandfly	350	12 million infected, 500,000 new cases per year[f]	Asia/Southern Europe/Africa/ Americas	+
Onchocerciasis (river blindness)	Blackfly	123	17.5 million	Africa/Latin America	++
American trypanosomiasis (Chagas' disease)	Triatomine bug	100	18 million	Central and South America	+
Dengue	Mosquito	1800	10–30 million per year	All tropical countries	++
Yellow fever	Mosquito	450	<5000 cases per year	Tropical South America and Africa	++

+ = likely, ++ = very likely, +++ = highly likely, ? = unknown.
(Source: McMichael AJ, Haines A, Sloof R, et al.[14])

Vegetation changes as the climate gets warmer. Among other consequences of this, several varieties of allergenic weeds may flourish in regions where they are now rare or nonexistent. This is expected to aggravate allergic respiratory diseases and may be partly responsible for the increasing prevalence of asthma.

The indirect effects of global warming include a sea-level rise of up to 50 cm by the year 2050, resulting from melting of polar and alpine ice caps and thermal expansion of the seawater mass. This could disrupt many coastal ecosystems, jeopardize coastal and perhaps some ocean fisheries, salinate river estuaries that are an important source of drinking water, and displace scores of millions of people from low-lying coastal regions in many parts of the world, including the Netherlands, Bangladesh, much of South China, parts of Japan, and small island states (Vanuatu, the Maldives, etc.), which face inundation and obliteration. As many as 20 to 25 million people along the eastern seaboard of the United States may be affected, mainly by salination of subsurface aquifers rather than by sea-level rise per se, although this would be a factor along seacoasts from north of Cape Hatteras to Florida. Many of those displaced are likely to become "environmental refugees" in third-world megacities or drift into urban squalor in the rich industrial nations. Sea-level rise during the 21st century could have adverse consequences for people in some of the largest cities and human settlements on earth. Up to half a billion people worldwide, now living at or very close to sea level on coastal plains and river estuaries, are at risk.

Another effect of global climate change with implications for human health is anomalous weather events, in particular more frequent and severe weather emergencies such as catastrophic floods, hurricanes and tornadoes, and heat waves. Atmospheric physicists and climatologists believe some unusual weather events in the 1986–1995 decade may be attributable to global climate change. These anomalous weather events have already extracted a heavy financial toll from the insurance industry and from national disaster funds in the United States and elsewhere (Table 11–4). They have both direct and indirect health impacts. Floods often disable sewage treatment and water purification plants, thus increasing the risk of fecal-oral transmission of pathogens. Disruption of people's homes, families, jobs, and lives as a result of floods and hurricanes can have serious and lasting psychologic consequences.[26]

The impact of global warming on food security could be very serious; here the interconnection of global warming with resource depletion and desertification is important. Global warming could jeopardize the viability of crops in some of the world's most important grain-growing regions because it will alter rainfall patterns and soil moisture levels and hasten desertification of marginal grazing and agricultural land. This has already happened in much of the West African Sahel, parts of northeast Brazil, and elsewhere in Africa (Ethiopia, Sudan, Angola, Zimbabwe, etc.). An increase in surface-level UVR flux, discussed below, will make matters worse if it impairs plant re-

TABLE 11–4.   Insured Losses from "Billion Dollar" Storm Events Since 1987

Year	Event	Insured Loss (billions of dollars)
1987	"Hurricane" (S.E. England, Brittany)	2.5
1988	Hurricane Gilbert (Jamaica, Mexico)	0.8
1989	Hurricane Hugo (Puerto Rico, South Carolina)	5.8
1990	European storms (4 total)	10.4
1991	Typhoon Mireille (Japan)	4.8
1992	Hurricane Andrew (Florida)	16.5
1993	"Storm of the Century" (Eastern United States)	1.7
1994	Winter storms in Germany	2.0

Source: Watson RT, Zinyowera MC, Moss RH, et al. (eds): Climate Change 1995—Impacts, Adaptations and Mitigation of Climate Change: Scientific-Technical Analysis. Cambridge: Cambridge University Press, 1996. (Contributions of Working Group II to the Second Assessment Report of the IPCC.)

production or growth. Predictions are difficult when so many variables are involved, but the models developed by agronomists suggest that while some grain crops might benefit from warmer climate and higher levels of atmospheric carbon dioxide, the overall impact is likely to be a decline in world grain crop production[27] (Table 11–5).

Desertification is made worse by unsound and inappropriate agricultural methods. The "green revolution" that dramatically increased agricultural output in the 40 years following the end of World War II is over: Many forms of agricultural output have remained stationary or have declined in the past 5 to 10 years, raising troubling questions about the earth's carrying capacity.

Global warming is the principal if not the only cause of the retreat of alpine glaciers that has been observed since the late 19th century. Eventually this could reduce the ice-melt component of many river systems that contribute by irrigation or seasonal flooding to productivity of food-producing regions. The deficit would be partly compensated by increased rainfall, but in the long term, river flow will decline. Shortages of fresh water for irrigation and drinking may prove to be the most critical limiting factor on further population growth in many parts of the world.

▶ STRATOSPHERIC OZONE ATTENUATION

In 1974, Rowland and Molina, two atmospheric physicists, predicted that chlorofluorocarbons (CFCs), a widely used class of chemicals, would permeate the upper atmosphere where they would break down under the influence of solar radiation to produce chlorine monoxide.[28] Chlorine monoxide destroys ozone; each molecule of chlorine monoxide is capable of destroying over 10,000 ozone molecules. Rowland and Molina were awarded the Nobel Prize for Physics in 1995 in recognition of their work. Other atmospheric

TABLE 11–5. Selected Crop Study Results for 2 × CO_2-Equivalent Equilibrium GCM Scenarios

Region	Crop	Yield Impact (%)	Comments
Latin America	Maize	−61 to increase	Data are from Argentina, Brazil, Chile, and Mexico; range is across GCM scenarios, with and without CO_2 effect.
	Wheat	−50 to −5	Data are from Argentina, Uruguay, and Brazil; range is across GCM scenarios, with and without CO_2 effect.
	Soybean	−10 to +40	Data are from Brazil; range is across GCM scenarios, with CO_2 effect.
Former Soviet Union	Wheat Grain	−19 to +41 −14 to +13	Range is across GCM scenarios and region, with CO_2 effect.
Europe	Maize	−30 to increase	Data are from France, Spain, and northern Europe; with adaptation and CO_2 effect; assumes longer season, irrigation efficiency loss, and northward shift.
	Wheat	increase or decrease	Data are from France, U.K., and northern Europe; with adaptation and CO_2 effect; assumes longer season, northward shift, increased pest damage, and lower risk of crop failure.
	Vegetables	increase	Data are from U.K. and northern Europe; assumes pest damage increased and lower risk of crop failure.
North America	Maize	−55 to +62	Data are from U.S. and Canada; range is across GCM scenarios and sites, with/without adaptation and with/without CO_2 effect.
	Wheat	−100 to +234	
	Soybean	−96 to +58	Data are from U.S.; less severe or increase with CO_2 and adaptation.
Africa	Maize	−65 to +6	Data are from Egypt, Kenya, South Africa, and Zimbabwe; range is over studies and climate scenarios, with CO_2 effect.
	Millet	−79 to −63	Data are from Senegal; carrying capacity fell 11–38%.
	Biomass	decrease	Data are from South Africa; agrozone shifts.
South Asia	Rice	−22 to +28	Data are from Bangladesh, India, Philippines, Thailand, Indonesia, Malaysia, and Myanmar; range is over GCM scenarios, with CO_2 effect; some studies also consider adaptation.
China	Rice	−78 to +28	Includes rain-fed and irrigated rice; range is across sites and GCM scenarios; genetic variation provides scope for adaptation.
Other Asia and Pacific Rim	Rice	−45 to +30	Data are from Japan and South Korea; range is across GCM scenarios; generally positive in north Japan and negative in south.
	Pasture	−1 to +35	Data are from Australia and New Zealand; regional variation.
	Wheat	−41 to +65	Data are from Australia and Japan; wide variation, depending on cultivar.

Note: For most regions, studies have focused on one or two principal grains. These studies strongly demonstrate the variability in estimated yield impacts among countries, scenarios, methods of analysis, and crops, making it difficult to generalize results across areas or for different climate scenarios.
CO_2 = carbon dioxide; GCM = Global Climate Model; U.K. = United Kingdom; U.S. = United States.
Source: Watson RT, Zinyowera MC, Moss RH, et al. (eds): Climate Change 1995—Impacts, Adaptations and Mitigation of Climate Change: Scientific-Technical Analysis. Cambridge: Cambridge University Press, 1996. (Contributions of Working Group II to the Second Assessment Report of the IPCC.)

contaminants that destroy stratospheric ozone include other halocarbons and perhaps oxides of nitrogen, e.g., in exhaust emissions of high-flying supersonic jet aircraft. Volcanic eruptions sometimes release chlorine compounds into the atmosphere, so natural as well as human-induced processes can contribute to stratospheric ozone attenuation.

Rowland and Molina's predictions soon began to come true. In 1985, Farman and others observed extensive attenuation (a "hole") in the stratospheric ozone layer over Antarctica during the southern hemisphere spring.[29] This has recurred annually; since 1990 seasonal ozone depletion has been observed in the northern hemisphere too; it is greatest over parts of Siberia and northeastern North America. Stratospheric ozone depletion was correlated with increased surface level UVR flux by Kerr and colleagues at the Canadian Climate Center in 1993.[30] Ozone depletion so far is about 3 to 4 percent of total stratospheric ozone and still increasing annually. Its extent varies regionally and seasonally. In the southern hemisphere spring of 1996, the area affected by stratospheric ozone depletion over Antarctica was greater than ever before and the thinning worse than ever.

The stratospheric ozone layer protects the biosphere from exposure to lethal levels of UVR. The gravity of this progressive loss of stratospheric ozone was recognized almost immediately and led many industrial nations to adopt the Montreal Protocol, calling for a moratorium on manufacture and use of CFCs.[31] CFCs were widely used as solvents in the manufacture of microprocessors for computers, foaming agents in polystyrene packing, propellants in spray cans, and as Freon gas in air conditioners and refrigerators; their supposed chemical inertness made them a popular choice. But because they are inert they have, on average, an atmospheric half-life of about 100 years, so stratospheric ozone depletion will continue to be a serious problem well into the 22nd century. Stratospheric ozone must not be confused with toxic, surface-level air pollution with ozone that contaminates fumes from some industrial processes or results from the action of sunlight on automobile exhaust fumes ("photochemical smog"). Although this partially protects large urban industrial centers from UVR, it does, of course, have other harmful effects on health.

Stratospheric ozone depletion permits greater amounts of harmful UVR to enter the biosphere, where it has adverse effects on many biologic systems and on human health (Table 11–6). The principal biologic effects of increased UVR are disruption of the reproductive capacity and vitality of small and single-celled organisms, notably phytoplankton at the base of marine food chains, pollen, amphibians' eggs, many insects, and the sensitive growing ends of green leaf plants. These biologic effects could threaten food security at several critical points in marine and terrestrial food chains.

Increased UVR also has direct adverse effects on human health. It increases the risk of ocular cataract, increases the risk of skin cancer, and impairs immune function.

The mechanism for cataract formation is believed to be UV radiation in the wavelength 300 to 380 nm, which disrupts repair processes. Other eye damage associated with sunlight and with UVR includes macular degeneration and pterygium formation.[32]

UVR is a known carcinogen.[33] The risk of both basal cell skin cancer and malignant melanoma is increased by higher levels of exposure to UVR. It is calculated that an average global stratospheric ozone depletion of 10 percent in midlatitudes, if sustained for the next 30 to 40 years (which seems likely)

TABLE 11-6. Adverse Effects of Ultraviolet Radiation

Biologic Effects of Ultraviolet Radiation
  DNA Damage:
    Ecologically important
      Impaired photosynthesis
      Impaired plant growth
      Impaired motility of phytoplankton
    Agriculturally important
      Impaired reproductive capacity
      Damage to nitrogen-fixing soil bacteria
      Impaired plant and animal health

Human Health Effects of Ultraviolet Radiation
  Immunosuppression
    Enhanced susceptibility to infection (epidemics)
    Cancer proneness
  Dermatologic
  Sunburn
    Loss of elasticity (Premature aging)
    Photosensitivity
  Neoplasia
    Melanocytic (malignant melanoma)
    Squamous and basal cell cancer
    ? Cancer of the lip
  Ocular
    Cataract
    ? Pterygium

will lead to approximately 250,000 additional cases per annum of non-melanoma skin cancer.[34] Similar calculations have not been made for malignant melanoma, but case-control studies have established evidence for a dose-response relationship as well as an increased risk associated with episodes of acute sunburn.[35] Another effect of UVR on skin is "premature aging"—wrinkles and skin creases that are due to loss of elasticity.

The damage to the immune system is due to the effect of UVR on Langerhans cells in the dermis, an essential component in cell-mediated immunity (see Chap. 4). This effect has been demonstrated in experimental animals and confirmed in humans.[36] One possible consequence that has been suggested but not confirmed is that herd immunity could be jeopardized. Routine immunizations might be less effective, and naturally acquired immunity might also be impaired. Either of these processes would increase the risk of spread of epidemic infections. At a time when vector-borne disease can be expected to extend into new territories and when migrations, short-term international travel movements, and shifting refugee populations, among other factors, all favor the spread of epidemic infections, impaired herd immunity could have serious consequences.

▶ RESOURCE DEPLETION

The more people there are, the greater the stress on finite and scarce resources. Two resources are essential for survival: fresh water for drinking and irrigation and food. Water shortages in some parts of the world are associated with conflicts, and in the next 50 years as the shortages spread to other countries and regions, these conflicts probably will be exacerbated (Table 11–7). Threats to water security are a primary cause of some of the most intractable conflicts in the world.[37] The IPCC "Summary for Policymakers" suggests that water shortage will be an important limiting factor on future population growth and economic development in some regions, notably much of the Middle East, southern Africa, parts of Brazil, and the Southwest of the United States.[38] Sea-level rise that is due to global warming and salination of river estuaries and water tables close to seacoasts will threaten some of the largest human settlements on earth such as Tokyo, Shanghai, Calcutta, Bombay, Jakarta, Lagos, among others, with 1995 populations of 10 million or more. There will be much population movement away from coastal zones that are now at, or only just above, sea level. Not only will some of this inhabited land be below sea level, its freshwater supplies will be compromised by

TABLE 11–7. Per Capita Water Availability (m³/year, per cap) in 2050

Country	1990	No Climate Change–2050	GFDL 2050	UKMO 2050	MPI 2050
Cyprus	1280	770	470	180	1100
El Salvador	3670	1570	210	1710	1250
Haiti	1700	650	840	280	820
Japan	4430	4260	4720	4800	4480
Kenya	640	170	210	250	210
Madagascar	3330	710	610	480	730
Mexico	4270	2100	1740	1980	2010
Peru	1860	880	830	690	1020
Poland	1470	1200	1160	1150	1140
Saudi Arabia	310	80	60	30	140
South Africa	1320	540	500	150	330
Spain	2850	2680	970	1370	1660

1) Assumptions about population growth are from the Intergovernmental Panel on Climate Change (IPCC) IS92a scenario based on the World Bank (1991) projections; the climate data are from the IPCC WGII TSU climate scenarios (based on transient model runs of Geophysics Fluid Dynamics Laboratory [GFDL], Max-Planck Institute [MPI] and United Kingdom Meteorological Office [UKMO]).
2) The results show that in all developing countries with high rate of population growth, future "per capita" water availability will decrease independently of the assumed climate scenario.
(Source: IPCC, 1996.)

seepage of seawater into subsurface aquifers; many heavily populated river es-tuaries will thus lose much of their carrying capacity. Desertification of graz-ing lands and marginal cultivated agricultural land would further threaten food security.

Another critical limiting factor is shortage of ocean and coastal fish stocks. This was seen in the early 1990s in dramatic form in the collapse of many of the world's ocean fisheries, mainly resulting from irresponsible over-fishing; but it was aggravated by changes in marine ecosystems accompanying disappearance of coastal wetlands, disruption of river outflows by massive dams (e.g., the Aswan High Dam), pollution with chemicals, oil spills, etc. Fish provide about 20 to 25 percent of human protein needs, considerably more in coastal-dwelling populations in South and Southeast Asia. It is not clear where replacement protein will come from.[39]

Other factors influencing the abundance of marine harvests include changes in ocean temperature and flow of currents such as El Niño, which can affect marine ecology in several ways. Fish harvests decline precipitously when there is a toxic algal bloom that kills off the fish or drives them to re-gions beyond the range of inshore fishermen.

Another effect of the El Niño southern oscillation of the late 1980s and early 1990s was associated with proliferation of zooplankton that feed on al-gae. These provided a symbiotic haven for cholera vibrio that had been intro-duced to the Pacific coast of South America in water used as ballast in ships from the Indian subcontinent. The consequence of this combination of events—global trade patterns, oceanic current fluctuation and warmer coastal seas, and symbiosis of cholera vibrio with algae and zooplankton—was a massive epidemic of cholera with over 300,000 cases in Peru, Ecuador, and the Pacific coast of Colombia.[40]

Shortage of energy in industrializing nations, especially India and China, is another form of resource depletion that adds further damaging factors to the complex pattern of events that I am describing. Rising energy needs in these industrializing nations have led to greatly increased and often ineffi-cient combustion of low-grade coal, which not only adds to the burden of greenhouse gases but causes considerable health-harming atmospheric pollu-tion. Energy production and combustion have diverse impacts on health, ranging from chronic respiratory damage from inhalation of smoke from cooking fires inside inadequately ventilated village huts in the developing world[41] to the after-effects of the Chernobyl nuclear reactor disaster and ill-defined and poorly understood effects of living close to high voltage electric power lines.[42]

▶ SPECIES EXTINCTION AND REDUCED BIODIVERSITY

As a result of human activity, unique animal and plant species are becoming extinct at an accelerating rate. Much of the discussion centers on the loss of species that might have some benefit for humans if they could be studied in detail and their properties exploited, e.g., as anticancer agents. This is a narrow anthropocentric view that considers only the possible direct benefits of biodiversity for humans. Subtle features of biodiversity matter more, especially loss of genetic diversity.[43] It could be hazardous to continue on our present course of increasing reliance on monocultures of high-yielding grain crops. Entire harvests could be wiped out by an epidemic plant disease to which that strain is vulnerable; the same danger may apply to genetically engineered crops. If a genetically diverse crop is struck by plant disease, some strains are likely to survive.

We have long understood that widespread pesticide use on weeds and insects that damage crops kills large numbers of useful arthropod species such as bees, and leads to the death or reproductive failure of many species of birds.[44] Fat-soluble polychlorinated hydrocarbons (polychlorinated biphenyls [PCBs], dioxins, some pesticides) that concentrate as they move through food chains can adversely affect reproductive outcomes, e.g., by causing lethal deformities (some of which might also occur in humans). There has been some concern about human spermatozoa counts[45]; pesticides have been accused of causing this, although the evidence is controversial. We have become aware of the interdependence among many diverse species that share an ecosystem. John Donne's phrase, "No man is an island," applies to the myriad species that share the biosphere; when the bell tolls for amphibia whose eggs are killed by rising UVR flux, or for monarch butterflies that die when their winter habitat disappears, the bell tolls for us all. Destruction of natural ecosystems could have lethal consequences for humans as well as for spotted owls.

▶ DESERTIFICATION

Conversion of marginal agricultural land into desert is a widespread problem. Land that was suitable for light grazing was inappropriately used in attempts to grow crops. Thin soil on mountain slopes that held native vegetation capable of resisting erosion in annual spring snow-melt was cleared and cultivated, leading to rapid erosion—the soil slid down steep mountain slopes leaving only bare rock on which nothing grows. Trees and shrubs have been stripped from arid zone savannah and from many mountain slopes to provide fuelwood, with the same result.[46] Sometimes the climate changed, as in parts of formerly tropical rain forest in Central and South America that have been cleared as grazing land for beef cattle or in attempts to grow wheat or rice. The hydrologic cycle from tropical rain forest to rivers and lakes to clouds that precipitate as heavy rain is disrupted when trees are cut. Within a decade or less, rainfall is reduced, and soil moisture levels decline sharply.[47] The Sahara Desert was at least partly covered with rain forest as recently as 3000 years ago; once the trees were gone, conversion to desert proceeded rapidly and has shown no signs of recovery. Similar processes are at work in many other parts of the world; the consequence is declining potential to produce food. Formerly bountiful land that desertifies can take from a few hundred to a few hundred thousand years to become fertile again.

▶ ENVIRONMENTAL POLLUTION

Environmental pollution can be localized, regional, or global; all forms adversely effect human health and the integrity of the environment (see Chap. 4). Those in the category of "global change" include major environmental disasters and catastrophes: the Chernobyl nuclear accident in the former Soviet Union[48]; massive oil spills in maritime accidents involving supertankers (*Torrey Canyon, Exxon Valdez,* etc.); and insidious permeation of the entire biosphere by stable toxic chemicals that enter and are transmitted from one species to another through marine and terrestrial food chains.

The collapse of the former Soviet Union and its satellites revealed gross environmental destruction that could take many centuries to recover. This has had many adverse effects on health, including occurrence of high levels of birth defects and severe respiratory damage.[49] There are very severe social and emotional costs, too, studied in most detail among people displaced by the Chernobyl nuclear reactor disaster,[50] but observed also among people affected by other long term environmental catastrophes in the former Soviet Union and elsewhere.

Some forms of chemical pollution are global in scope: PCBs, dioxins, and dichlorodiphenyltrichloroethane (DDT), fat-soluble chemicals that travel through food chains, have permeated the entire world. Lead and mercury occur in trace amounts in emissions from coal-burning power generators and ore-smelting plants (which emit other toxic chemicals such as arsenic). The total burden worldwide, falling on land and into the sea, amounts to millions of metric tons annually. Lead and mercury concentration in cormorants' feathers has been assayed in museum specimens prepared by taxidermists before the industrial revolution and compared to present-day levels; modern levels are as much as 1000 to 10,000 times greater than before the industrial revolution.[51] Low-level lead poisoning does long-term, possibly permanent damage to intellectual development.[52] This may have contributed to the fall of the Roman Empire.

▶ DEMOGRAPHIC CHANGES

Underlying all the above features of global change are several aspects of population dynamics. The most obvious is population growth, which since approximately the 1950s has accelerated in an unprecedented surge in much, though not all, of the world.[53] Most western European nations have not experienced this population explosion, and in the former Soviet Union there has been a decline in numbers (and a reduction in life expectancy). Most of the world, including the United States, has had sustained population growth; in parts of Africa, Latin America, and Asia, growth rates have been up to 5 percent per annum, a population doubling time of about 17 years. After many millennia of stable population in the hunter-gatherer era, development of agriculture about 10,000 years ago led to the first surge in population growth and subsequently to slow and generally steady arithmetical increase in numbers. Roughly coinciding with the industrial revolution and European colonization of the Americas and Oceania, another population surge began. Population growth became approximately exponential about 200 years ago, leading to the sharp increase of the last 100 years. This was followed by a hypergeometric population explosion that coincided with, and was probably in part caused by, the "green revolution" and greatly increased agricultural productivity in the two to three decades after World War II (see Fig. 9–2). A crude simplification is that populations expand to meet the available food supply. In the 19th and early 20th centuries, agricultural development led to abundant food; the population expanded to reach the available supply. Some reasons for population growth are complex and controversial and others are simply not understood. Since about the 1950s, the efficacy of public health measures (vaccination, environmental sanitation, oral rehydration therapy, etc.) has played a part, but behavioral factors such as optimism about the future and earlier age at marriage and childbearing may have been equally important. UN population projections show the growth rate declining after the middle of the 21st century, when there will be higher proportions of older people beyond reproductive ages, but these forecasts may be based more on hope than honest expectation (see Fig. 11–4).

As well as increased numbers, unprecedented movements of people have occurred since the late 19th century. Long-term migration has been very large, an estimated 30 to 40 million people from Europe to the Americas and Australia in the period from 1850 to 1910 and perhaps larger undocumented migrations within Asia, e.g., of ethnic Chinese into many parts of Southeast Asia over a longer period.[54] Perpetual wars and widespread political unrest have contributed to migrations, but the main factors have been economic: Many migrants have perceived that their opportunities for work and a good life would be better elsewhere than where they were born and raised.

Rapid urban and industrial growth is an important parallel sociodemographic phenomenon. The proportion of the world's population living in cities will exceed 50% before the year 2000.[55] In rich industrial nations, urban land shortage, real estate values, new building techniques, and personal preferences have led to spectacular growth of high-rise apartment dwelling. In developing nations, movement of people from rural to urban regions is attributable to industrialization, mechanization of agriculture, attraction of rural subsistence farmers and landless peasants to prospects for more lucrative work in cities, and in many countries, flight from oppression by powerful

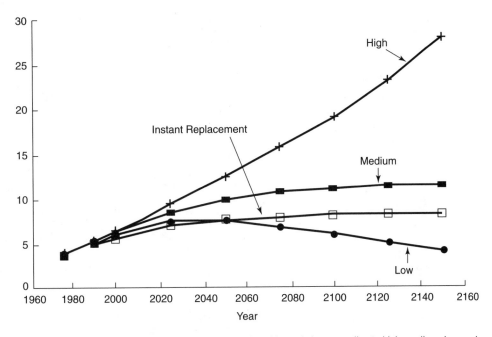

Figure 11–4. United Nations' projections of world population, according to high, medium, low, and instant replacement scenarios. *(Source: Cohen, JE.[53])*

landowners, banditry, or armed conflict. Megacity shantytown slums with populations of 10 million or more have proliferated (Table 11–8); these lack sanitary and other essential services and create an ideal breeding ground for disease and social unrest. This aspect of global change has far-reaching effects on health.

We could regard these migrations as a biological process, a form of tropism that has attracted people toward places where they can grow and develop, away from places where growth and development were inhibited. This perspective comes close to considering humans as a parasitic infestation of the biosphere,[56] a harsh judgment, but one for which there is some empirical support.

Another form of movement with important health implications is international air travel. In the early 1990s, about 600 to 700 million persons per annum traveled by air between countries and continents, on business or pleasure, or for seasonal employment.[57] Rapid air movement allows people who may be incubating serious communicable diseases to travel to destinations where large numbers of people could be susceptible to pathogens introduced in this way.

TABLE 11-8. The World's Twenty-Five Largest Cities, 1995

	Population (millions)	Average Annual Growth Rate 1990–1995 (Percent)
Tokyo, Japan	26.8	1.41
Sao Paulo, Brazil	16.4	2.01
New York, United States	16.3	0.34
Mexico City, Mexico	15.6	0.73
Bombay, India	15.1	4.22
Shanghai, China	15.1	2.29
Los Angeles, United States	12.4	1.60
Beijing, China	12.4	2.57
Calcutta, India	11.7	1.67
Seoul, Republic of Korea	11.6	1.95
Jakarta, Indonesia	11.5	4.35
Buenos Aires, Argentina	11.0	0.68
Tianjin, China	10.7	2.88
Osaka, Japan	10.6	0.23
Lagos, Nigeria	10.3	5.68
Rio de Janeiro, Brazil	9.9	0.77
Delhi, India	9.9	3.80
Karachi, Pakistan	9.9	4.27
Cairo, Egypt	9.7	2.24
Paris, France	9.5	0.29
Manila, Philippines	9.3	3.05
Moscow, Russia	9.2	0.40
Dhaka, Bangladesh	7.8	5.74
Istanbul, Turkey	7.8	3.67
Lima, Peru	7.5	2.81

(Source: United Nations Population Division, 1996.)

► EMERGING AND REEMERGING INFECTIONS

Another way in which the world has changed is the emergence and reemergence of lethal infectious pathogens.[58] The human immunodeficiency virus (HIV) pandemic is the most obvious; since its recognition in the United States in 1981, HIV and acquired immunodeficiency syndrome (AIDS) has rapidly become a worldwide pandemic. All over the world, with variations dependent on ecologic and social themes, circumstances have conspired to facilitate the rapid spread of HIV/AIDS. African nations that were poised in the 1970s for a great developmental leap forward were hit particularly hard: The ranks of urban white-collar workers who engaged in promiscuity have been decimated; men from rural areas who sought work in cities were infected by prostitutes with whom they consorted, leaving widows to die in their turn and a generation of orphans to be reared by grandparents. A similar sequence is unfolding in the Indian subcontinent. In Thailand, village girls who go to Bangkok to earn their dowry by prostitution return instead with HIV disease. In the United States, what was seen originally as a gay white male disease is increasingly often transmitted heterosexually, and as noted elsewhere, attitudes toward sexuality and sex education peculiar to the United States are hindering efforts at control.[59] In western European nations where there is less hypocrisy about human sexuality, control is challenging but at least feasible.

HIV/AIDS is linked to the resurgence of two old plagues, tuberculosis and syphilis, which find fertile soil in immunocompromised hosts and often now are due to resistant strains of pathogens. These three diseases are endemic in megacity slums in the developing world, and in the counterpart of these slums in rich industrial nations among the homeless disenfranchised urban underclass.

Other emerging infections are due to organisms such as Ebola virus, hantavirus, *Borrelia burgdorferi* (Lyme disease), *Legionella pneumophila* (Legionnaires' disease), etc. Others are due to expansion of old diseases like hemorrhagic dengue into regions from which such diseases had been eliminated generations ago, only to return now because of the combination of climate change and the introduction of hardy vector species like *Aedes albopictus*, already described. Some see a deadly combination of rising and shifting populations in periurban slums with no public health services, deteriorating nutritional status that reduces resistance to infection, high levels of UVR flux that impair cell-mediated immunity, antibiotic-resistant pathogens, and pesticide-resistant disease vectors. The stage is set for epidemic, even pandemic disease[60] (see Chap. 3).

Other classes of infections are neither emerging nor reemerging, just different. These are infections caused by very dangerous, sometimes lethal strains of common microorganisms such as the hemolytic streptococcus, which responded well to antibiotics when these first came into use in the 1950s, but have become resistant to all commonly used contemporary antibiotics. This problem merits mention as a feature of global change because it is caused by human-induced changes in microbial ecosystems that are truly global in scope. Antibiotics of all kinds have been used all over the world, often indiscriminately, prescribed for sometimes trivial time-limited conditions like the common cold, and in some countries in South and East Asia and Latin America, readily available without prescription in open market stalls. The same and other antibiotics have been as widely used, and misused, in animal husbandry where the aim is to promote faster and healthier growth of animals intended for slaughter. After innumerable bacterial generations have been exposed to the whole gamut of antibiotics, it is hardly to be wondered at that many bacteria, responding to the inexorable laws of evolution, have bred strains that are impervious to virtually every one of the weapons the microbe-hunters can deploy. This further enhances our vulnerability to epidemics.

► OTHER RELEVANT CHANGES

Important economic, social, industrial, and political factors accompany the above processes and contribute to the difficulty of finding solutions. Global economies have supplanted national and regional ones; transnational corporations owing allegiance to no nation, seemingly driven by the desire for a profitable balance sheet in the next quarterly report, move capital and production from places where obsolete plant and equipment, labor and environmental laws, and political systems may impede them, to countries without these restraining influences to maximize short-term profits.[61]

Political revolts against local and regional taxation have undermined the effectiveness and efficiency of public health and other essential infrastructures in some rich industrial nations, most of all in the United States. For years there have been no new investments, no maintenance, no salary increases (sometimes reductions of pay and benefits), and serious staff reductions in many public health services. A nation that neglects its defenses against dangers to health, such as gastrointestinal disease outbreaks resulting from inadequate food and water safety measures, puts its citizens at greater risk than a nation that fails to maintain defense forces and police services. Unfortunately it could take a major outbreak of a preventable epidemic disease to bring this reality to the attention of enough voters in the United States to prompt a return to saner tax policies.

Television sound bites and irresponsible fragmentary news reporting deprive many people of information that is essential to enable them to make intelligent decisions about such matters as public health services and environmental sustainability. Aspiring political leaders are subjected to character assassination that discourages all but the most mendacious and meretricious from seeking political office and leads many people to regard elected officials with contempt and deters them from voting—a dangerous trend that has the potential for capture of the political agenda by determined single-issue interests such as religious right-wing factions in the United States and neofascists in some European nations.

Almost all those who are elected lack the political courage to make the tough decisions—such as imposing deterrent taxes on fossil fuels—that the state of the world demands if the climatic trends are to be halted before irreversible harm is done. No political leader in the world seems capable of planning with a time horizon of 50 to 100 years. Anyone who tried in a democracy would almost certainly face overwhelming defeat in the next election, because policies such as higher taxes on fossil fuels would be unacceptable to almost all voters.

► PUBLIC HEALTH RESPONSES

Perhaps never before have public health workers and their services faced such challenges as they do now. Actions of several kinds are required (Table

11–9). Some obvious and quite simple measures can be initiated at once, e.g., protection, especially of fair-skinned infants and children, against excessive sun exposure. We need to establish or strengthen our surveillance of insect vectors and the pathogens they can carry.

New research strategies and innovative approaches to research are required. We need to narrow the gap between research and policy. The Health Issues panel of the Canadian Global Change Program surveyed prominent biomedical scientists across Canada in 1993, seeking opinions and advice on

TABLE 11–9. Public Health Responses to Global Change

Monitoring
    Food production and distribution
    Heat-related illnesses
    Migrant and refugee populations

Epidemiologic surveillance
    Water quality
    Vectors, pathogens
    Infectious diseases
        Fecal-oral
        Respiratory
        Vectorborne
    Acute sunburn
    Heat-related illnesses
    Cancer
        Malignant melanoma
        Nonmelanoma skin cancer
        Other cancer
    Cataract

Surveys and Epidemiologic Studies
    Sun-seeking and sun-avoiding behavior
    Attitudes to sustainability
    Case-control and cohort studies of skin cancer
    Cohort and follow-up studies (risk assessment)
    Clinical trials of protective sunscreens, etc.

Public Health Action
    Advisory messages about safe sun exposure
    Standard setting for protective clothing, etc.
    Health education aimed at behavior change
    Health care of migrant groups
    Disaster plans and preparedness

Public Health Policies
    Food and nutrition policies
    Research policies and priorities
        Population studies
        Environmental health research
        Cause-effect relationships
        Transdisciplinary research

what the research priorities should be and what strategies should be used to conduct the necessary research.[62] The priorities were perceived to be *population-related* (health impacts, effects, and mitigation of urbanization, population growth, migration, and crowding); *pollution-related* (health impacts of air and other forms of pollution, global warming, and stratospheric ozone depletion; much of what is required is surveillance and monitoring as well as research); and *behavioral* (stimulating value changes; women's health and birth control). A consensus emerged that we must break out of the reductionist and departmentalized approach to biomedical, behavioral, and social research; we need to form new coalitions among biomedical, behavioral, and social scientists to address our problems in innovative ways. Others have similar thoughts and doubts about the reductionist approach that breaks problems down into many small parts to be tackled by discipline-circumscribed teams.[63]

Effective responses are hampered by many factors. In many public health departments, the decay of infrastructures and erosion of morale as dedicated staff are laid off and salaries frozen or cut have inhibited meaningful efforts to prepare for any but immediate emergencies. Yet some obvious preparations to cope would cost little. Disaster planning must be maintained at a high level of preparedness; nothing is more certain than that there will be more, more frequent, and probably more severe weather emergencies. Large human settlements on floodplains or in places where there can be tidal surges are increasingly vulnerable. Insurance companies have recognized this by reluctance to insure against some natural disasters. Some public health agencies and local government departments have disaster plans, but many do not or have not revised them for many years.

There are many simple actions that public health services can carry out to mitigate the adverse effects of global change on human health. For instance, weather reports now often mention the level of UVR flux and offer advice about sun avoidance.

► GROUNDS FOR OPTIMISM

Faced with the array of problems I have outlined, it would be easy to admit defeat. But there are grounds for optimism about our situation. Humans are robust, a very hardy species: We have demonstrated considerable ability to adapt to a wide range of harsh environments. We are resourceful, intelligent, and often at our best in a crisis. We are now, perhaps, entering the greatest crisis we have ever faced. Its insidious onset has lulled us into complacency, if indeed we think at all about the nature of the global changes that endanger us. There is also an element of denial, akin to the reluctance of a cancer patient to accept the seriousness of the condition or of the risk-taking adolescent to whom death or permanent disability as a result of dangerous behavior is unimaginable.

Epidemiology and other public health sciences can do much to induce greater recognition of the need for changes in values and behavior. Precedents in the history of public health since the second half of the 19th century[64] are encouraging. I described and discussed in Chapter 1 the necessary sequence for control of any public health problem: awareness that the problem exists, understanding what causes it, capability to control it, a sense of values that the problem matters, and political will. All but the last of these exists now. We have the basic scientific evidence that enables us to predict what will happen; empirical evidence to support the predictions is rapidly mounting. Soon it will constitute an incontrovertable body of knowledge and understanding that even the most obtuse self-interested group will be unable to deny or rebut. Increasing numbers of important interest groups, such as the insurance industry and leaders in some resource-based industries, are recognizing the need for action. Increasing numbers of thoughtful people are aware of the need to conserve resources rather than squandering them wantonly as we did in the 1950s and 1960s with many "disposable" products. A few more dramatic disasters resulting from the collapse or major disruption of established weather systems would help to galvanize public opinion and lead to pressure for change that even the most complacent political leaders would be unable to ignore. It is encouraging to recall that when the "Republican revolution" of 1994 led to changes in political priorities, the new Republican majority in the U.S. Congress that had planned to reverse decades of environmental protection were sharply brought to heel by the complaints of their constituents; environmental protection laws and regulations have remained substantially intact. This suggests that the change of values required as a necessary prerequisite for action to mitigate global change is already beginning. It will undoubtedly help if the health impacts of global change are given greater attention in the media. Public health workers and epidemiologists can contribute by emphasizing the health effects of global change and actions needed to minimize their impact.

▶ ENVIRONMENTAL ETHICS AND THE PRECAUTIONARY PRINCIPLE

The change of values that I believe is already underway is leading to recognition of the need to observe a code of conduct for the environment, an ethic of environmental sustainability.[65] Environmental movements are gathering strength in many countries and "green" parties are seen increasingly as respectable and in the mainstream of politics. They are beginning to influence the political agenda despite pressure from powerful industrial and commercial interest groups that have long been able to achieve their ends by control of political decisions. The pressure often comes first from grass-roots levels, perhaps because of a proposal to establish a toxic waste dump or a polluting industry; but its origins may matter less than its increasingly successful efforts to influence the outcome.

Another hopeful sign is recognition of the so-called Precautionary Principle. When there is doubt about the possible environmental harm that may arise from an industrial or commercial development, a nuclear power station, an oil refinery, an opencut coal mine, or other environmentally damaging activities, people and communities who will be most affected are increasingly given the benefit of the doubt because of the Precautionary Principle. This is, of course, the ethical principle of nonmaleficence (see Chap. 10).

► **MITIGATION OPTIONS**

The 1995 IPCC Report discusses several mitigation options (Table 11–10): energy-efficient industrial processes and methods of transportation; reduction of human settlement emissions; sound agricultural conservation and rehabilitation policies; forest management policies and strategies, etc. The Framework Convention on Climate Change that was adopted by most national leaders early in 1996 spells out ways in which industries that contribute heavily to greenhouse gas accumulation can and must change. These changes are not without cost, although experience has often demonstrated that conserving energy, like all other conservation measures, is cost-effective. An obvious change that would benefit all who share the earth is introduction of deterrent taxes that would discourage use of private cars for all but truly essential purposes. Political leaders everywhere are reluctant to enact this unpopular measure and are equally reluctant to spend large capital sums on new or upgraded public transport systems in an era when reducing taxes is what got many of them elected in the first place. This is unlikely to change until a climatic emergency or other environmental crisis forces large numbers to come to their senses and realize that the time for action, rather than rhetoric, has arrived. Public health workers should be preparing to take the initiative in the event of climatic emergencies or environmental crises and should have cogent arguments ready to state the case for action toward environmental sustainability.

Our situation resembles that depicted by the clock on the cover of the *Bulletin of the Atomic Scientists,* with hands pointing to a few minutes before midnight. The analogy is a calendar from which all but a few days near the end of the year have been torn. The imperative need for action is urgent.

Human actions have caused the interconnected phenomena of global change that collectively present unprecedented threats to human health and well-being. Effective countermeasures will require intervention on an almost superhuman scale. Fundamental changes in human values and human behavior are essential prerequisites.

We can prevail if there is widespread, indeed virtually universal, recognition that our present actions threaten our own and our descendents' prospects for survival; if we desist from unsustainable "development" policies and actions; if we adopt nurturing, conserving behaviors, recognizing that all

TABLE 11–10. Mitigation Options

Energy supply
Reduce greenhouse emissions:
  Efficient conversion
  Suppress emissions
  Decarbonize fuels
  Switch to nuclear fuel
  Switch to renewable sources of energy

Industry
Technical abatement options:
  Fuel substitution (low carbon, electric, renewable, hydrogen fuel, energy-efficient fuel, etc.)
Policy options:
  Fostering technology transfer
  Energy audits
  Technical innovations through research and development
  Recycling, etc.

Transportation
Reducing emissions
  Energy-intensive innovations
  Alternative fuels
Transport policy shifts

Human settlements
Residential buildings
  Space conditioning (heating, cooling)
  Water heating, lighting, cooking, appliances
  Potential for residential energy savings
Commercial buildings
  Space conditioning
  Lighting, heating, office equipment, etc.
  Potential for energy savings

Community-level
  Reducing heat islands
  Methane emissions from waste dumps

Policy options for buildings, heat islands, etc.

Agricultural and forestry options
  Carbon dioxide, methane, etc. abatement
  Conservation, reforestation, etc.

of us must make some concessions to the reality of finite resources in a finite world. We must acknowledge that global ecosystems are mortally sick; and if these ecosystems fail and die, so will we all. If we all work together, our beautiful blue planet will go on spinning with the rich and wonderful diversity of life that makes life worth living.

► **REFERENCES**

1. Tudge C: *The Time Before History.* New York: Scribner's, 1996.
2. Eddy JA: *Climate and the role of the sun.* In Rotberg RI, Rabb TK (eds): Climate and History. Princeton, NJ: Princeton University Press, 1981, pp. 145–167.
3. Houghton JT, Filho LGM, Callander BA, et al. (eds): *Climate Change 1995—the Science of Climate Change.* Cambridge: Cambridge University Press, 1996. (Vol. 1 of the *Report of the Intergovernmental Panel on Climate Change*).
4. McMichael AJ: The health of persons, populations and planets. Epidemiology comes full circle. *Epidemiology* 6:633–636, 1995.
5. *Canadian Global Change Program.* Ottawa: Royal Society of Canada, 1992.
6. McMichael AJ: *Planetary Overload; Global Environmental Change and the Health of the Human Species.* Cambridge: Cambridge University Press, 1993.
7. *Annual Population Statistics and Projections.* New York: UN Statistical Office, 1995.
8. Cohen JE: *How Many People Can the Earth Support?* New York: Norton, 1995.
9. *Our Planet, Our Health; Report of the WHO Commission on Health and Environment.* Geneva: WHO, 1992; with Annexes on *Food and Agriculture, Energy, Urbanization,* and *Industry.*
10. See, for example, Silver CS, DeFries RS (eds): *One Earth, One Future.* Washington, DC: National Academy Press, 1990; and Yoda S (ed): *Trilemma; Three Major Problems Threatening the World Survival.* Report of the Committee for Research on Global Problems. Tokyo: Central Research Institute of Electric Power Industry, 1995.
11. Intergovernmental Panel on Climate Change: *Scientific Assessment of Climate Change, a Report by Working Group I.* Geneva: WHO and UNEP, 1990.
12. Intergovernmental Panel on Climate Change: *Impact Assessment; A Report to IPCC from Working Group II:* Canberra: Australian Government Printing Office, 1990.
13. Watson RT, Zinyowera MC, Moss RH, et al. (eds): *Climate Change 1995—Impacts, Adaptations and Mitigation of Climate Change: Scientific-Technical Analysis.* Cambridge: Cambridge University Press, 1996. (Contributions of Working Group II to the Second Assessment Report of the IPCC.)
14. McMichael AJ, Haines A, Sloof R, et al. (eds): *Climate Change and Human Health.* Geneva: WHO, WMO, UNEP, 1996.
15. Government-sponsored scientific committees in the United Kingdom, the Netherlands, Canada, Sweden, Australia have all produced multiple reports since approximately 1985. In the United States, the National Academy of Sciences has produced several reports.
16. See Haines A, Fuchs C: Potential impacts on health of atmospheric change. *J Pub Health Med* 13:69–80, 1991; Last JM: Global change; ozone depletion, greenhouse warming and public health. *Annu Rev Pub Health* 14:115–136, 1993.
17. Union of Concerned Scientists: *World Scientists' Warning Briefing Book.* Cambridge, MA: UCS, 1993.
18. Worldwatch Institute: *State of the World.* Washington, DC. (Annual reports since 1985.)
19. Brookes WT: The global warming panic. *Forbes* 144:14:96–102, 1989.
20. Lindzen RS: Some remarks on global warming. *Environ Sci Technol* 24:424–426, 1990.
21. Milne A: *Beyond the Warming.* Sturminster, UK, Prism Press, 1996.

22. United Nations Conference on Environment and Development (the Rio Summit). New York: United Nations, 1992. ("Agenda 21").

23. Patz JA, Epstein PR, Burke TA, et al. Global climate change and emerging infectious diseases. *JAMA* 275:217–223, 1996.

24. Semenza JC, Rubin CH, Falter KH, et al.: Heat-related deaths during the July 1995 heat wave in Chicago. *N Engl J Med* 335:84–90, 1996.

25. Reilly J, Baethgen W, Chege FE, et al.: Agriculture in a changing climate: Impacts and adaptation. In *Climate Change 1995—Impacts, Adaptations and Mitigation Options*. Scientific-Technical Analysis. Cambridge: Cambridge University Press, 1996, pp. 427–467. (Contribution of Working Group II to the Second Assessment Report of IPCC).

26. Duffy JC (ed): *Health and Medical Aspects of Disaster Preparedness.* New York: Plenum, 1990: 14 NATO Series on Challenges of Modern Society.

27. Parry ML, Rosenzweig C: Health and climate change; food supply and risk of hunger. Lancet 342:1345–1347, 1993.

28. Molina MJ, Rowland FS: Stratospheric sink for chloro-fluoro-methanes; chlorine atom-catalyzed destruction of ozone. *Nature* 249:810–814, 1974; see also Rowland FS, Molina MJ: Estimated future atmospheric concentrations of CCl_3F (fluorocarbon-11) for various hypothetical tropospheric removal rates. *J Phys Chem* 80:2049–2056, 1976.

29. Farman JC, Gardiner BG, Shanklin JD: Large losses of total ozone in Antarctica reveal seasonal ClO_x/NO_x interaction. *Nature* 315:207–210, 1985.

30. Kerr JB, McElroy CT: Evidence for large upward trends of ultraviolet-B radiation linked to ozone depletion. *Science* 262:523–524, 1993.

31. United Nations Environmental Programme (UNEP): *Montreal Protocol on Substances That Deplete the Ozone Layer.* Montreal, September 16, 1987.

32. World Health Organization: *The Effects of Solar UV Radiation on the Eye. Report of an Informal Consultation.* Geneva: WHO, 1994.

33. International Agency for Research on Cancer: *Solar and Ultraviolet Radiation.* Lyon, France: IARC, WHO, 1992: 55 IARC Monographs on the Evaluation of Carcinogenic Risks to Humans.

34. United Nations Environmental Programme: *Environmental Effects of Ozone Depletion; 1991 Update.* Nairobi: UNEP, 1991.

35. Elwood JM, Whitehead SM, Gallagher RP: Epidemiology of human malignant skin tumors with special reference to natural and artificial ultraviolet radiation exposures. *Carcinog Compr Surv* 11:55–84, 1989; see also Evans RD, Kopf AW, Lew RA, et al.: Risk factors for the development of malignant melanomas. A review of case-control studies. *J Dermatol Surg Oncol* 14:393–408, 1988.

36. Kripke ML: Ultraviolet radiation and immunology. Something new under the sun. *Cancer Res* 54:6102–6105, 1994.

37. Homer-Dixon TF, Percival V: *Environmental Scarcity and Violent Conflict; Briefing Book.* Washington, DC, and Toronto: AAAS and University of Toronto, 1996.

38. Intergovernmental Panel on Climate Change: *Climate Change 1995; Impacts, Adapatations and Mitigation; Summary for Policymakers.* Geneva: WMO, WHO, UNEP, 1995.

39. Food and Agriculture Organization: *State of the World's Fisheries.* Rome: FAO, 1995. (Annual Report)

40. Epstein PR: Emerging diseases and ecosystem instability: New threats to public health. *Am J Public Health* 85:168–172, 1995.

41. de Koning HW, Smith KR, Last JM: Biomass fuel combustion and health. *Bull World Health Organ* 63:11–26, 1985.

42. WHO Commission on Health and Environment: *Report of the Panel on Energy.* Geneva: WHO, 1992; see also Nakicenovic N, et al.: Energy primer. In Watson RT, Zinyowera MC, Moss RH, et al.: *Climate Change 1995, Cambridge: Cambridge University Press,* 1996, pp. 75–92.

43. Wilson EO: *The Diversity of Life.* Cambridge, MA: Harvard University Press, 1992.

44. Carson R: *Silent Spring.* Boston: Houghton Mifflin, 1962.

45. Colborn T, Myers JP, Dumanoski D: *Our Stolen Future: Are We Threatening Our Own Fertility, Intelligence and Survival? A Scientific Detective Story.* New York: Dutton, 1996 [Although this book is tendentious and poorly researched, it contains enough truthful, disturbing information to be worth glancing at.]

46. Agarwal B: *Cold Hearths and Barren Slopes; The Woodfuel Crisis in the Third World.* London: Zed Books, 1986.

47. Almandares J, Anderson PK, Epstein PR: Critical regions. A profile of Honduras. Lancet 342:1400–1402, 1993.

48. Anderson TW: *Health Problems in Ukraine Related to the Chernobyl Accident.* Washington, DC: World Bank, Natural Resources Management Division, 1992.

49. Herzman C: *Environment and Health in Central and Eastern Europe. A Report for the Environmental Action Programme for Central and Eastern Europe.* Washington, DC: The World Bank, 1995.

50. Marples DR: *The Social Impact of the Chernobyl Disaster.* Edmonton: University of Alberta Press, 1988.

51. Nriagu JO: A history of global metal pollution. *Science* 272:223–26, 1996.

52. Tong S, Baghurst P, McMichael A, et al.: Lifetime exposure to environmental lead and children's intelligence at 11–13 years: The Port Pirie cohort study. *Br Med J* 312:1569–1575, 1996.

53. Cohen JE: *How Many People Can the Earth Support?* New York: Norton, 1995, pp. 25–31.

54. *UN Demographic Yearbooks* and historical demographic records; Brass W: *Historical Demography.* London: Macmillan, 1960; Cohen JE: *How Many People Can the Earth Support?* New York: Norton, 1995.

55. UN Statistical Office, World Bank, and *UN Demographic Yearbooks* give details.

56. Hern WM: Why are there so many of us? Description and diagnosis of a planetary ecopathological process. *Popul Environment* 12:1:9–37, 1990.

57. International Air Transport Authority: *Annual Air Movements Statistics.* Montreal, 1995.

58. Lederberg J: Infection emergent. JAMA 275:243–244, 1996; see also Roizman B (ed): *Infectious Diseases in an Age of Change. The Impact of Human Ecology and Behavior on Disease Transmission.* Washington, DC: National Academy Press 1995; see also Horton R: The infected metropolis. Lancet 347:134–135, 1996.

59. Cates WJr: Contraception, unintended pregnancies and sexually transmitted diseases: Why isn't a simple solution possible? *Am J Epidemiol* 143:311–318, 1996.

60. Garrett L: *The Coming Plague; Newly Emerging Diseases in a World Out of Balance.* New York: Farrar, Straus & Giroux, 1994.

61. Kennedy P: *Preparing for the 21st Century.* New York: Random House, 1993.

62. *Implications of Global Change for Human Health; Final Report of the Health Issues Panel of the Canadian Global Change Program.* Ottawa: Royal Society of Canada, 1995.

63. McMichael AJ, Bolin B, Costanza R, et al.: Sustainable health in a globalizing world: An emerging conceptual shift. Discussion paper no 87. *International Institute of Ecological Economics*. Royal Swedish Academy: Stockholm, 1996.
64. Last J: New pathways in an age of ethical and ecological concern. *Int J Epidemiol* 23:1:1–4, 1994.
65. Schrader-Frechette K: Ethics and the environment. *World Health Forum* 12:3:311–321, 1991.

Epilogue

One of life's ironies is that as my personal future shrinks I become more pre-occupied about the really long-term future. What will the world be like for you, my student reader, when you are my age? What will the world be like for those who come after you?

I belong to the generation that has lived through three-quarters of the 20th century, a period of unprecedented change, of great turbulence and strife, and yet a very exciting time to be alive. Many of the changes in my life-time have improved the human condition. The three that I believe matter most in medicine and health care are the dismantling, in most nations, of economic barriers between sick people and the care they need; feminizing of the medical profession that has infused our calling with renewed values; and advances in medical science and technology that, costly though they may be, make it possi-ble to prevent or treat many conditions that were previously hopeless. Some changes have diminished prospects for a civilized and happy life, for instance nuclear weapons and forces that subvert democracy, such as the growing power of transnational corporations and intolerant religious fundamentalism.

During my lifetime my fellow humans and I have done terrible damage to the earth's life-supporting ecosystems; much of the damage, outlined in the last chapter, is irreparable or at best will take thousands of years to heal. In some countries the evil of ethnic nationalism prevails and people continue to kill each other. There have been countless outbursts of murderous sav-agery among people who have not differed from one another even in lan-guage, let alone in possession or lack of land and worldly goods. There have been almost incessant wars, with rising death rates among noncombatant children and women, and vicious genocides that have caused indescribable suffering for many millions. War and its effects on everyone, especially on in-nocent children and women, are the worst of all public health problems.[1]

The collapse of the Soviet Union and its satellites and the end of the Cold War—events not even imaginable when I wrote the first edition of this book—have reduced the risk that our species will destroy itself and many oth-ers with us; but the threat has not vanished.

Yet the changes for the better outweigh those for the worse. The world has become a global village that can be traversed from end to end in much less time than from one sunrise to the next. Telephones, radio, television, faxes, the Internet and the World Wide Web can put us in instant contact with others anywhere else on earth.

These unprecedented advances in communications technology are not only of immense educational and scientific value, they are also the most pow-erful tool we have ever had to help us understand and get along better with each other.

Ten years ago, in the Epilogue to the first edition, I discussed two dangers facing us, global ecosystem collapse because of our uncontrolled population growth and the ultimate interpersonal violence, destruction of all or most of us in a nuclear war. The risks remain, but the balance has shifted; our world seems more likely to end the way T. S. Eliot[2] suggested, "Not with a bang but a whimper."

This Epilogue, however, is a message of hope. Consider progress in the health sciences since the beginning of the 20th century, or if you prefer, just in the last 10 years. The pace of advances in diagnostics and therapeutics has been stunning. Molecular biology is advancing too rapidly for anyone to keep up with it; in my field, molecular epidemiology, is evolving into a branch of biomedical science. Other biomedical scientists around the world are mapping the human genome, with consequences that will surely be more good than bad. Advances in the science, art, and practice of public health have been less spectacular but nonetheless impressive, and they are often cost-free and subtle, like the shifting values that have reduced, and in some respects eliminated, health-harming behavior.

Recent Advances in Learning Theory and Practice

Other advances are underway. You, my student reader, are the beneficiary of an advance in learning theory and practice. We used to say that a quarter of the knowledge a student acquired in medical school would be obsolete or proved wrong within 10 years (but we couldn't predict which quarter it would be). The numbers have changed: Now it is half of all medical knowledge that has to be reappraised, revised, or discarded, and in 5 years, not 10. Medical schools everywhere have moved in the same direction as the one where I work, scrapping endless hours of lectures and replacing them with problem-based learning, or PBL. A friend who, like me, endured the old way, called that "BBL," or bottom-based learning—learning by the application of the bottom to a seat in an auditorium and being lectured at for as much as 8 hours a day. It took my brain at least 5 years to recover from the damage it suffered in medical school. PBL, in contrast, begins with a real-life problem and challenges you to find out for yourself all that you consider relevant to solve this problem, using whatever means seem most appropriate to do so. Not only is this better than the old way to learn, it is much more fun. We have begun to insist, too, that medical decisions must be based on evidence,[3] not rule of thumb. More and more of the evidence and therefore the solutions to our problems in clinical and preventive medicine can be found at your fingertips and displayed on a computer screen.

Our Wired World

The speed of this explosion in communications technology takes my breath away. One day in December of 1996 I spoke to an audience of about a hundred middle-aged people; they were mostly churchgoing and city-dwelling, not affluent, about half of them with no more than a high school education. I asked how many were "wired"—using the Internet. Only a handful were not. A year or two earlier very few of the people in the room would have understood the question.

The Internet allows instantaneous worldwide communication of important public health information, such as notification of dangerous outbreaks of infectious disease.[4] It is a superb educational tool at every level from kindergarten to advanced postgraduate study. It has been embraced enthusiastically for the continuing professional education of specialist physicians in Canada,[5] Australia, and other countries where distances are great and resources concentrated in a few urban centers. It has equal or greater value as an educational tool in public health and preventive medicine.[6] The World Wide Web, a prodigious interactive information system developed at the high-energy particle physics laboratory near Geneva, Switzerland, expanded from a few thousand web sites in 1993 to over 1.6 million by early 1996. Some of the best web sites are those of the U.S. Centers for Disease Control and Prevention and the World Health Organization. The web is so vast that no one could ever catalogue it, let alone provide a comprehensive list of health-related web sites, but in the Appendix I offer a few to get you started.

I believe I have preserved my youthful enthusiasm and zest for life by an ongoing process of lifelong learning. As I enter my eighth decade I continue to learn as eagerly as I did in my eighth year, if perhaps a little more slowly. All praise be to electronic communication! I have made the revisions for this book in the comfort of my office at home. I have hardly set foot in the medical library except to socialize with colleagues. Seated at my computer I have visited medical libraries and other rich learning resources all over the world, restricted only by my lack of imagination and energy, and unfamiliarity with the key words required to find all, rather than just some, of the information that could have made this book as current as today's newspaper.

Ideas Are Better Than Facts

The book is not, of course, as current as today's newspaper, nor do I want it to be; it does not need to be. There are a great many facts in it, but I mean it to be a book of ideas, rather than the latest (dare I say my last?) word on the subjects I care about and have tried to cover. Anyway, today's last word on anything is obsolete tomorrow, or next week, or next year. If you want to know the last word on anything, look for it on the World Wide Web and you will surely find it there—though sometimes you must be cautious, and always you must critically appraise the quality of the evidence you find at web sites.

The advantage of a book is that it contains ideas as well as facts. That is why tyrants and mindless mobs ban and burn books—not for the facts they contain, but for the ideas in them. I was encouraged to revise this book into a new edition by friends and former students who asked me to do it. Because, they said, the ideas that they liked in it would carry more weight if supported by up-to-date facts. Quite right of course. Once I had accepted that, it became a pleasure to write this revision, not at all the chore I dreaded and had put off for so long.

Advice to a Young Student

What final messages do I have for you, my student reader? In the last chapter and the Epilogue of the first edition, I offered a few guesses about aspects of the future of health; most remain valid. Rather than updating and refurbishing those scenarios and educated guesses, I will ask you two more questions:

What kind of future do *you* want?

What must *you* do to make that future happen?

Serious answers to these questions make use of a method called Visioning.[7,8] The futurist who employs visioning considers probable, possible, and desirable futures and plans to make the desirable future happen. It is not difficult to envision a probable, even a possible future—although I doubt whether many practitioners of this art guessed right about the geopolitical changes and the technologic advances of the decade from 1987 to 1996. Visioning, and scenarios about alternative futures based on a set of realistic assumptions,[9] can guide our thoughts and plans about future patterns of health in the population and much else that is relevant to health and the human condition.

Reader, I like to think that you have values resembling mine—or that if you don't already, some of the facts I have offered will lead to conclusions that cause you to develop values like mine. I am encouraged to believe this because I have observed in my lifetime how values can and do change: for example, regarding what seemed when I was young to be an immutable social custom, offering a cigarette as a token of friendship when introduced to strangers. That custom is as extinct now for all but a small minority as flicking a horse's rump with a buggy whip.

Now I see around me encouraging signs of a change in values that relate to care and concern for the environment. We have a long way to go in this regard in North America, where much green and pleasant land is still sacrificed to the insatiable demands of the motorcar for ever more space to speed from one city to the next and to park there on arrival. So I have hopes that you will acquire soon, if you do not already possess, values that lead you to respect, care for, and sustain the environment, our planetary life support system.

I hope you will desire a future of harmony among people and harmony between people and other living things with which we share the earth and whose future is intertwined with our own. When I included *Ecology* in the title of this book, I had this hope in mind. The most compelling definition of health that I can offer is "a sustainable state of harmony among humans and the other living things with which we share the earth." I like the notion of health as harmony; I hope you do too.

Other values trouble my student friends nowadays. For 30 years, when my young colleagues have sought my advice about what they should do with their lives, I have urged them to keep their options open for as long as they can. Avoid a precipitate, premature, or enforced choice of a specialty or a place to practice. The final choice about these two essential ultimate decisions can be made, I have always suggested, any time up to or even beyond, 10 years after graduating. Alas, this seems no longer to be feasible for most new medical graduates or for many graduates of other programs of health professional education. Extraneous values and politics have led to relentless and often irresistible pressure to choose a specialty as early as halfway through medical school, or even sooner. The consequence is ever increasing specialization— and fragmentation, balkanization of the health professions. It is becoming increasingly difficult for members of these proliferating and centrifugal specialties to communicate with their colleagues in other fields, not to mention their patients, and for patients to navigate a confident pathway among this bewildering array of specialized branches of practice, each with its unique and dazzling high-tech impedimenta. It is very difficult, too, for a medical graduate, once embarked on a particular specialist track, to back off and begin a new career in another specialty, as I and many of my contemporaries did. There is a lesson here from evolution: A species that specializes in order to cope with a particular environment is endangered when that environment changes. The fiscal and managerial environment of medical practice in the United States, and similar nations, is changing rapidly and radically. Specialists should be wary, superspecialists should be super wary.

One specialty that has never lost sight of the aims of medicine that I set out in the first paragraph of this book, that has a broad, all-encompassing vision of people and their health, and has retained its human touch is public health, including its medical branch of preventive medicine. So, my dear student friend and reader, consider this for your life's work.

► **REFERENCES**

1. Levy BS, Sidel VW (eds): *War and Public Health*. New York: Oxford University Press, 1997.
2. Eliot TS: *The Hollow Men*. London: Faber, 1925.
3. Sackett DL, Richardson WS, Rosenberg W, et al.: *Evidence-based Medicine—How to Practice and Teach EBM*. London: Churchill-Livingstone, 1996. [Available on line on the Internet, at **http://www.bmj.com/archive/7069c.htm**]
4. Laporte RE, Akazawa S, Hellmonds P, et al.: Global public health and the information superhighway. *Br Med J* 308:1651–1652, 1994.
5. Campbell CM, Parboosingh JT, Gondocz ST, et al.: Self-education for professionals; study of physicians' use of a software program to create a portfolio of their self-directed learning. *Acad Med* 71;10(suppl):S49–S51, 1996.
6. Laporte RE: Telepreventive medicine—the autobahn to health. *Br Med J* 313: 1383–1384, 1996.

7. Taket A (ed): *Visioning: Health Futures in Support of Health for All; Report of an International Consultation.* Geneva: WHO/HST/93.4 (WHO Mimeograph publication) 1993.
8. Health Futures Research. *World Health Stat Q* 47;3/4:98–184, 1994. [This volume contains several important papers. See in particular Garrett MJ: An introduction to national futures studies for policymakers in the health sector, pp. 101–117; Bezold C: Scenarios for 21st-century healthcare in the United States of America: Perspectives on time and change, pp. 126–139; Banta HD, Gelijns AC: The future and health care technology: Implications of a system for early identification, pp. 140–148; and Wolfson MJ: POHEM—a framework for understanding and modelling the health of human populations, pp. 157–176. But the entire volume merits careful study.]
9. Brouwer JJ, Schreuder RF (eds): *Scenarios and Other Methods to Support Long-term Health Planning; Proceedings and Outcome of a STG/WHO Workshop, Noordwijk, the Netherlands, 14–16 October 1986.* Utrecht: Van Arkel, 1990.

Appendix

▶ **RECOMMENDED ADDITIONAL READING**

Public Health, Preventive Medicine, Health Promotion

Canadian Task Force on the Periodic Health Examination: *Canadian Guide to Clinical Preventive Services*. Ottawa: Ministry of Supply and Services, 1994.
The Canadian Task Force worked closely with the U.S. Preventive Services Task Force; this report has over 1000 pages (compared with the U.S. Task Force's 400); discussions of screening and counseling procedures and their evaluation.

Clinician's Handbook of Preventive Services. Washington, DC: U.S. Department of Health and Human Services, 1994.
An update and expansion of the 1989 U.S. Preventive Services Task Force report.

Detels R, Holland WW, McEwen J, Omenn GS (eds): *Oxford Textbook of Public Health*. 3rd ed. New York: Oxford University Press, 1997.
A three-volume comprehensive reference textbook with contributions by experts in many parts of the world on all aspects of the theory and practice of public health; its size and price make it suitable mainly for libraries.

Scutchfield FD, Keck CW (eds): *Principles of Public Health Practice*. Albany, NY: Delmar, 1997.
An anthology describing the main features of public health services in the United States, including chapters on the history; legal basis; federal, state, and local services; public health associations; and "how to do it" considered from several perspectives.

U.S. Preventive Services Task Force: *Guide to Clinical Preventive Services: An Assessment of the Effectiveness of 169 Interventions*. Baltimore: Williams & Wilkins, 1989.
Leading health problems; screening, counseling, immunizations, etc., summarized on plasticized cards for quick reference.

Wallace RB (ed): *Maxcy-Rosenau-Last Public Health and Preventive Medicine*. 14th ed. Stamford, CT: Appleton & Lange, 1998.
The North American one-volume reference text, most of which is equally relevant elsewhere in the world.

Woolf SH, Jonas S, Lawrence RS (eds): *Health Promotion and Disease Prevention in Clinical Practice*. Baltimore: Williams & Wilkins, 1996.
A comprehensive account of clinical preventive medicine, i.e., a compendium for clinicians. Puts flesh on the bones of the U.S. Preventive Services Task Force Report.

Epidemiology

There are so many books that it is impossible to select a few without omitting others equally good; I apologize for many omissions.

Beaglehole R, Bonita R, Kjellström T: *Basic Epidemiology*. Geneva: WHO, 1993.
Fundamental principles and practice of epidemiology; intended for beginners but advanced students can learn from it.

Evans AS: *Causation and Disease: A Chronological Journey*. New York: Plenum, 1993.
Etiologic discoveries with pictures of many of the men and women who made them.

Gordis L: *Epidemiology*. Philadelphia: Saunders, 1996.
By a master teacher at Johns Hopkins School of Hygiene and Public Health.

Gregg M (ed): *Field Epidemiology*. New York: Oxford University Press, 1996.
Contributions by many authorities at the U.S. Centers for Disease Control and Prevention.

Kelsey JL, Whittemore AS, Evans AS, et al.: *Methods in Observational Epidemiology*. 2nd ed. New York: Oxford University Press, 1996.
A very good account of common methods.

Last JM (ed): *A Dictionary of Epidemiology*. 3rd ed. New York: Oxford University Press, 1995.
Many people tell me they regard this as a textbook as well as a source of definitions, both authoritative and, in a few instances, offbeat.

MacMahon B, Trichopoulos D: *Epidemiology: Principles and Methods*. 2nd ed. Boston: Little, Brown, 1996.
A new book more than a new edition; lucid, terse, and comprehensive.

Logic and Reasoning in Medicine and Epidemiology

Murphy EA: *The Logic of Medicine*. Baltimore: Johns Hopkins University Press, 1976.
Cuts through the foggy thinking that often prevails in medical practice and public health.

Sackett DL, Richardson WS, Rosenberg W, et al.: *Evidence-based Medicine—How to Practice and Teach EBM*. London: Churchill-Livingstone, 1996.
Available online via the electronic library of the British Medical Association, at **http://www.bmj.com/archive/7069c.htm**

Popper KR: *The Logic of Scientific Discovery*. New York: Science Editions, 1961.

Susser MW: *Causal Thinking in the Health Sciences*. New York: Oxford University Press, 1973.
A very thoughtful book that has become a classic.

Warren KS (ed): *Coping with the Biomedical Literature: A Primer for the Scientist and the Clinician*. New York: Praeger, 1981.

Communicable Diseases

Ewald PW: *Evolution of Infectious Disease.* New York: Oxford University Press, 1994.
On the ecology of infectious pathogens.

Garrett L: *The Coming Plague; Newly Emerging Diseases in a World Out of Balance.* New
York: Farrar, Straus, & Giroux, 1994.
A science writer's account of some new and emerging infectious disease threats.
Highly recommended.

Kunitz SJ: *Disease and Social Diversity; the European Impact on the Health of Non-Europeans.*
New York: Oxford University Press, 1994.
Explores the genetic basis for susceptibility and resistance to infection and the social
and cultural factors contributing to disease when one civilization overwhelms another.
Very highly recommended.

Manson-Bahr PEC (ed): *Manson's Tropical Diseases.* 20th ed. Philadelphia: Saunders,
1996.

Morse SS (ed): *Emerging Viruses.* New York: Oxford University Press, 1993.
History, ecology, evolution of virus diseases with contributions by many of the world's
leading authorities.

International Health

Jamison DT, Mosley WH, Measham AR, et al.: *Disease Control Priorities in Developing
Countries.* New York: Oxford University Press, 1993.
This book is sponsored by the World Bank; offers a detailed analysis of a wide range of
health problems.

Social Demography

Cohen JL: *How Many People Can the Earth Support?* New York: Norton, 1995.
An objective analysis of the present state and possible futures of human populations
on earth. Neither alarmist nor complacent, and very thoughtful. Highly recommended.

Social, Behavioral Sciences, etc

Ader R, Felten DL, Cohen N (eds): *Psychoneuroimmunology.* 2nd ed. New York: Academic Press 1990.

Helman C: *Culture, Health and Illness.* 2nd ed. Oxford: Butterworth-Heinemann, 1990.

Nichter M: *Anthropology and International Health.* Boston: Kluwer, 1989.
Two excellent monographs on medical anthropology.

Sigerist H: *On the Sociology of Medicine.* Roemer M (ed). Chicago: MD Publications,
1960.

Susser MW, Watson W, Hopper K: *Sociology in Medicine.* 3rd ed. New York: Oxford University Press, 1985.
A richly referenced sourcebook.

▶ PUBLIC HEALTH INFORMATION ON THE INTERNET

The following are some useful sites on the World Wide Web; innumerable others are accessible via links.

Websites at U.S. Government Agencies

Centers for Disease Control and Prevention: **http://www.cdc.gov**
Links to many agencies, e.g., CDC Wonder on the Web, National Center for Health Statistics, Agency for Toxic Substances and Disease Registries, state health agencies, bibliographic sources, and health-related search engines.

Environmental Protection Agency: **http://www.epa.gov**
National Institutes of Health: **http://www.nih.gov**
Links to NIH agencies, including National Library of Medicine **(http://www. nlm.nih.gov)**, bibliographic sources, and search engines.

UN Agencies and Government Sites in Other Countries

World Health Organization: **http://www.who.ch**
The WHO Information Service (WHOIS) is very useful and user-friendly. Links to many national health departments, NGOs, and health-related agencies.

U.K. Department of Health: **http://www.open.gov.uk/doh/dhhome.htm**
U.K. Office of National Statistics (formerly Office of Population, Censuses and Surveys): **http://www.open.gov.uk/lmsd/onsbackg.htm**

Health Canada: **http://www.hwc.ca**

Nongovernmental Organizations and Others

Global Health Network: **http://www.pitt.edu/home/GHNet/GHNet.html**
World Wide Web Virtual Medical Library has pages in many fields; epidemiology is at **http://chanane.ucsf.edu/epidem/epidem.html**

American Public Health Association: **http://www.apha.org**
E-Med News Home Page: **http://www.pjbpubs.co.uk/a/emedhome.html**
Achoo! On-line Healthcare Services: **http://www.achoo.co**
A search engine that lists nearly 8000 health-related internet sites, discussion groups, etc.

An online source for many medical journals, some books, and other publications is **http://biomednet.com**

Internet Discussion Groups

A great deal of health-related information is accessible in internet discussion groups and by gopher searches. Look also at your local e-mail bulletin boards to find out what is going on where you live.

Index

A page number in *italic* indicates that the information on that page is only in a box, figure, or table.

Benzene *158*, 170, *171*
Benzidine 157, *158*
Benzo[a]pyrene *158*
Benzoic acid 213
Beriberi 217–18, 221
Beryllium *158*, 162
Bias
   epidemiology 380–81
   in case-control studies 77–79
   in cohort studies 81
   types 97–100
Biodiversity 409–10
Biofeedback 252
Biologic determinants 7
Biomedical ethics *see* Ethics
Bipyridine 177
Birth
   as vital statistic 39, *42*, 280
   stressful 250, *251*
Birth defects
   causes *15*, *132*, 174, *260*
   mortality statistics *271–72*
   and postneonatal mortality rate 52
Bis(chloromethyl) ethers 157, *158*
Black lung 167, *168*
Blindness *see* Visual impairment
Blood, and disease transmission 121, 145, 148–49, 371–72
Bottle feeding (infants) 224, 353, 387
Botulism *123*, *135*, 210–11, 214
Boys *see* Children
Brazil
   communicable diseases 113
   desertification 403
   industrial development 398
   smoking prevalence *258*
   water shortage predicted 408
Breastfeeding 224, 227, 353
Britain *see* United Kingdom
Bromine *179*
Bronchitis
   causes 171, 181, 256
   occupational hazard 164, 167
Brucella abortus 210
Brucellosis 122, *123*
Bubonic plague 122
Built environment 197–98
Bulimia 226
Burma 146

Cadmium 162, *163*
Campylobacter jejuni 122, *136*
Canada
   aging of population *281*
   cancer 157
   carbon dioxide emissions 399
   chemical disasters *328*
   chemical use and testing 174–75
   communicable diseases 63, 126, 138–39, 371
   health laws and policies 22, 330, 372, 377
   health statistics 67, 89, 237–38, *239*
   heart disease 227, 284
   pollution 183, 197
   recommended dietary allowances 214
   silicosis 167
   smoking prevalence *258*
   subcultures 241
   suicides 298, *299*
Canadian Addiction Research Foundation 340
Canadian Climate Center 406
Canadian Global Change Program 417–18
Canadian International Development Agency 340
Cancer
   causes and risk factors *15*, 289–90, *292–93*
     air pollution 181–82
     alcohol *260*
     asbestos 156, 165–66
     chemicals 156–58, 161, 170, 172, 174, 214
     diet 222, 223, 283
     drugs 77, *79*
     hepatitis 139
     industrial processes *158*
     ionizing radiation 81, 185–86, *188*, 196, 289–90, 291
     metals 162–63
     pathogens *132*, *143*
     smoking 80, *83*, 84, 104–5, 181–82, 256, *257*, 282, 380–81
     STDs 131, *132*
     ultraviolet radiation 186–87, *188*, 406–7, *417*
   defined 289
   epidemiological study 76, 77
   in children 71, 81, *84*, 156
   incidence 290–91

About the Author

John Last was born and educated in Australia. He graduated in medicine (MB, BS) from the University of Adelaide in 1949 and proceeded to the MD with a thesis on epidemiologic studies in Australia, the United States, and the United Kingdom. He has worked in Australia, England, Scotland, and the United States and for the World Health Organization and other agencies in several developing countries. He has been professor of epidemiology and community medicine at the University of Ottawa, Canada, since 1969. He was editor-in-chief of the 11th, 12th, and 13th editions of *Public Health and Preventive Medicine* ("Maxcy-Rosenau-Last"); editor of the first, second, and third editions of *A Dictionary of Epidemiology;* scientific editor of the *Canadian Journal of Public Health,* 1981–1991; editor of *Annals* of the Royal College of Physicians and Surgeons of Canada, 1990–1997; and he has served as editor or a member of the editorial board of several other medical journals. He is the author of chapters in 36 books and over 200 original articles in journals of medicine, epidemiology, and public health.

Dr. Last was president of the American College of Preventive Medicine from 1987 to 1989 and Canadian Vice President of the American Public Health Association in 1988–1989. He has held office in several other professional associations and colleges and is an honorary life member of the International Epidemiological Association. He was the Wade Hampton Frost Lecturer to the Epidemiology Section, American Public Health Association, in 1989; he received the MD degree *honoris causa* from Uppsala University, Sweden, in 1993; the Duncan Clark Award of the Association of Teachers of Preventive Medicine for lifetime achievement in preventive medicine in 1994, and the Abraham M. Lilienfeld Award of the American College of Epidemiology in 1997.